THE
CARNIVORE
COOKBOOK

The Complete Guide to Success on the Carnivore Diet
with Over 100 Recipes, Meal Plans, and Science

Maria Emmerich & Craig Emmerich

VICTORY BELT PUBLISHING INC.
Las Vegas

Front and back cover photos and copyright page photo by Hayley Mason and Bill Staley

Cover design by Kat Lannom

Interior design and illustrations by Kat Lannom, Justin-Aaron Velasco, Yordan Terziev, and Boryana Yordanova

Recipe photos by Jenny Ross

TC 0120

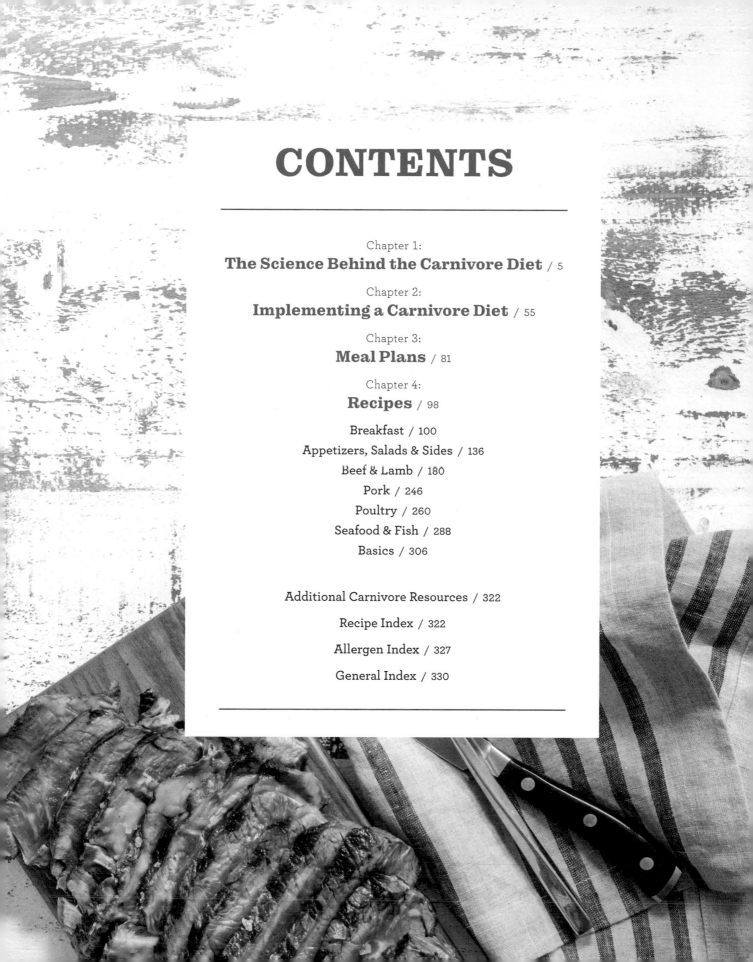

CONTENTS

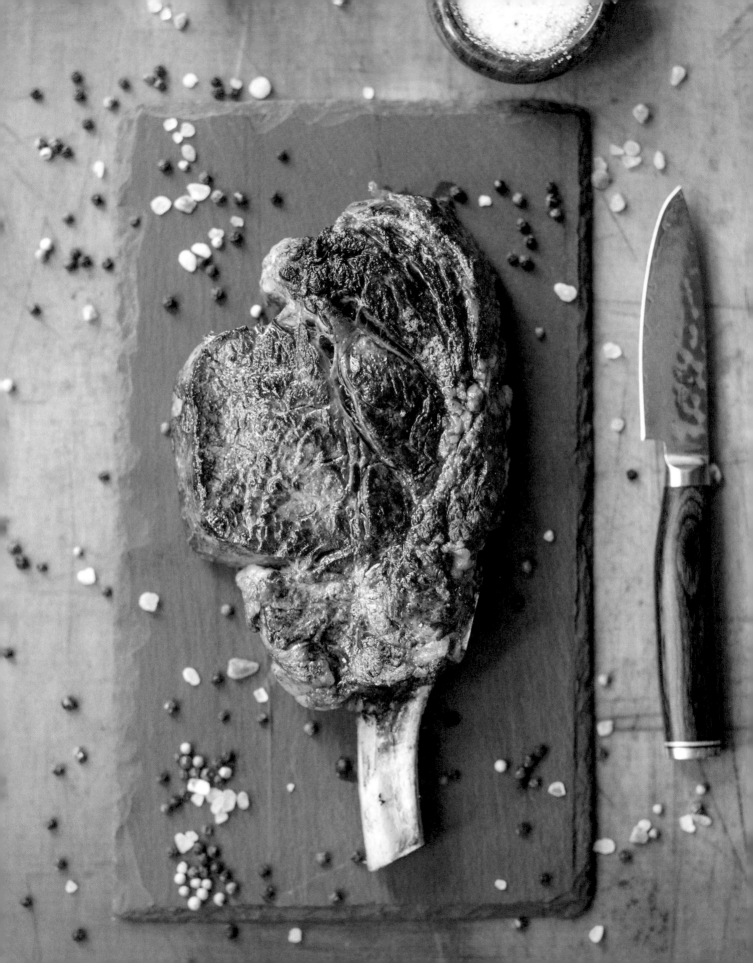

Chapter 1:
The Science Behind the Carnivore Diet

The carnivore diet has many benefits. There are numerous reasons why this diet can be so helpful for weight loss and healing:

1. It cuts out inflammatory sugars and other sweeteners.

   - Sugar, whether it comes in the form of natural fruit sugar or refined sugar, is one of the biggest causes of inflammation in the body. The carnivore diet eliminates almost all sugars, which lowers inflammation.

   - High sugar intake leads to the formation of advanced glycation end products (a sort of crust that forms on cells and prevents them from responding properly), glycated LDL particles (oxidized LDL particles that increase atherosclerotic risk), and insulin resistance (see page 6).

   - Avoiding all sweeteners, even zero-calorie natural sweeteners, helps reduce and even eliminate sugar cravings and sweet tooth. It also shifts the palate toward more savory flavors.

2. It eliminates inflammatory grains. Grains are one of the top causes of sensitivity or allergy, which can lead to leaky gut and inflammation. Cutting out grains helps reverse these problems.

3. It removes omega-6 vegetable and seed oils. Omega-6 fats are easily oxidized and should be limited in any diet. When they become oxidized, they cause inflammation and damage (free radicals) in the body.

4. It can cure leaky gut, which is a condition in which gut permeability is compromised and toxins are allowed to "leak" through the intestinal wall and get into the bloodstream. This can lead to an autoimmune response to these foreign substances in the blood and other issues.

   - Paleomedicina Hungary has shown that a carnivore diet can reverse intestinal permeability.[1]

   - Reducing inflammation also helps heal the gut.

   - The carnivore diet doesn't include many of the causes of leaky gut, such as oxalates, lectins, and gluten (all from plants).

5. It reverses insulin resistance, which is dysfunction of insulin signaling in the body. The most common cause of insulin resistance is exceeding your personal fat threshold. This means that most of the fat cells you have are overstuffed and inflamed.

- Carnivore is a powerful way to lose body fat, which is the best way to reverse insulin resistance.

- Carnivore promotes gains in lean mass, which helps reverse insulin resistance by giving the body more places to store glucose.

- Protein has the highest thermic effect of food (see page 63), which means that more of the calories you eat don't count as much, also helping with fat loss.

6. It increases nutrient density. Animal proteins have some of the highest nutrient density of any food. They are also among the most bioavailable; this means the body gets a huge dose of nutrients from a carnivore diet, ensuring that it has all the nutrients it needs to heal itself.

7. It simplifies eating. Most people don't have to worry about counting macros or carbs. Given how satiating animal proteins are, you typically need to eat only one or two meals a day. Most meals take 10 minutes or less to prep and cook, and cleanup is minimal.

8. It provides the body with the food it is designed to digest. Our bodies are made to eat primarily animal proteins. Avoiding plant matter eliminates many of the causes of gastrointestinal issues and leaky gut.

9. It helps with autoimmune diseases. All of the above improvements help the body reverse disease, especially autoimmune disease.

Let's begin by taking a look at what our ancestors ate and what our bodies are designed to consume.

> Maria had the opportunity to be a speaker on the Low Carb Cruise in 2019. One of the other speakers talked about her eating disorder and her constant thoughts of food. The reason eating carnivore is so therapeutic for disordered eating is that you are eating to live, not living to eat. Carnivores are known to think about food the least; compared to other diets, carnivore is simple, satisfying, and filling. Carnivores enjoy food, yet stop eating when they are full. This fact is freeing in many ways; you can live a life filled with adventure rather than being plagued by thoughts of food.

---

[1]Csaba Tóth, Andrea Dabóczi, Mark Howard, Nicholas J. Miller, and Zsófia Clemens, "Crohn's Disease Successfully Treated with the Paleolithic Ketogenic Diet," *International Journal of Case Reports and Images* 7, no. 6 (2016): 570–8.

WHAT DID OUR ANCESTORS EAT?

The carnivore diet is representative of our ancestral diet. Many of our ancestors ate some plants seasonally, such as in late summer and fall when fruits were ripe and some vegetation was plentiful. However, for most of the year, they ate primarily animal proteins. Eating fruits and veggies seasonally was a mechanism to store fat in order to prepare for the leaner winter months when food was scarce.

One of the best scientific tools for identifying the amount of animal protein our ancestors consumed is isotope analysis. This sensitive tool can detect how much animal protein the Neolithic-era Neanderthals ate. Testing showed that Neanderthals were top-level carnivores, and their main protein source was large herbivores.[2]

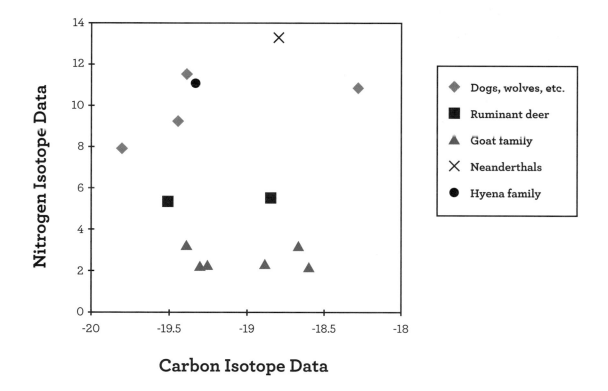

The higher up and farther to the right a group is on this chart, the more apex carnivore or top of the food chain it was. As you can see, Neanderthals were higher-level carnivores than even wolves or hyenas. They sustained themselves primarily by eating animal proteins.

---

[2]Michael P. Richards and Erik Trinkaus, "Isotopic Evidence for the Diets of European Neanderthals and Early Modern Humans," *Proceedings of the National Academy of Sciences of the United States of America* 106, no. 38 (2009): 16034–9.

Another study looked at weaning profiles and how they could predict the animal dietary profile. The researchers stated, "Our findings highlight the emergence of carnivory as a process fundamentally determining human evolution."[3]

A third study using the same methods of isotope analysis showed that Upper Pleistocene Modern Humans ate largely the same diet as the Neanderthals. They were top-level carnivores.[4] These early humans lived just 30,000 to 45,000 years ago, which isn't that long ago in our history. Agriculture and farming didn't start until around 7,000 to 10,000 years ago.

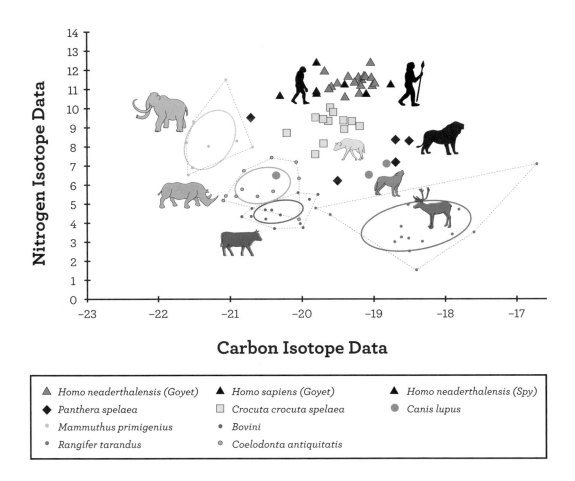

Symbol	Species	Symbol	Species	Symbol	Species
▲	*Homo neaderthalensis* (Goyet)	▲	*Homo sapiens* (Goyet)	▲	*Homo neaderthalensis* (Spy)
◆	*Panthera spelaea*	◻	*Crocuta crocuta spelaea*	●	*Canis lupus*
•	*Mammuthus primigenius*	•	*Bovini*		
•	*Rangifer tarandus*	•	*Coelodonta antiquitatis*		

For tens of thousands of years, early humans were eating a primarily carnivore diet. Both early humans and Neanderthals were higher-level carnivores than lions, wolves, and hyenas from the same time frame. Most of their protein came from large animals, including *Mammuthus* (wooly mammoths), *Rangifer* (reindeer), and *Coelodonta* (early rhinoceros).

[3]Elia Psouni, Axel Janke, and Martin Garwicz, "Impact of Carnivory on Human Development and Evolution Revealed by a New Unifying Model of Weaning in Mammals," *PLOS One* 7, no. 4 (2012): e32452.

[4]Cristoph Wissing, Hélène Rougier, Chris Baumann, Alexander Comeyne, Isabelle Crevecoeur, Dorothée G. Drucker, Sabine Gaudzinki-Windheuser, et al, "Stable Isotopes Reveal Patterns of Diet and Mobility in the Last Neandertals and First Modern Humans in Europe," *Scientific Reports* 9, no 1 (2019): 4433.

These early humans were direct ancestors of us humans living today. During this critical time in our history, our ancestors relied heavily on animal proteins to support the growing brain. We believe it was the nutrient-dense animal proteins that made up the majority of their diet that enabled the human brain to grow.

THE HUMAN DIGESTIVE TRACT

The digestive tract can be a good indicator of what an animal is designed to eat. Let's look at the modern human digestive tract and see if there are clues that point to us being primarily carnivores by design.

If humans are omnivores, as many people claim, then we should be able to process plant and animal matter equally well. To investigate this possibility, we'll compare the human digestive tract to the digestive tracts of other species.

Humans have the same components of digestion as other primates. We have a stomach, small intestine, cecum with appendix, and colon. But let's look closer at these components of digestion, starting with the large differences in the small intestine and colon.

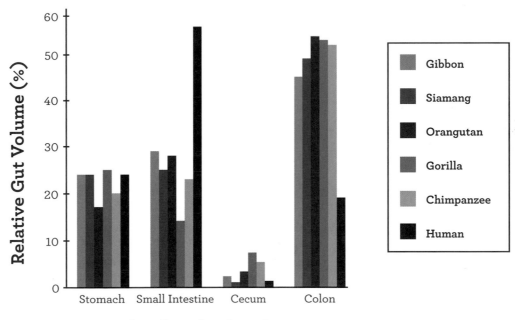

As you can see in this chart[5], the human small intestine is much larger than that of other primates, and the colon is much smaller. What does this mean? A large colon is good for handling low-quality food sources such as plant leaves, stems, and stalks and fibrous fruits that require a lot of digestive work to break down. Primates also have cecum's that enable them to ferment plant matter (cellulose or fiber) into energy (fatty acids). Humans don't have a cecum large enough to do this, and that's why we don't digest plant fiber; it just goes right through us. Meanwhile, the large human small intestine is great for digesting high-quality foods that are energy and nutrient dense and easy to break down, which are primarily animal proteins, fish, and eggs, along with some cooked plants.

Another part of the digestive system that is smaller in humans than in other primates is the cecum, a pouch that stores plant fibers to be fermented and turned into energy. The human cecum is found at the start of the colon.

The Human Bowel

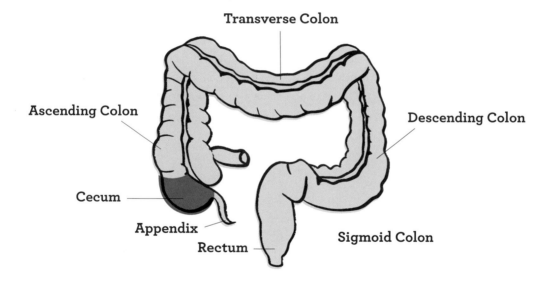

A true omnivore or herbivore would have a much larger cecum. For comparison, the cecum of a koala—an herbivore—is a long, curled pouch in which plant fiber sits to be fermented and digested. The lack of a long cecum is another reason why we humans can't turn fiber into fuel.

---

[5]Katharine Milton, "Nutritional Characteristics of Wild Primate Foods: Do the Diets of Our Closest Living Relatives Have Lessons for Us?" *Nutrition* 15, no. 6 (1999): 488–9.

Digestive System of a Koala

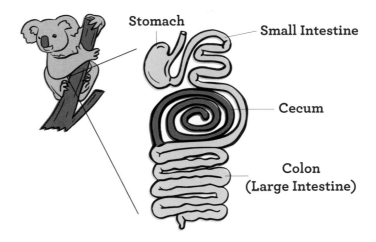

Our human biology dictates that we are primarily carnivores. Does this mean we can't digest plant foods? No, but our bodies are not designed to digest significant amounts of them, either. As humans evolved, our brains became larger and larger, and that required some trade offs. The brain is an energy and nutrient hog. Supplying our large brains with the necessary nutrients required us to eat more and more nutrient- and energy-dense foods. To do so, our ancestors had to shift their diets to more and more animal food sources. We traded big guts for big brains, and that required us to be primarily carnivores.

Plant Fiber: Do We Need It to Have a Healthy Gut?

You might be thinking, "But I thought we needed fiber to be regular and feed our gut flora." (Gut flora are the microorganisms living in our digestive tract.) Let's take a closer look at human digestion and fiber's role.

There are two types of dietary fiber: insoluble and soluble.

Insoluble fiber doesn't dissolve in water. It is the tough stuff that makes up tree bark and nutshells. There is a lot of it in grains, seeds, nuts, vegetables, and certain fruits. It passes through our entire digestive tract practically untouched. Not even the bacteria in our gut flora can easily digest it. Insoluble fiber is said to be good for us because it can "bulk up our stool" and help "keep things moving," but there is growing evidence that it can actually be detrimental to digestive health. It can elongate and irritate the bowel, which can cause issues.[6]

---

[6]Konstantin Monastyrsky, *The Fiber Menace* (Sarasota, FL: Ageless Press, 2011).

Studies have shown that reducing fiber consumption actually *reduces* constipation.[7] A high-fiber diet also has been shown to make diverticulosis (a condition that causes small, bulging pouches to form in the digestive tract) worse, not better.[8] There even is a study that refutes the supposed heart-healthy claims about fiber; the subjects of this study showed no reduction in heart issues with increased fiber intake.[9]

Soluble fiber dissolves in water. It gels when added to liquid—think Metamucil. It also feeds some of your gut flora, as it is fermentable by the microbes in the gut, and thus is thought to be good for the health of the gut microbiome. But is dietary fiber necessary for a healthy gut microbiome?

First, the cellulose and fructooligosaccharides (FOS) in plants are not the only fermentables that can feed the gut flora (aka prebiotics). There are many others, including many animal sources.

Foods with the Highest Prebiotic Content[10]

Substrate	Total Short-Chain Fatty Acids
Casein	7.42 mmol/g
Cellulose	1.53 mmol/g
Chicken cartilage	5.50 mmol/g
Collagen	7.96 mmol/g
Fructooligosaccharides (FOS)	10.37 mmol/g
Glucosamine	7.11 mmol/g
Glucosamine chondroitin	5.36 mmol/g

[7]Kok-Sun Ho, Chamaine Yu Mei Tan, Muhd A. Mohd Daud, and Francis Seow-Choen, "Stopping or Reducing Dietary Fiber Intake Reduces Constipation and Its Associated Symptoms," *World Journal of Gastroenterology* 18, no. 33 (2012): 4593–6.

[8]Anne F. Peery, Patrick R. Barrett, Doyun Park, Albert J. Rogers, Joseph A. Galanko, Christopher F. Martin, and Robert S. Sandler, "A High-Fiber Diet Does Not Protect Against Asymptomatic Diverticulosis," *Gastroenterology* 142, no. 2 (2012): 266–72.e1.

[9]M. L. Burr, A. M. Fehily, J. F. Gilbert, S. Rogers, R. M. Holliday, P. M. Sweetnam, P. C. Elwood, and N. M. Deadman, "Effects of Changes in Fat, Fish, and Fibre Intakes on Death and Myocardial Reinfarction: Diet and Reinfarction Trial (DART)," *Lancet* 2, no. 8666 (1989): 757–61.

[10]S. Depauw, G. Bosch, M. Hesta, K. Whitehouse-Tedd, W. H. Hendriks, J. Kaandorp, and G. P. Janssens, "Fermentation of Animal Components in Strict Carnivores: A Comparative Study of Cheetah Fecal Inoculum," *Journal of Animal Science* 90, no. 8 (2012): 2540–8.

As you can see in the table, fructooligosaccharides (FOS) are the most fermentable foods. But FOS are found only in certain vegetables and fruits, and typically in small amounts. Tomatoes, zucchini, bell peppers, eggplant, carrots, cauliflower, and many other types of produce contain no FOS. The highest FOS contents are found in foods like scallions and white onions. White onions have 2 grams of FOS per 100 grams (about the size of one medium onion). Most other vegetables and fruits, if they contain any FOS, contain less than 1 gram per 100 grams. There are other prebiotics in plants, but they are much less fermentable. (Cellulose is 1.53 compared to FOS at 10.37.)

After FOS, the next most fermentable products are animal sources:

- Collagen (found in connective parts and joints of animals)

- Casein (milk protein)

- Glucosamine (found in cartilage)

- Chicken cartilage

- Glucosamine chondroitin (found in cartilage)

These animal sources are not far behind FOS in their ability to feed the gut flora. So you *can* feed your gut flora with animal foods. In addition to the above, butyric acid (found in butter and cheese) feeds the gut flora along, as do other animal sources. Therefore, we can safely say that eating carnivore doesn't mean depriving your gut flora of food, as many people would lead you to believe.

There is growing evidence that large amounts of plant fiber are not only unnecessary but may actually be detrimental to health. We don't see how shoving loads of a nutrient that our bodies largely cannot digest through the GI tract, causing elongation of the bowel as well as irritation, could possibly be healthy.

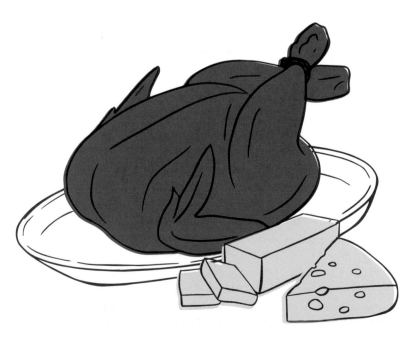

The Flexibility of the Gut Microbiome

Ultimately, the question is, "What is a healthy gut?" Is a healthy gut for a carnivore different from a healthy gut for a vegetarian? And can the gut microbiome change based on what we eat? Let's look at an interesting study comparing vegetarian and carnivore diets and how they alter the gut microbiome.[11]

First, how quickly can the gut microbiome change? It turns out that it can change based on diet in just one day! Take a look at this chart:

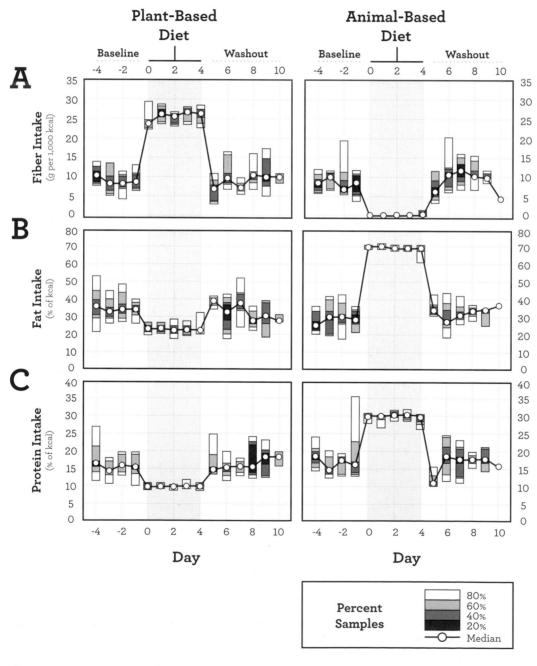

The chart opposite shows the changes in fiber (section A), fat (section B), and protein (section C) intake for each of the two groups studied—one that ate a plant-based diet and one that ate an animal-based diet—during the four-day experiment. The subjects ate a standard American–type diet before and after the test.

Sections D and E in the chart below show the changes in the gut microbiome during the test. Alpha diversity (section D) represents the changes in the types of gut flora present. Beta diversity (section E) represents the changes in the amounts of specific strains. The blue arrows in section E indicate when the change in diet actually hits the bowels for digestion.

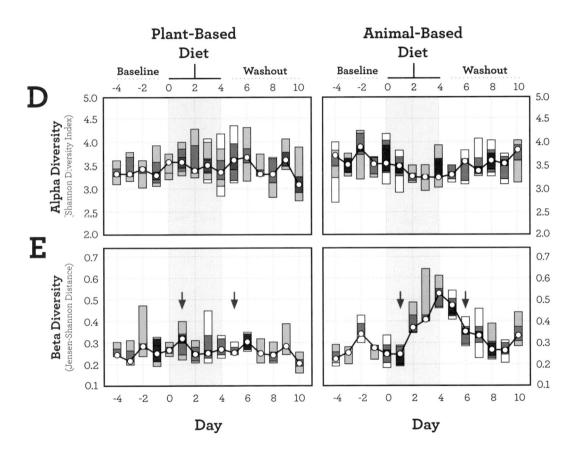

As you can see, just one day after an animal-based diet hits the gut, the microbiome changes significantly (section E). There are two other important things to learn from this chart. First, section D shows that there were no significant changes in the diversity of a given sample for either diet. This means that all the same strains of gut microbes were still present. But the total numbers of certain types of microbes compared to baseline (prior to the test), shown in section E, saw bigger movement on the animal-based diet. The chart on the next page shows that movement in more detail.

[11]L. A. David, C. F. Maurice, R. N. Carmody, D. B. Gootenberg, J. E. Button, B. E. Wolfe, A. V. Ling, et al, "Diet Rapidly and Reproducibly Alters the Human Gut Microbiome," *Nature* 505, no. 7484 (2014): 559–63.

Changes in Bacteria Clusters in Response to Diet[11]

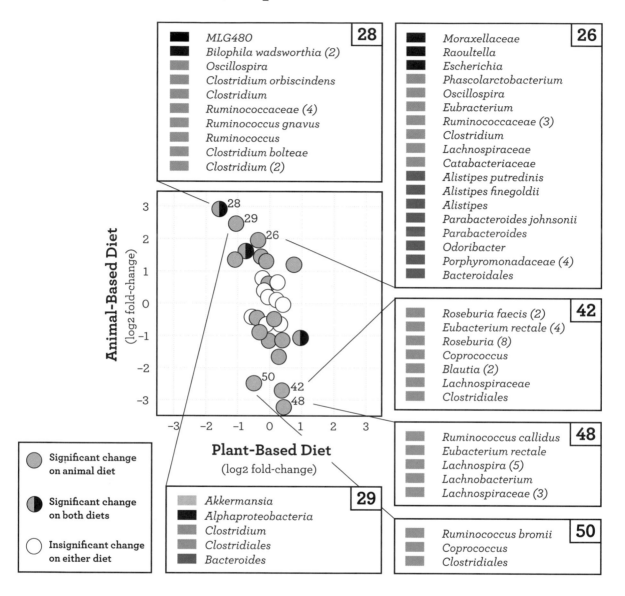

28
- MLG480
- Bilophila wadsworthia (2)
- Oscillospira
- Clostridium orbiscindens
- Clostridium
- Ruminococcaceae (4)
- Ruminococcus gnavus
- Ruminococcus
- Clostridium bolteae
- Clostridium (2)

26
- Moraxellaceae
- Raoultella
- Escherichia
- Phascolarctobacterium
- Oscillospira
- Eubracterium
- Ruminococcaceae (3)
- Clostridium
- Lachnospiraceae
- Catabacteriaceae
- Alistipes putredinis
- Alistipes finegoldii
- Alistipes
- Parabacteroides johnsonii
- Parabacteroides
- Odoribacter
- Porphyromonadaceae (4)
- Bacteroidales

42
- Roseburia faecis (2)
- Eubacterium rectale (4)
- Roseburia (8)
- Coprococcus
- Blautia (2)
- Lachnospiraceae
- Clostridiales

48
- Ruminococcus callidus
- Eubacterium rectale
- Lachnospira (5)
- Lachnobacterium
- Lachnospiraceae (3)

50
- Ruminococcus bromii
- Coprococcus
- Clostridiales

29
- Akkermansia
- Alphaproteobacteria
- Clostridium
- Clostridiales
- Bacteroides

Animal-Based Diet (log2 fold-change)

Plant-Based Diet (log2 fold-change)

- ● Significant change on animal diet
- ◑ Significant change on both diets
- ○ Insignificant change on either diet

While the diversity of the microbes was the same, the numbers of clusters of different microbes (represented by the numbered groups in the chart above) shifted more on a carnivore diet. In other words, you have almost all the same types of microbes in your gut, but some types are more or less prevalent depending on what you are eating. Also significant here is that just two days after returning to the standard diet, the subjects for both diets had returned to baseline (shown on the previous page in section E, in the washout section after the diet changed back to baseline). This demonstrates how rapidly the microbiome can change based on diet.

Response to Dietary Changes in (C) Genes for Vitamin Biosynthesis

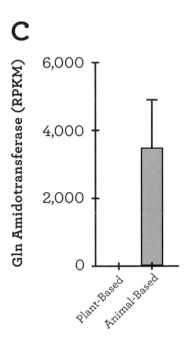

In this study, the researchers also looked at changes in microbial activity and gene expression.

One of the biggest changes in gene expression with the carnivore diet was a large increase in the genes vital for vitamin biosynthesis (section C in the chart on page 14). This means there is a large increase in the synthesis of vitamins when a person is eating a carnivore diet compared to eating a vegetarian diet. This is likely due to the more abundant and bioavailable nutrients that come from animal proteins (see the section "The Case for a Meat-Based Diet: Nutrient Density of Animal Proteins" later in this chapter).

Remember, these changes occurred in just a day or two. Our gut microbiome is very good at adapting to what we eat. We think this stems from our hunter-gatherer ancestors' need to adapt quickly to the different seasons. As mentioned earlier, they needed to eat fruit to put on weight in the fall and then eat primarily meat in the winter when plant foods were unavailable.

The best microbiome for your body is one that is well adapted to the diet you are eating and plan to eat in the future. The microbiome of someone eating plants will have different amounts of certain microbes than that of someone eating carnivore, and it should; there are different jobs to do. A carnivore needs to process more bioavailable nutrients, more protein, and more fat, and the microbiome will reflect that. The microbes that help with plant processing are still present, just at lower levels. But carnivores and vegetarians will have similar diversity, or numbers of different microbes. When switching from one way of eating to the other, the body just shifts the amounts of the different types of microbes accordingly, and in just a day or two.

In long-term carnivores, will the microbes that process grains or other plants be reduced or eventually even eliminated over time? That is hard to say. We have not eaten gluten or wheat in over ten years. Are the microbes that are good at processing it gone? We likely still have some of the microbes that are good at processing it, but even if they are all gone at this point, do we even care if we never plan on eating wheat again? We have seen some N=1 (individual) examples of carnivores who have eaten just meat for one to two years or more and tested their gut microbiome. They found that they still had all the same major strains or diversity of microbes present in their gut.

Stomach Acid pH

A final point of interest is stomach acid pH. In general, herbivores have a stomach pH of 5 to 6. Omnivores have a stomach pH of 3 to 4, while carnivores have a stomach pH of 2 to 3. Scavengers have a stomach pH of 1 to 1.5. Humans have a stomach pH of 1 to 2, typically around 1.5.[12] A more acidic stomach (that is, a lower pH number) is better for digesting meats, and a very acidic stomach helps digest meats that are starting to decay. This supports the theory that early humans ate primarily large herbivores like woolly mammoths. These massive animals would feed a group for a long time, and with primitive preservation techniques, the meat would be turning as they consumed it over a period of months. This is likely why humans evolved to have stomachs almost as acidic as those of many scavengers.

In summary, leveraging our bodies' natural design can be a powerful tool for healing and weight loss. It is especially powerful for managing chronic health issues, as eating carnivore acts as the perfect elimination diet, removing common allergens and plant antinutrients (see page 25) that cause so many of the problems people deal with today.

Can humans eat some plants and thrive? Yes, we can. Can we eat only plants and thrive? We don't think so. There are many cases of inadequate protein and nutrient deficiencies in a plant-only diet (B12, D3, iron, etc.). If we want to thrive, and especially if we want to reverse chronic disease, we need to return to the diet our ancestors ate, and the evidence points to that being mostly a carnivorous diet.

---

[12]G. McLauchlan, G. M. Fullarton, G. P. Crean, and K. E. McColl, "Comparison of Gastric Body and Antral pH: A 24 Hour Ambulatory Study in Healthy Volunteers," *Gut* 30, no. 5 (1989): 573–8.

THE CASE AGAINST PRODUCE

One of the common arguments against a carnivore lifestyle is that our ancestors ate fruits and vegetables, so why shouldn't we? This argument is flawed for a few reasons:

- As we have demonstrated, our bodies are designed to be primarily carnivorous. Just because we can eat fruits and vegetables doesn't mean that they are ideal for our bodies in large amounts.

- Modern produce looks nothing like what our ancestors ate.

- Our ancestors had access to these fruits and vegetables only in the summer months in most climates.

- All plants come with antinutrients, which can damage our health, cause leaky gut, and allow autoimmune issues to develop.

In this section, we examine each of these points, beginning with why the produce we eat today is nothing like the vegetables and fruits our Paleolithic ancestors ate.

Hybridization and Cross-Breeding

Modern produce is bred to be larger and much higher in sugar or starch than the fruits and vegetables our ancestors consumed. Many of the fruits and vegetables found in Paleolithic times would not even be recognizable today. Let's take a look at a few examples.

Wild Watermelon	Modern Watermelon
	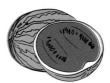
Based on seventeenth-century paintings, wild watermelon may once have had seeds arranged in a swirly geometric pattern. It was less than 2 inches across and had to be opened with a hammer or sharp object. It had an extremely bitter taste. There were six known varieties found only in Namibia and Botswana. The fruit was ripe and ready to eat for only a couple of weeks. It was 80% water, 1.9% sugar, and 18.1% other (mostly starch and fat).	The modern watermelon measures 26 inches across—over 10 times bigger. It is very sweet and juicy and is easy to open. More than 1,200 varieties are grown year-round in 15-plus countries, producing 95 million tons of fruit. These fruits are 91.5% water (14 times juicier), 6.2% sugar (3.3 times as sweet), and 2.3% other (with almost no fat or starch).

Wild Banana	Modern Banana

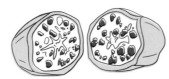 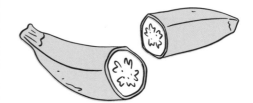

The first bananas were cultivated over 7,000 years ago in what is now Papua New Guinea. There were two varieties: *Musa acuminta* and *Musa balbisiana*. The fruits were stocky and hard with large, tough seeds throughout their interior. Most of the flesh was inedible.

Modern bananas are grown all over the world, and 80 million tons of bananas are produced per year. The original plants would sometimes produce mutant variants without seeds. These variants were hybridized over the years to create the fruit we consume today. Bananas are now nearly seedless, three times longer, and over 21% sugar.

Wild Carrot	Modern Carrot

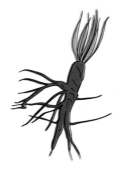 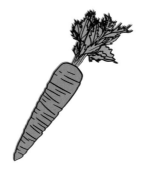

The wild carrot was very thin with a distinct and powerful flavor. It was originally purple or white and originated in Persia and Asia Minor in the tenth century. It was a biennial plant, meaning that it took two years to complete the biological cycle.

The modern carrot is the result of years of manipulating mutant strains of purple carrots through experimentation done by the Dutch in the sixteenth century. The bright orange variety we see today is much sweeter and is grown year-round all over the world.

Wild Corn	Modern Corn

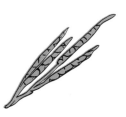 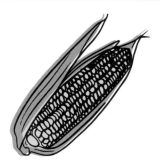

About 10,000 years ago, wild corn was a grass called teosintes. It was barely edible and as dry as a potato. It was about ¾ inch long with just 5 to 10 very hard kernels. A hammer or sharp object was needed to peel it. There were 8 known varieties, and it was found only in Central America. It was 75% water, 1.9% sugar, and 23% other (mostly starch).

Modern corn is 7½ inches long with over 800 kernels per ear (1,000 times larger in volume). More than 200 varieties are grown in 69 countries, which produce over 790 million tons per year. It is very sweet and juicy is made up of 73% water, 6.6% sugar (3.5 times sweeter), and 20% other (mostly starch).

Wild Peach	Modern Peach

 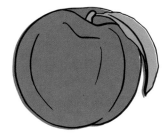

The wild peach measured less than 1 inch across. About 36% of the fruit was stone (pit); only 64% was edible. There were 3 known varieties, and they were found only in China in 4000 BCE. The peach tasted earthy with a sweet, sour, and salty flavor, almost like a lentil. It was 71% water, 8% sugar, and 20% other.

The modern peach is about 4 inches across, or 67 times larger in volume, and the stone comprises only 10% of the fruit, leaving 90% edible. It is very sweet and juicy. More than 200 varieties are produced in more than 80 countries. It is 89% water, 8.4% sugar (4 times sweeter by volume), and 1.7% other.

Wild Strawberry	Modern Strawberry
  Wild strawberries were very small at less than ¼ inch across. They were sweet and tart. It would take a day of foraging to collect a handful.	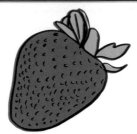 The strawberry was first hybridized by French botanists in the 1300s. They managed to make the fruit 15 to 20 times larger, but still much smaller than today's berry. In 1764, the pine strawberry was hybridized. It wasn't until 1806 when, by accident during hybridization experiments, the huge modern strawberry was developed. Strawberries are now grown year-round all over the world, with over 9 million tons produced each year.

Wild Tomato	Modern Tomato
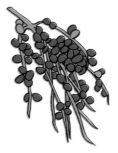 The tomato originated in Peru and was a small, almost berrylike fruit that measured about ⅓ inch across. The wild variety was avoided for years for fear of it being poisonous. It looked like a deadly nightshade plant, and every part of the plant was poisonous except for the fruit.	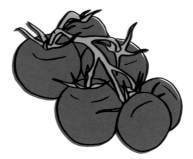 The modern tomato is hundreds of times bigger than its wild ancestor at over 4 inches across. It was hybridized in Mexico and was introduced to Europe (Spain and Italy) in the sixteenth century. It didn't become popular in America until the 1840s. Today, 3,000 varieties are grown all over the world, with 160 million tons of tomatoes produced each year.

This list could go on to encompass pretty much all the produce we eat today—all fruits, along with most vegetables, are the result of massive hybridization and cross-breeding over just the last few hundred years. Kohlrabi, kale, broccoli, Brussels sprouts, cabbage, and cauliflower were all hybridized from one plant, *Brassica oleracea*. Each exploited one part of the plant. Expansion of the flowers created broccoli and cauliflower. Expansion of the stem made kohlrabi. Expansion of the leaves gave us kale, collard greens, and Chinese broccoli. Expansion of the axillary buds gave us Brussels sprouts. Expansion of the terminal bud gave us cabbage. This all started around the fifth century for kale, the fifteenth century for cauliflower, and the eighteenth century for Brussels sprouts—only about 300 years ago.

A great example of how hybridization is aimed at making produce sweeter and sweeter is the recent introduction of cotton candy grapes. One serving has 100 calories and 28 grams of sugar, compared to 62 calories and 15 grams of sugar in one serving of regular grapes. That is almost double the sugar content of an already sugar-laden fruit!

In some cases, like tomatoes and strawberries, it was only about 100 years ago that they were adapted into the modern forms eaten today. As a result, people are consuming far more natural sugars and starches than ever before in human history. And as the sugar and starch content goes up, the nutrient density goes down, meaning that we get fewer vitamins and minerals per caloric.

Seasonality of Produce

In addition to hybridization, we now have a global food supply supported by technologies that allow us to grow fruits and vegetables year-round. This also is fairly new in human history. Let's take a closer look at the seasonality of produce.

As little as 100 years ago, fresh produce was not nearly as available as it is today. The first refrigerators were invented in 1834, with the first home refrigerators appearing in 1913. Frozen produce began appearing in the 1930s. The canning process dates back to 1809 and is credited to a French inventor named Nicolas Appert.

Fresh produce didn't become commonly available in the wintertime in most of North America until the late 1910s with the launch of an industrialized fresh food icon: iceberg lettuce. Lettuce entrepreneurs used California's year-round growing season and state-of-the-art refrigeration technology along with an extensive rail system for distribution to make iceberg one of America's most consumed vegetables. Chosen for its travel hardiness rather than its taste, iceberg lettuce set the precedent for the modern fresh produce industry. From this one product evolved the entire produce section of the grocery store that we see today as refrigeration technologies and year-round growing techniques were developed over the last 100 years.

As discussed earlier, our ancestors didn't eat fruits and vegetables all year long. Most of it was eaten in late summer and fall. What function did this serve for our hunter-gatherer ancestors?

Consuming more carbohydrates meant that less body fat was used for fuel and more dietary fat was stored. (This is due to oxidative priority, or the order in which our bodies process fuels, which we talk about in detail in the "Carnivore for Weight Loss" section on page 59.) From an evolutionary perspective, this makes sense: they were adding body fat, and preserving the fat they had, in the fall in order to prepare for the lean winter months when food was scarce. But today, we no longer have lean winter months. We can eat huge fresh strawberries in January. This puts us in a situation that our bodies have not yet evolved to deal with: we are constantly in fat preservation and storage mode.

Food Additives

One other concern about our modern food supply is all the additives being put into foods. Millions of new additives have crept in over just the last 30 to 40 years. Sure, our ancestors likely could eat root vegetables and more starch than people do today, but our ancestors did not eat like we do in modern times. After years of consuming "food" filled with ever higher amounts of fructose, food dyes, MSG, pesticides, and other chemicals, our cells are so damaged that we need a stricter approach to allow our bodies to heal.

It is important to understand scale when it comes to evolution. When we talk about human evolution, we speak in millennia, not centuries. It takes thousands of years to adapt to major changes in our food supply, not 100. Here's a good analogy: Imagine that human history spans the length of a football field, and you are standing at the goal line looking back to the beginning (about 2.4 million years). Agriculture and farming started just 15 inches away from you (10,000 years ago). This is the first time humans ate grains.

The majority of the changes in our food supply—the hybridization and cross-breeding of fruits and vegetables, the year-round availability of produce, and the introduction of millions of food additives—have occurred in the last 100 years or so. That is 0.15 inch away from you, or about the size of one or two blades of grass. The implementation of millions of food additives and chemicals over the last 40 years is just 0.06 inch away, or about the width of a sewing needle. Our bodies have not yet evolved to handle these changes properly, and it has led to an epidemic of obesity and disease. The carnivore diet is a great way to steer clear of these changes to which our bodies haven't adapted.

Plant Antinutrients

Growing up, we were told that we should eat unlimited amounts of fruits and veggies. There were no negatives to them, only positives, so to be healthy, we wanted to eat as many of them as possible. But it turns out that this isn't true. Fruits are just glorified candy loaded with sugar. And all plants come with compounds that can negatively affect our health.

Plants are not defenseless things; they are actually pretty smart and have natural defenses. When they need our help to disperse seeds, they package the seeds in colorful and appealing fruit and fill it with sugar to entice us to eat it. But that is the only part of itself that the plant wants you to eat. If you ate the leaves, stems, or roots, you would kill the plant. Since plants can't growl, bite, or run away like other animals, they have evolved their own weapons to defend themselves against those who might try to eat them.

All vegetables have antinutrients. These compounds are meant to protect the plant from insects and other pests that might eat them. They are natural pesticides. Some appear to be fairly benign when ingested by humans, but others are not. And it can depend on the individual's metabolic health and immune status. Some people with depressed immune systems (caused by Lyme disease and so on) are more sensitive to these natural pesticides. Other metabolically healthy people may be less sensitive.

There are thousands of plant antinutrients. Cabbage alone contains 49 natural pesticides and similar compounds. Of those, maybe three of have been studied in humans to analyze their effects on health. One of them is glucosinolate. Glucosinolate combines with myrosinase (an enzyme) to make sulforaphane, which is a natural pesticide that can be particularly harmful, as we will explain in the next section. So there are tons of compounds in plants that can affect our health, and many that have never even been studied to see how they could affect us.

These natural pesticides serve no function in the human body. That is why they are called antinutrients. The body sends them to the detoxification pathway to be removed. Some are even lethal in large doses. Let's go over some of the more harmful known antinutrients in plants.

Glucosinolate and Sulforaphane

Cruciferous vegetables belong to a family of plants that use isothiocyanates to protect themselves. Included in the cruciferous family are arugula, bok choy, broccoli, Brussels sprouts, cabbage, cauliflower, collard greens, kale, kohlrabi, mustard greens, mustard seeds, radishes, rutabagas, turnips, wasabi, and watercress, among others. Let's take a look at broccoli, one of the most popular cruciferous vegetables.

The isothiocyanate (naturally occurring small molecules that are formed from glucosinolate precursors of cruciferous vegetables) that the broccoli plant uses to defend itself is sulforaphane. But it doesn't sit in the field with sulforaphane on its surface. Sulforaphane is so toxic that if the broccoli sat there with sulforaphane on it, it would kill its own cells. This is where the plant is clever: it stores the two harmless ingredients for making sulforaphane, glucosinolate and myosinase, in separate compartments in its cells, which keeps them from combining and killing the plant. But when the plant is attacked or eaten, those compartments break open, and the two ingredients mix to form sulforaphane, which can kill insects, worms, and bacteria.[13]

You might be saying, "I'm not an insect or a worm, so why should I care?" Well, this toxin does the same thing in our bodies as it does in insects. It poisons mitochondria, inhibits enzymes that help us detoxify, generates reactive oxygen species (ROS), interferes with iodine absorption, can poke tiny holes in the sheaths or outer parts of our cells, and can deplete levels of glutathione, an important antioxidant. Sulforaphane can kill small animals via these mechanisms.

There are studies out there indicating that sulforaphane is actually helpful. They point to its ability to kill cancer cells. But sulforaphane is like chemotherapy in that way: it doesn't target cancer cells; it just kills every cell it encounters. The studies pointing to this "benefit" are epidemiological studies that are weak correlations at best.

All cruciferous vegetables contain sulforaphane-generating compounds, but there are ways to reduce the effects. Sprouts can have 20 to 100 times the amounts found in mature plants. Freezing or boiling the vegetables for 10 minutes can reduce the sulforaphane by about 50 percent. Steaming them reduces the amounts by about 65 percent. But you will still be getting some sulforaphane, which your system then has to detox. This may be okay for someone with a strong immune system, but for someone with Lyme disease or another chronic disease that suppresses the immune system, it can cause problems.

Oxalates

One of the most damaging types of antinutrients found in almost all plants is oxalates. Oxalates are tiny crystals that can act like tiny glass shards or spears in the body when they accumulate. Check out these photos of the oxalates in kiwi fruit.[14]

---

[13]Georgia Ede, "Is Broccoli Good for You? Meet the Crucifer Family…" Diagnosis Diet website, accessed October 30, 2019, www.diagnosisdiet.com/is-broccoli-good-for-you

[14]K. Konno, T. A. Inoue, and M. Nakamura, "Synergistic Defensive Function of Raphides and Protease Through the Needle Effect," *PLOS One* 9, no. 3 (2014): e91341.

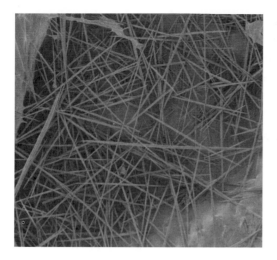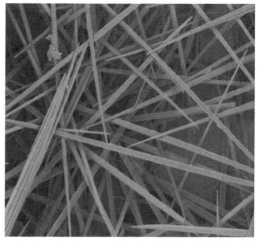

"Synergistic Defensive Function of Raphides and Protease through the Needle Effect" by Kotaro Konno, Takashi A. Inoue, Masatoshi Nakamura is licensed under CC BY 4.0.

These irritants can really bother our bodies when consumed in large amounts. The tiny spears damage cells throughout the digestive tract and in the body when they are absorbed, which can lead to leaky gut and many other issues. These oxalates are toxins and need to be detoxed from the body.

Some plants have high levels of oxalates, while others have less. Some of the highest oxalate levels are found in spinach, Swiss chard, curly kale, chocolate, almonds and other nuts, sesame seeds and other seeds, potatoes, sweet potatoes, cinnamon, turmeric, peanuts and other legumes, green tea, beets, rhubarb, figs, kiwi, blackberries, grains, and plantains, with peanuts, almonds, potatoes, and spinach being some of the worst. Lower levels of oxalates are found in arugula, bok choy, endive, cabbage, lettuce, cauliflower, cucumbers, radishes, mustard greens, garlic, avocado, mushrooms, peas, and watercress.[15]

The safe limit of oxalates for humans depends on a lot of factors. For most people, 100 milligrams a day or less is probably okay, but for people with digestive issues, suppressed immune systems, and other health conditions, the limit can be lower. The lethal level—the level that will kill you—has a wide range of 3.5 to 30 grams. In those who are vulnerable, just 3.5 grams can be deadly. That is only three of the green smoothies that are so popular these days. One 52-year-old man in Barcelona, Spain, died after eating three bowls of sorrel soup (which has about 3.5 grams of oxalates).[16] He had diabetes, which likely caused his tolerance level to be on the lower side. But others have died from ingesting too much oxalate at one time.

---

[15]Sally K. Norton, "Lost Seasonality and Overconsumption of Plants: Risking Oxalate Toxicity," *Journal of Evolution and Health* 2, no. 3 (2017): 4. jevohealth.com/journal/vol2/iss3/4/

[16]See note 15 above.

In addition to eating high amounts of foods with oxalates, people with digestive issues (celiac disease, small intestinal bacteria overgrowth, Crohn's disease, irritable bowel syndrome, and so on), a history of extended use of antibiotics, or a history of kidney problems and kidney stones are all at higher risk for oxalate accumulation. Oxalates can attach to cells throughout the body and disrupt the normal function of nerves, glands, bones, eyes, heart, and other cells.[17] They are primarily detoxed through the kidneys, causing irritation of the kidneys; oxalate buildup causes over 80 percent of kidney stones.[18]

Oxalate accumulation over time can cause many of the common symptoms of aging, including fragile bones, hormone imbalances, joint problems, nerve damage, headaches, sleep disorders, and restless legs.[19] A 1993 study out of Japan found that 85 percent of samples from people over 50 contained oxalate deposits. Upwards of 80 percent of people with thyroid problems have oxalates in their thyroid.[20] Microcalcification of calcium oxalates in the breasts has been shown to be a potential early indicator of breast cancer.[21] Even gout has been linked to oxalates.

Oxalates also deplete the body of many minerals—especially iron, calcium, and magnesium. This is part of the danger in thinking that because certain plants are high in minerals, eating them will improve our health. For example, spinach is high in calcium, but it is also high in oxalates, which grab onto calcium and steal it from the body.

Unfortunately, unlike other antinutrients in plants, there isn't much you can do to reduce the oxalate content in foods. Boiling, soaking, fermenting, and cooking don't reduce oxalate content significantly. The best thing you can do is to avoid high-oxalate foods, especially green smoothies, which can contain high concentrations of oxalates.

When dealing with excess oxalates, it's a good idea to up your mineral consumption with nutrient-dense foods like beef (see the section "The Case for a Meat-Based Diet: Nutrient Density of Animal Proteins"). Spending time in a sauna is another good way to remove oxalates from the body. Citrates help, too, so taking potassium citrate and magnesium citrate supplements can be helpful.

---

[17]M. Broyer, P. Jouvet, P. Niaudet, M. Daudon, and Y. Revillon, "Management of Oxalosis," *Kidney International Supplements* 53 (1996): S93–98.

[18]V. Butterweck and S. R. Khan, "Herbal Medicines in the Management of Urolithiasis: Alternative or Complementary?" *Planta Medica* 75, no. 10 (2017): 1095–103.

[19]N. Rahman and R. Hitchcock, "Case Report of Paediatric Oxalate, Urolithiasis and a Review of Enteric Hyperoxaluria," *Journal of Pediatric Urology* 6, no. 2 (2010): 112–6.

[20]J. D. Reid, C. H. Choi, and N. O. Oldroyd, "Calcium Oxylate Crystals in the Thyroid. Their Identification, Prevalence, Origin, and Possible Significance," *American Journal of Clinical Pathology* 87, no. 4 (1987): 443–54.

[21]A. M. Castellaro, A. Tonda, H. H. Cejas, H. Ferreyra, B. L. Caputto, O. A. Pucci, and G. A. Gil, "Oxalate Induces Breast Cancer," *BMC Cancer* 15 (2015): 761.

Phytate (Phytic Acid)

Phytic acid is a plant acid that can be found in all parts of plants but mostly occupies the bran-rich outer coating of seeds, beans, nuts, and grains. It is not found in animals.

Phytic acid acts like a sponge, soaking up minerals and preventing their absorption into the body. It is particularly good at preventing iron, calcium, zinc, copper, and magnesium from being absorbed. Phytic acid itself doesn't appear to be absorbed into our bodies; it leaves the body intact once detoxed. But with the phytic acid go the vital minerals that have bound to it, which causes mineral deficiencies. This may be one of the reasons vegans, who tend to get their protein from plant sources like beans and nuts, tend to have low levels of these minerals.

Removing the bran from nuts and seeds can eliminate much of their phytic acid. Phytic acid levels also can be reduced by soaking, sprouting, and fermenting foods.

Glycoalkaloids

You may not have heard of glycoalkaloids, but you probably have heard of nightshades. Nightshades are a family of plants that contain glycoalkaloids and include tomatoes, eggplant, potatoes, and peppers, as well as tobacco.

Glycoalkaloids are natural pesticides made by plants for protection. They defend the plants against bacteria, fungi, viruses, and insects. Glycoalkaloids bind with cholesterol in cell membranes, which disrupts the structure of the membranes and causes the cells to leak or burst. They act also as neurotoxins by blocking the enzyme cholinesterase. Cholinesterase breaks down acetylcholine, which is a vital neurotransmitter. This breakdown enables acetylcholine to accumulate in the brain, potentially causing mental health issues.

Since studies have shown that glycoalkaloids destroy cell membranes, some researchers have wondered if glycoalkaloids could be one of the causes of leaky gut.[22]

Glycoalkaloid toxicity can cause neurological symptoms including apathy, restlessness, drowsiness, mental confusion, rambling, incoherence, stupor, hallucinations, dizziness, trembling, and visual disturbances.[23] One potential cause of anxiety and insomnia is eating too many nightshades.

---

[22]B. Patel, R. Schutte, P. Sporns, J. Doyle, L. Jewel, and R. N. Fedorak, "Potato Glycoalkaloids Adversely Affect Intestinal Permeability and Aggravate Inflammatory Bowel Disease," *Inflammatory Bowel Diseases* 8, no. 5 (2002): 340–6.

[23]S. E. Milner, N. P. Brunton, P. W. Jones, N. M. O'Brien, S. G. Collins, and A. R. Maguire, "Bioactivities of Glycoalkaloids and Their Aglycones from Solanum Species," *Journal of Agricultural and Food Chemistry* 59, no. 8 (2011): 3454–84.

It is predicted that in the year 2020, depression will be the leading cause of disability in the United States. You decide what you put on the end of your fork. Let food be thy medicine.

The potato has the highest concentration of glycoalkaloids. Boiling potatoes reduces the amount of glycoalkaloids by only a few percentage points. Deep-frying them at 300°F has no effect at all; at 410°F, you can reduce glycoalkaloids by 40 percent. However, baking and other cooking methods don't reduce the amounts significantly. Studies have shown that as little as 1 milligram of glycoalkaloids per kilogram of body weight can be toxic, and as little as 3 milligrams per kilogram of body weight can be fatal. The FDA stipulates that the glycoalkaloids in potatoes cannot exceed 91 milligrams per pound.[24]

Let's look at potato chips as an example. A 1-ounce bag (single-serving size) contains roughly 2.7 to 12.4 milligrams of glycoalkaloids.[25] That small bag—the smallest one available—is enough for glycoalkaloids to reach toxicity levels in a 26-pound child. How many adults can easily throw down an 8-ounce bag of chips? That portion can supply up to 100 milligrams of glycoalkaloids, which is enough to reach the lower end of the toxicity range for a 200-pound person. When you consider that potatoes are also one of the foods highest in oxalates, could Americans' love of potatoes and french fries be what has led to the epidemic of leaky gut and resulting autoimmune disorders?

In summary, we have covered just a few of the most studied antinutrients in plants. There are hundreds of compounds in fruits and vegetables, and we don't even know what many of them do in the human body. But we do know that lectins and saponins can cause leaky gut, tannins and resveratrol can damage cell membranes, goitrogens disrupt thyroid function, polyphenols are estrogenic and deplete iron, and salicylates can cause allergy-like symptoms. Many more natural pesticides are present in plants, and there haven't been studies in humans to know their real effects.

When you consider the ever-increasing sizes of fruits and vegetables along with their year-round availability, it is clear that we are getting more and more of these natural pesticides in our bodies, and they can negatively affect our health. This may be one of the reasons we are seeing a large increase in leaky gut and related autoimmune diseases.

---

[24]Georgia Ede, "How Deadly Are Nightshades?" Diagnosis Diet website, accessed November 13, 2019, www.diagnosisdiet.com/nightshades/

[25]See note 23 above.

THE CASE FOR A MEAT-BASED DIET: NUTRIENT DENSITY OF ANIMAL PROTEINS

An important aspect of a healthy diet that enables weight loss and healing is eating the most nutrient-dense foods possible. Getting all the vitamins and minerals your body needs while consuming the fewest calories to get them is essential for healing and long-term health.

Many people wonder how to get enough vitamins and minerals when eating carnivore. The popular belief is that you get your vitamins and minerals from fruits and vegetables. But is that really true? Let's dive into this a bit further and see where vitamins and minerals come from.

Animal Proteins versus Plants

We often hear about the latest "superfood," such as apples, blueberries, and kale. But are these really superfoods? A superfood should be one that has the most nutrients across the widest range of nutrients possible. Take a look at the following chart. It compares the micronutrients in apples, blueberries, kale, beef, and beef liver, with the highest scoring highlighted the darker color and the second place finishers highlighted in the lighter color.

Nutrients in "Superfoods" Compared to Animal Protein

Per Serving	Apples	Blueberries	Kale	Beef	Beef Liver
Calcium (mg)	9.1	4.5	63.4	11.0	11.0
Magnesium (mg)	7.3	4.5	15.0	19.0	18.0
Phosphorus (mg)	20.0	9.0	24.6	175.0	387.0
Potassium (mg)	163.8	57.8	200.6	370.0	380.0
Iron (mg)	0.2	0.2	0.8	3.3	8.8
Zinc (mg)	0.2	0.2	0.2	4.5	4.0
Selenium (mcg)	0	0.1	0.4	14.2	39.7
Vitamin A (IU)	69.2	40.5	13,530.9	40.0	53,400.0
Vitamin B6 (mg)	0	0.1	0.1	0.4	1.1
Vitamin B12 (mg)	0	0	0	2.0	11.0
Vitamin C (mg)	7.3	7.3	36.1	2.0	27.0
Vitamin D (IU)	0	0	0	7.0	19.0
Vitamin E (mg)	0.2	0.5	0.8	1.7	0.6
Niacin (mg)	0.2	0.3	0.4	4.8	17.0
Folate (mcg)	0	4.5	11.4	6.0	145.0

As you can see, the real superfood is beef liver. It is one of the most nutrient-dense foods on the planet. Of the others, only kale scores any first- or second-place finishes, and one is vitamin C, which you don't need as much of when eating carnivore—you can find more on this in the section "Bioavailability and Recommended Daily Allowances (RDA)." In second place overall is regular beef—like a sirloin steak. Yes, we are telling you to look at your steak like it is a piece of kale, loaded with nutrients.

You may be wary of liver, but we encourage you to incorporate it into your carnivore diet. There are ways to sneak it in, such as by adding it to ground beef (one part liver per four to five parts ground beef) for tasty, nutrient-dense burgers. In the meantime, let's look at how that steak measures up against kale, blueberries, and apples.

(per 100g)	Apples	Blueberries	Kale	Beef
Calcium (mg)	5.0	6.0	72.0	11.0
Magnesium (mg)	4.0	6.0	17.0	19.0
Phosphorus (mg)	11.0	12.0	28.0	175.0
Potassium (mg)	90.0	77.0	228.0	370.0
Iron (mg)	0.1	0.3	0.9	3.3
Zinc (mg)	0.1	0.2	0.2	4.5
Selenium (mcg)	0	0.1	0.5	14.2
Vitamin A (IU)	38.0	54.0	769.0	40.0
Vitamin B6 (mg)	0	0.1	0.1	0.4
Vitamin B12 (mg)	0	0	0	2.0
Vitamin C (mg)	4.0	9.7	41.0	2.0
Vitamin D (IU)	0	0	0	7.0
Vitamin E (mg)	0.1	0.6	0.9	1.7
Niacin (mg)	0.1	0.4	0.5	4.8
Folate (mcg)	0	6.0	13.0	6.0

Beef ranks number one in 11 out of 15 vitamins and minerals and number two in another two of them. So instead of telling our kids to eat their veggies, we should be telling them to eat their steak! (And believe us, in our house we do.)

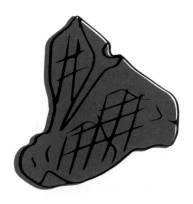

Per Serving	Chicken	Pork	Eggs	Salmon	Beef	Beef Liver
Calcium (mg)	11.0	5.0	53.0	9.0	11.0	11.0
Magnesium (mg)	28.0	24.0	12.0	27.0	19.0	18.0
Phosphorus (mg)	196.0	296.0	191.0	240.0	175.0	387.0
Potassium (mg)	255.0	489.0	134.0	363.0	370.0	380.0
Iron (mg)	0.7	0.4	1.8	0.3	3.3	8.8
Zinc (mg)	0.8	1.4	1.1	0.4	4.5	4.0
Selenium (mcg)	17.8	40.6	31.7	24.0	14.2	39.7
Vitamin A (IU)	21.0	0	487.0	50.0	40.0	53,400.0
Vitamin B6 (mg)	0.5	0.7	0.1	0.6	0.4	1.1
Vitamin B12 (mg)	0.4	0.5	1.3	3.2	2.0	111.0
Vitamin C (mg)	1.2	0	0	3.9	2.0	27.0
Vitamin D (IU)	2.0	53.0	35.0	526.0	7.0	19.0
Vitamin E (mg)	0.1	0.1	1.0	3.6	1.7	0.63
Niacin (mg)	11.2	8.8	0.1	8.7	4.8	17.0
Folate (mcg)	4.0	0	47.0	26.0	6.0	145.0

Looking across a range of animal proteins, you can see that some are even higher in certain nutrients than beef. For example, pork is higher in potassium and selenium. Chicken is higher in magnesium. Salmon is higher in vitamins D and E. Eggs are higher in calcium. Eating a variety of animal proteins can provide you with all the nutrients your body needs, especially if you include organ meats.

Even with these numbers showing that animal proteins are champions of nutrient density, there is another factor that makes them even more dominant: the bioavailability of those nutrients.

Bioavailability of Nutrients

Bioavailability refers to how well the body can absorb and utilize nutrients. It doesn't help us much if a food is extremely high in a given nutrient but our bodies can't make use of that nutrient and it goes right through us. Antinutrients, which we discussed earlier in the section "Plant Antinutrients," are a big culprit when it comes to reducing bioavailability. Oxalates bind to minerals like calcium, magnesium, and potassium, depriving our bodies of these nutrients, and phytates block the absorption of critical nutrients like calcium, iron, and zinc.

A study of zinc absorption found that when plant foods were substituted for meat, zinc absorption was reduced by almost half. The researchers concluded that "those consuming vegetarian diets…may require as much as 50 percent more zinc than nonvegetarians."[26] They also found that "vegetarians need to increase dietary iron by 80% to compensate for an estimated lower iron bioavailability of 10% from a vegetarian diet, compared with 18% from a mixed Western diet."

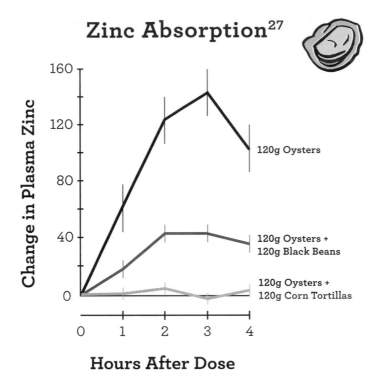

Zinc Absorption[27]

Change in Plasma Zinc

160

120

80

40

0

120g Oysters

120g Oysters + 120g Black Beans

120g Oysters + 120g Corn Tortillas

0   1   2   3   4

Hours After Dose

In another study, researchers compared zinc absorption in the body when oysters were eaten by themselves versus with black beans or corn tortillas. As you can see in the chart above, zinc absorption was cut by 75 percent when the oysters were eaten with black beans and completed disrupted when they were eaten with corn tortillas. All of the zinc from the oysters was robbed from the body because of the antinutrients in the corn tortillas.

A study on iron found that eating red meat increased nonheme iron absorption by 85 percent.[28] Another study showed that iron absorption from legumes was as low as 0.84 percent even in those who were very iron deficient.[29] This is in part to phytates blocking absorption, but the study also found that "even after complete degradation of phytic acid, soybean protein still inhibits iron absorption." For reference, iron absorption from eggs ranges from 5 to 9 percent, or as much as ten times higher. Iron absorption from beef is 7 to 8 percent.[30]

---

[26]J. R. Hunt, S. K. Gallagher, L. K. Johnson, and G. I. Lykken, "High- Versus Low-Meat Diets: Effects on Zinc Absorption, Iron Status, and Calcium, Copper, Iron, Magnesium, Manganese, Nitrogen, Phosphorus, and Zinc Balance in Postmenopausal Women," *American Journal of Clinical Nutrition* 62, no. 3 (1995): 621-32.

[27]N. W. Solomons and R. A. Jacob, "Studies on the Bioavailability of Zinc in Humans: Effects of Heme and Nonheme Iron on the Absorption of Zinc," *American Journal of Clinical Nutrition* 34, no. 4 (1981): 475-82. Georgia Ede, "Your Brain on Plants: Micronutrients and Mental Health," Diagnosis Diet website, September 5, 2017, www.diagnosisdiet.com/micronutrients-mental-health/.

[28]L. Hallberg, M. Hoppe, M. Andersson, and L. Hulthén, "The Role of Meat to Improve the Critical Iron Balance During Weaning," *Pediatrics* 111, no. 4 (2003): 864-70.

[29]S. R. Lynch, J. L. Beard, S. A. Bassenko, and J. D. Cook, "Iron Absorption from Legumes in Humans," *American Journal of Clinical Nutrition* 40, no. 1 (1984): 42-7.

[30]P. Etcheverry, K. M. Hawthorne, L. K. Liang, S. A. Abrams, and I. J. Griffin, "Effect of Beef and Soy Proteins on the Absorption of Non-Heme Iron and Inorganic Zinc in Children," *Journal of the American College of Nutrition* 25, no. 1 (2006): 34–40.

There are many more examples of this effect, including vitamin A. Animal foods have about 20 times the bioavailability of vitamin A as plant sources.[31] It is also important to note that vitamins B12, D3, and K2 do not exist in plant foods.[32]

Bioavailability and Recommended Daily Allowances (RDA)

An important factor to note when looking at the Recommended Daily Allowances (RDA) for vitamins and minerals is that the guidelines represent what is needed when someone is eating a standard American diet. The RDA was meant to encompass all people and ensure that no one is deficient in any nutrients. That means person A may need ten units of something (because of diet and other factors), whereas person B needs only one unit. However, the recommendation will be ten units to ensure that everyone is covered. That still doesn't mean person B needs ten units; they need only one. Diet can have a big impact on what's needed. A person who eats more bioavailable foods that don't contain antinutrients will require far fewer nutrients than someone who eats plants that have a lot of antinutrients and nutrients that are less bioavailable.

Several examples show how someone eating a low-carb or carnivore diet requires different levels of micronutrients than someone eating a standard American diet. One example is iodine. The thyroid slows down when eating keto: T3 drops by 40 to 50 percent.[33] But this isn't hypothyroid. Our bodies get more efficient at using T3 and thus need less. The thyroid is an iodine hog, so a slower thyroid means that less iodine is needed. T3 levels correlate to the level of carbohydrates consumed. This means that a normal T3 level for someone eating lots of carbs is much higher than a normal T3 level for someone eating low to no carbs. And artificially pumping up T3 when carbohydrate consumption is low can cause issues as the body thinks carbs are available when they aren't.

Zinc is another example. As discussed in the section "Plant Antinutrients," antinutrients like phytates block zinc absorption. This means that someone who eats primarily vegetarian or plant foods may require 50 percent or more zinc than the average person. Someone who eats no plants needs far less zinc.

---

[31]Marjorie J. Haskell, "The Challenge to Reach Nutritional Adequacy for Vitamin A ß-carotene Bioavailability ad Conversion—Evidence in Humans," *American Journal of Clinical Nutrition* 96, no. 5 (2012): 1193S-1203S.

[32]L. J. Black, R. M. Lucas, J. L. Sherriff, L. O. Björn, and J. F. Bornman, "In Pursuit of Vitamin D in Plants," *Nutrients* 9, no. 2 (2017): 136.

[33]E. Danforth, Jr., E. S. Horton, M. O'Connell, E. A. Sims, A. G. Burger, S. H. Ingbar, L. Braverman, and A. G. Vagenakis, "Dietary-Induced Alterations in Thyroid Hormone Metabolism During Overnutrition," *Journal of Clinical Investigation* 64, no. 5 (1979): 1336–47.

Yet another example is vitamin C. If you don't get enough vitamin C, you can get scurvy. Diets low in fruit are often criticized because they don't provide enough vitamin C to prevent scurvy. As it turns out, however, your carbohydrate intake directly affects your vitamin C needs. The fewer carbs you eat, the less vitamin C you need.[34]

Also, the level of vitamin C needed to prevent scurvy is quite small—about 6.5 to 10 milligrams per day.[35] Contrary to what you might see listed in the nutritional information on product packaging, meats contain enough vitamin C to prevent scurvy. The USDA labs have a practice of entering 0 grams for vitamin C when testing protein,[36] which means that the nutritional information always says 0 grams, even though meat does contain some vitamin C. According to a study done in 2013, for example, ox protein has about 1.6 milligrams of vitamin C per 100 grams.[37] (The amount of vitamin C in beef could be higher.)

There are plenty of examples of people being carnivore for 20 years without any issues of scurvy or low vitamin C levels. Eating essentially zero carbs makes our requirement for C very low, and we get enough from meat, especially if we include organ meat like beef liver. Just make sure to include lots of fresh meats that are cooked properly, including an occasional serving of liver (if you enjoy it—or hide it in ground beef, as described on page 32), to ensure you get the vitamin C your body needs. Meats that aren't fresh, like cured or overcooked meats, are depleted of their vitamin C, so make sure to include some fresh meats in your diet.

We believe that you can get all the nutrients your body needs from animal foods. Animal foods contain no antinutrients to leach or block the absorption of nutrients, and they are much more bioavailable. This is reflected in people who have eaten carnivore for 20-plus years and are thriving, with none of the symptoms they had experienced prior to going carnivore (bipolar disorder, Lyme disease, etc.).

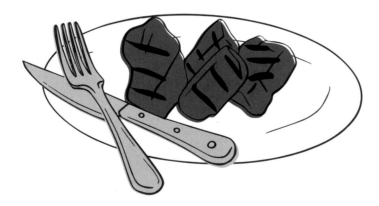

[34] Amber O'Hearn, "Ketogenic Diet and Vitamin C: The 101," BreakNutrition website, February 21, 2017, breaknutrition.com/ketogenic-dietvitamin-c-101/

[35] Institute of Medicine, "2, Vitamin C: Needs and Functions," in *Vitamin C Fortification of Food Aid Commodities: Final Report* (Washington, DC: National Academies Press, 1997).

[36] Amber O'Hearn, "C Is for Carnivore," Empirica blog, February 21, 2017, www.empiri.ca/2017/02/cis-for-carnivore.html

[37] Helmut Matzner and Geoffrey H. Bourne, "*Die Ascorbinsäure in der Pflanzenzelle* [Vitamin C in the Animal Cell]," Springer-Verlag, Mar 8, 2013: 1–70.

Not only does eating a carnivore diet supply the foods our bodies were designed to eat, but it also provides us with some of the most nutrient-dense foods available. You will supply your body with tons of bioavailable nutrients that it needs to heal and thrive.

HOW MUCH PROTEIN DOES YOUR BODY NEED?

Our bodies need amino acids to survive. Quality animal proteins supply us with all the amino acids we require. But what is the minimum amount of protein needed? It is based on your lean mass. The more lean mass you have, the more amino acids are required to maintain it.

For the average person, a good goal is to eat at least 0.8 times your lean mass (in pounds) in grams of protein a day. But this goal varies by age. Younger children need more protein to fuel growth. People over about 60 years old need more protein just to maintain, as the body's needs for protein increase (called leucine shift). You can find more information on page 48.

You calculate your lean mass by subtracting body fat from total weight. For example, a woman who is 5-foot-4 and 180 pounds with 40 percent body fat has 108 pounds of lean mass:

$$180 - (180 \times 0.4) = 108 \text{ pounds}$$

Therefore, she should eat at least 86 grams of protein a day:

$$108 \times 0.8 = 86 \text{ grams}$$

When eating carnivore, hitting this goal shouldn't be a problem. If you are doing a protein-sparing modified fast (see page 64), try to get at least this amount of protein per day.

Bioavailability of Proteins

Different protein sources have different amino acid compositions. The specific proteins you consume also affect how many grams of protein you need each day to maintain your lean mass.

There are nine essential amino acids that the body cannot make on its own. When a protein source includes all nine of those amino acids, it is considered a complete protein. On a carnivore diet, the proteins you eat are complete proteins; therefore, you can simply count the total grams of protein consumed. Many plant proteins are incomplete, which means that you need more of them to maintain or hit your protein goal. The lower the Amino Acid Score, the more protein from that source you will need to meet your protein goal for the day. The following chart lists the amino acid scores for common proteins.[38] As you can see, eating non-animal proteins can mean that you need many more grams of protein each day just to maintain your lean mass.

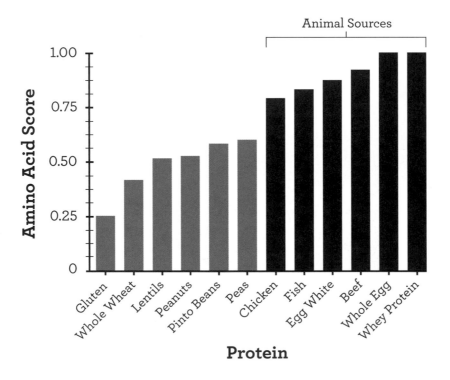

Protein Digestibility Corrected Amino Acid Score (PDCAAS)

---

[38]J. R. Hoffman and M. J. Falvo, "Protein—Which Is Best?" *Journal of Sports Science & Medicine* 3, no. 3 (2004): 118–30.

Lentil proteins, for example, have an Amino Acid Score of 0.51, which means that they are about half as bioavailable as egg or beef proteins. If your protein goal was 85 grams a day and you were relying on plant sources like lentils for protein, then you would need to consume about 170 grams of lentil protein a day. Eating carnivore ensures that you get the most bioavailable proteins that help you build and maintain lean mass and can reach your protein goal with the least calories, which is great for fat loss.

Protein Sources

Here are some charts of various animal proteins. The first few charts show you different cuts of meat and their fat and protein composition. The latter tables are sorted by the ratio of fat to protein, or protein/energy (P/E) ratio. This information is convenient when adjusting your diet for weight loss or maintenance. If you want to lose weight, go up the tables to the protein sources that are lower in fat and higher in protein. If you want to maintain, move down the tables and pick proteins that have more fat and less protein. In either situation, make sure to at least meet your protein requirement each day.

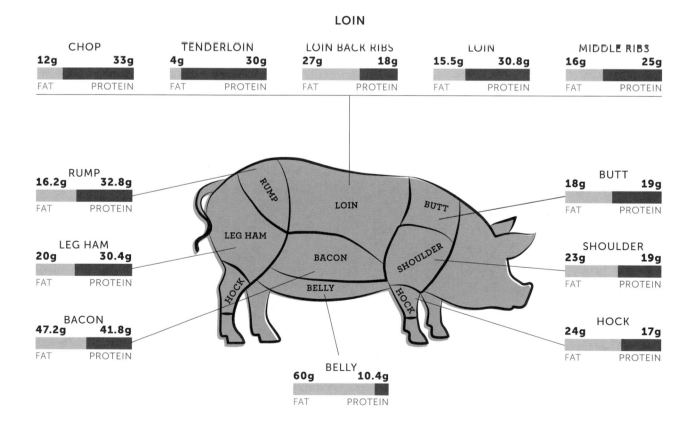

LOIN

CHOP		TENDERLOIN		LOIN BACK RIBS		LOIN		MIDDLE RIBS	
12g	33g	4g	30g	27g	18g	15.5g	30.8g	16g	25g
FAT	PROTEIN	FAT	PROTEIN	FAT	PROTEIN	FAT	PROTEIN	FAT	PROTEIN

RUMP			BUTT
16.2g	32.8g	18g	19g
FAT	PROTEIN	FAT	PROTEIN

LEG HAM			SHOULDER
20g	30.4g	23g	19g
FAT	PROTEIN	FAT	PROTEIN

BACON			HOCK
47.2g	41.8g	24g	17g
FAT	PROTEIN	FAT	PROTEIN

BELLY	
60g	10.4g
FAT	PROTEIN

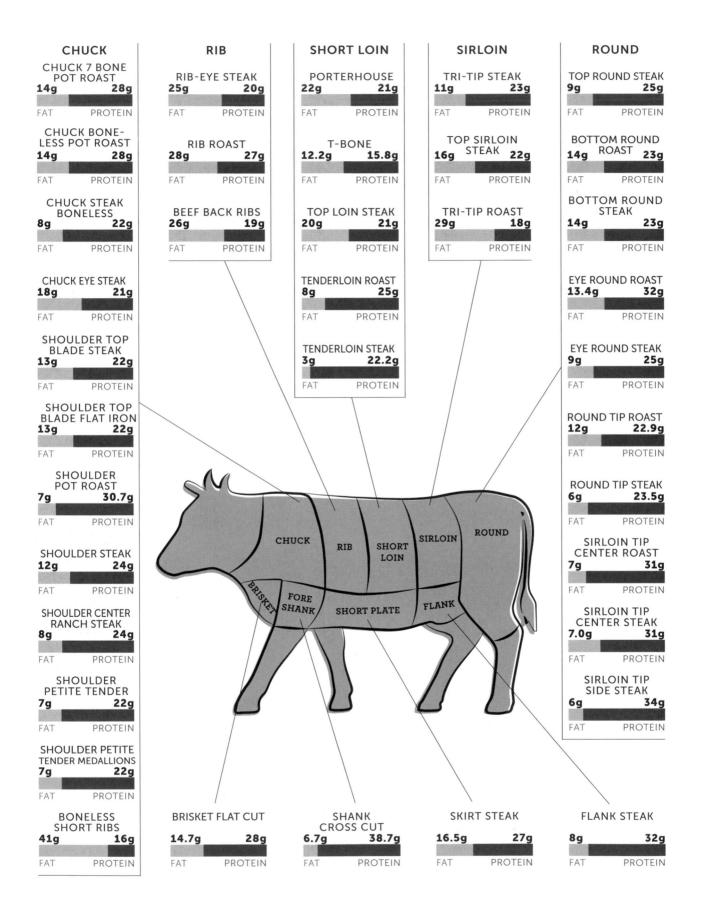

CHUCK

CHUCK 7 BONE POT ROAST
14g FAT | 28g PROTEIN

CHUCK BONELESS POT ROAST
14g FAT | 28g PROTEIN

CHUCK STEAK BONELESS
8g FAT | 22g PROTEIN

CHUCK EYE STEAK
18g FAT | 21g PROTEIN

SHOULDER TOP BLADE STEAK
13g FAT | 22g PROTEIN

SHOULDER TOP BLADE FLAT IRON
13g FAT | 22g PROTEIN

SHOULDER POT ROAST
7g FAT | 30.7g PROTEIN

SHOULDER STEAK
12g FAT | 24g PROTEIN

SHOULDER CENTER RANCH STEAK
8g FAT | 24g PROTEIN

SHOULDER PETITE TENDER
7g FAT | 22g PROTEIN

SHOULDER PETITE TENDER MEDALLIONS
7g FAT | 22g PROTEIN

BONELESS SHORT RIBS
41g FAT | 16g PROTEIN

RIB

RIB-EYE STEAK
25g FAT | 20g PROTEIN

RIB ROAST
28g FAT | 27g PROTEIN

BEEF BACK RIBS
26g FAT | 19g PROTEIN

BRISKET FLAT CUT
14.7g FAT | 28g PROTEIN

SHORT LOIN

PORTERHOUSE
22g FAT | 21g PROTEIN

T-BONE
12.2g FAT | 15.8g PROTEIN

TOP LOIN STEAK
20g FAT | 21g PROTEIN

TENDERLOIN ROAST
8g FAT | 25g PROTEIN

TENDERLOIN STEAK
3g FAT | 22.2g PROTEIN

SHANK CROSS CUT
6.7g FAT | 38.7g PROTEIN

SIRLOIN

TRI-TIP STEAK
11g FAT | 23g PROTEIN

TOP SIRLOIN STEAK
16g FAT | 22g PROTEIN

TRI-TIP ROAST
29g FAT | 18g PROTEIN

SKIRT STEAK
16.5g FAT | 27g PROTEIN

ROUND

TOP ROUND STEAK
9g FAT | 25g PROTEIN

BOTTOM ROUND ROAST
14g FAT | 23g PROTEIN

BOTTOM ROUND STEAK
14g FAT | 23g PROTEIN

EYE ROUND ROAST
13.4g FAT | 32g PROTEIN

EYE ROUND STEAK
9g FAT | 25g PROTEIN

ROUND TIP ROAST
12g FAT | 22.9g PROTEIN

ROUND TIP STEAK
6g FAT | 23.5g PROTEIN

SIRLOIN TIP CENTER ROAST
7g FAT | 31g PROTEIN

SIRLOIN TIP CENTER STEAK
7.0g FAT | 31g PROTEIN

SIRLOIN TIP SIDE STEAK
6g FAT | 34g PROTEIN

FLANK STEAK
8g FAT | 32g PROTEIN

Cow diagram labels: CHUCK, RIB, SHORT LOIN, SIRLOIN, ROUND, BRISKET, FORE SHANK, SHORT PLATE, FLANK

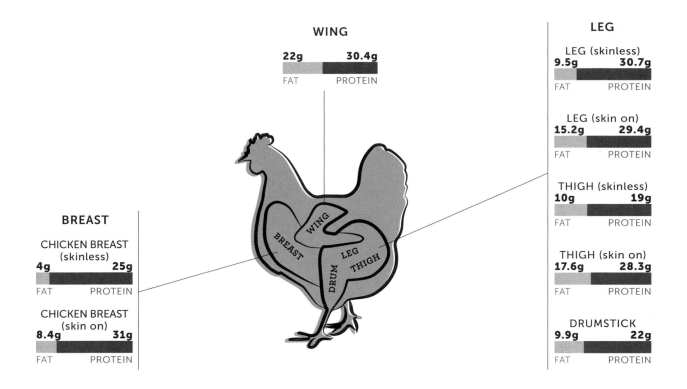

WING

22g   30.4g
FAT   PROTEIN

LEG

LEG (skinless)
9.5g   30.7g
FAT   PROTEIN

LEG (skin on)
15.2g   29.4g
FAT   PROTEIN

THIGH (skinless)
10g   19g
FAT   PROTEIN

THIGH (skin on)
17.6g   28.3g
FAT   PROTEIN

DRUMSTICK
9.9g   22g
FAT   PROTEIN

BREAST

CHICKEN BREAST
(skinless)
4g   25g
FAT   PROTEIN

CHICKEN BREAST
(skin on)
8.4g   31g
FAT   PROTEIN

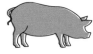

Pork (4 ounces)	Calories	Fat	Protein	Carbs	P/E Ratio
Belly	588	60.0	10.4	0	0.17
Loin back ribs (baby back ribs)	315	27.0	18.0	0	0.67
Hocks	285	24.0	17.0	0	0.71
Shoulder	285	23.0	19.0	0	0.83
Bacon	600	47.2	41.8	0	0.89
Cracklings (pork rinds)	530	40.0	39.0	1.9	0.98
Butt	240	18.0	19.0	0	1.06
Brains	156	11.0	14.0	0	1.27
Tongue	307	21.0	27.3	0	1.30
Ears	188	12.3	18.0	0.2	1.46
Leg ham	305	20.0	30.4	0	1.52
Middle ribs (country style)	245	16.0	25.0	0	1.56
Loin	265	15.5	30.8	0	1.99
Rump	280	16.2	32.8	0	2.02
Chop	241	12.0	33.0	0	2.75
Heart	168	5.7	26.8	0.5	4.70
Kidney	171	5.3	28.8	0	5.43
Liver	187	5.0	29.5	4.3	5.90
Tenderloin	158	4.0	30.0	0	7.50

Beef (4 ounces)	Calories	Fat	Protein	Carbs	P/E Ratio
Short ribs, boneless	440	41.0	16.0	0	0.39
Tri-tip roast	340	29.0	18.0	0	0.62
Back ribs	310	26.0	19.0	0	0.73
Rib-eye steak	310	25.0	20.0	0	0.80
Tongue	322	25.3	22.0	0	0.87
Sweetbreads	362	28.3	25.0	0	0.88
Porterhouse	280	22.0	21.0	0	0.95
Rib roast	373	28.0	27.0	0	0.96
Top loin steak, boneless	270	20.0	21.0	0	1.05
Top loin steak, bone-in	270	20.0	21.0	0	1.05
Brains	171	11.9	13.2	1.7	1.11
Chuck eye steak	250	18.0	21.0	0	1.17
T-bone	170	12.2	15.8	0	1.30
Top sirloin steak	240	16.0	22.0	0	1.38
Skirt steak	255	16.5	27.0	0	1.64
Bottom round steak	220	14.0	23.0	0	1.64
Bottom round roast	220	14.0	23.0	0	1.64
Shoulder top blade flat iron steak	204	13.0	22.0	0	1.69
Shoulder top blade steak	204	13.0	22.0	0	1.69
Round tip roast	199	12.0	22.9	0	1.91
Brisket, flat cut	245	14.7	28.0	0	1.91
Shoulder steak	204	12.0	24.0	0	2.00
Chuck pot roast, 7-bone	240	14.0	28.0	0	2.00
Chuck pot roast, boneless	240	14.0	28.0	0	2.00
Tri-tip steak	200	11.0	23.0	0	2.09
Eye of round roast	253	13.4	32.0	0	2.39
Chuck steak, boneless	160	8.0	22.0	0	2.75
Top round steak	180	9.0	25.0	0	2.78
Eye of round steak	182	9.0	25.0	0	2.78
Tripe (intestines)	107	4.6	13.3	2.3	2.89
Shoulder center ranch steak	152	8.0	24.0	0	3.00
Tenderloin roast	180	8.0	25.0	0	3.13
Shoulder petite tender	150	7.0	22.0	0	3.14
Shoulder petite tender medallions	150	7.0	22.0	0	3.14
Round tip steak	150	6.0	23.5	0	3.92
Flank steak	200	8.0	32.0	0	4.00
Shoulder pot roast	185	7.0	30.7	0	4.38
Sirloin tip center roast	190	7.0	31.0	0	4.43
Sirloin tip center steak	190	7.0	31.0	0	4.43
Liver	216	6.0	33.0	5.8	5.50
Sirloin tip side steak	190	6.0	34.0	0	5.67
Shank cross cut	215	6.7	38.7	0	5.80
Kidney	179	5.3	31.0	0	5.85
Heart	187	5.4	32.2	0.2	5.96
Testicles	154	3.4	29.7	1.14	6.54
Tenderloin steak	115	3.0	22.2	0	7.40

Fish & Seafood (4 ounces)	Calories	Fat	Protein	Carbs	P/E Ratio
Escargot	21.6	0.2	1.3	3.5	0.35
Caviar	299	20.3	27.9	4.54	1.12
Herring	283.5	20.2	23.8	0.0	1.18
Oysters	92	2.6	10.7	5.6	1.30
Mackerel	290	20.3	27.0	0	1.33
Eel	267	17.0	26.8	0	1.58
Anchovies	256	15.9	28.0	0	1.76
Sea urchin	137	5.6	18.3	3.9	1.93
Mussels	195	5.0	27.0	8.38	2.02
Clams	161	6.7	27.5	6.7	2.05
Sardines	139	7.5	18.0	0.0	2.40
Fish livers	118	5.0	12.5	5.8	2.50
Cockle	90	0.8	15.3	5.3	
Arctic char	208	10.0	29.0	0	2.90
Walleye	156	7.5	22.0	0	2.93
Swordfish	195	9.0	26.6	0	2.96
Trout	190	8.6	28.0	0	3.26
Scallops	126	1.0	23.0	6.0	3.29
Salmon	206	9.0	31.0	0	3.44
Squid	119	1.8	20.3	4.0	3.50
Octopus	186	2.4	33.8	5.0	4.57
Turbot	138	4.3	23.3	0	5.42
Flounder	97.5	2.7	17.3	0	6.41
Catfish	119	3.2	20.9	0	6.53
Salmon roe (ikura)	185	4.0	34.3	0	8.58
Halibut	155	3.5	30.7	0	8.77
Sea bass	135	3.0	27.0	0	9.00
Monkfish	110	2.2	21.1	0	9.59
Tilapia	145	3.0	29.7	0	9.90
Barramundi	110	2.0	23.0	0	11.50
Crayfish (crawfish)	93	1.4	19.0	0	13.57
Grouper	134	1.5	28.2	0	18.80
Mahi mahi	100	1.0	21.0	0	21.00
Crappie	132	1.34	28.2	0	21.04
Bluegill	133	1.34	28.2	0	21.04
Perch	132	1.34	28.2	0	22.00
Lobster	101	1.0	22	0	22.67
Tuna (yellowfin)	150	1.5	34	0	22.67
Crab	94	0.84	20.28	0	24.14
Orange roughy	119	1.0	25.7	0	25.70
Cod	113	1.0	26	0	26.00
Northern pike	128	1.0	28	0	28.00
Tuna (canned)	149	1.06	32.91	0	31.05
Langostino	93	0.67	21.3	0	31.79
Shrimp	112	0.32	27.2	0.23	49.45

Chicken & Poultry (4 ounces)	Calories	Fat	Protein	Carbs	P/E Ratio
Chicken skin	514	46.0	23.0	0	0.50
Goose	340	24.9	28.5	0	1.14
Game hen	220	16.0	19.0	0	1.19
Chicken feet	244	16.6	22.0	0.2	1.33
Wings	320	22.0	30.4	0	1.38
Thigh, skin-on	275	17.6	28.3	0	1.61
Duck	228	13.9	26.3	0	1.89
Thigh, skinless	165	10.0	19.0	0	1.90
Leg, skin-on	255	15.2	29.4	0	1.93
Turkey	175	9.9	21.0	0	2.12
Drums	178	9.9	22.0	0	2.22
Pheasant	200	10.5	25.7	0	2.45
Leg, skinless	210	9.5	30.7	0	3.23
Chicken heart	210	9.0	30.0	0.1	3.33
Chicken breast, skin-on	200	8.4	31.0	0	3.69
Chicken liver	189	7.4	27.7	1.0	3.74
Chicken giblets (kidney)	178	5.1	30.8	0	6.04
Chicken breast, skinless	138	4.0	25.0	0	6.25
Chicken gizzards	175	3.0	34.5	0	11.50

Wild Game (4 ounces)	Calories	Fat	Protein	Carbs	P/E Ratio
Bison heart	239	16.0	22.7	0	1.42
Bear meat	186	9.4	22.8	0	2.43
Bison liver	241	5.3	33.3	6.7	2.78
Bison, ground	166	8.2	23.0	0	2.80
Elk, ground	219	9.9	30.2	0	3.05
Venison, ground	212	9.3	30.0	0	3.23
Venison liver	196	8.0	28.0	0	3.50
Bison top sirloin	194	6.4	31.8	0	4.97
Bison rib-eye	200	6.4	33.4	0	5.22
Venison heart	187	5.4	32.3	0	5.80
Bison chuck shoulder	219	6.0	38.3	0	6.38
Elk loin	189	4.4	35.0	0	7.95
Rabbit meat	196	4.0	37.4	0	9.35
Bison top round steak	138	2.8	26.4	0	9.43
Venison roast	179	3.6	34.3	0	9.53
Venison steak	179	3.6	34.3	0	9.53
Elk steak	168	3.2	34.7	0	10.84
Venison loin*	169.3	2.7	34.3	0	12.85

Venison refers specifically to deer in this case.

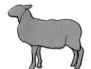

Goat & Lamb (4 ounces)	Calories	Fat	Protein	Carbs	Fiber	P/E Ratio
Lamb chops	313	22.7	25.5	0	0	1.12
Lamb, ground	313	22.7	25.5	0	0	1.12
Lamb liver	250	10.0	34.7	2.87	0	2.70
Goat liver	217	5.9	33.0	5.8	0	2.82
Goat oysters (testicles)	154	3.4	29.7	1.14	0	6.54
Lamb oysters (testicles)	154	3.4	29.7	1.14	0	6.54
Goat meat	162	3.4	30.7	0	0	9.03
Goat ribs	162	3.4	30.7	0	0	9.03

Eggs & Dairy (per ounce unless noted)	Calories	Fat	Protein	Carbs	P/E Ratio
Ghee	248	28.2	0.08	0	0
Butter	203	23.0	0.24	0.02	0.01
Mascarpone	121	12.83	0.95	1.12	0.07
Sour cream	28.5	2.78	0.35	0.67	0.10
Cream cheese	99	9.76	1.74	1.56	0.15
Egg yolks (1 large)	47	3.87	2.32	0.52	0.53
Feta	74.8	6.0	4.0	1.16	0.56
Asiago	130	11.0	7.0	0.94	0.59
Roquefort	104.6	8.7	6.1	0.57	0.66
Stilton	116	9.9	6.72	0.03	0.68
Cheddar	114	9.44	6.48	0	0.69
Blue	100	8.15	6.07	0.66	0.69
Gorgonzola	100	8.15	6.1	0.66	0.69
Ricotta (whole milk)	49.3	3.68	3.19	0.86	0.70
Brie	94.7	7.85	5.88	0.13	0.74
Mozzarella (whole milk)	90	7.0	6.12	0.7	0.79
Swiss	82.5	6.51	5.66	0.3	0.83
Gouda	101	7.78	7.07	0.63	0.84
Goat cheese	74.8	6.0	5.25	0	0.88
Provolone	99.5	7.55	7.25	0.61	0.89
Gruyère	117	9.17	8.45	0.1	0.91
Mozzarella (part-skim)	83.6	5.61	6.73	1.58	0.94
Romano	109.7	7.64	9.0	1.03	1.04
Egg (1 large)	68.2	4.7	5.5	0.5	1.07
Plain Greek yogurt (whole milk, per cup) *	230	11	22.0	9.0	1.10
Parmesan	111	7.32	10.13	0.91	1.23
Cottage cheese (4% fat) *	206	9.0	23.35	7.10	1.45
Plain Greek yogurt (0% fat, per cup) *	144.6	0.96	25.0	9.0	2.51
Egg white (1 large)	17.4	0.06	3.64	0.24	12.13

These products are higher in carbs, so you should limit or avoid them for best results.

But Doesn't Eating Too Much Protein Cause Blood Sugar to Spike?

A common misconception in the keto community is that eating too much protein spikes blood sugar. Obviously, the carnivore diet involves eating a lot of protein, so we'd like to take a minute to dispel this myth.

Our bodies are always making glucose to maintain a steady blood glucose level and to replenish liver and muscle glycogen (see page 60) when we aren't eating carbs. They are really good at this task.

One source of glucose is body fat. Fat is stored as triglyceride molecules. A triglyceride molecule is made up of three free fatty acid (FFA) molecules linked by a glycerol molecule. When the body needs fat for fuel, it cleaves, or separates, the glycerol from the three FFA molecules, and the FFA molecules bind to albumin (a protein made by the liver), which enables the FFA to enter the bloodstream. Your body can burn this FFA directly in the muscles and other cells. This is where the majority of your fuel comes from when you are keto adapted, not from ketones. Some FFA goes to the liver and is converted to ketones to power parts of the body that can't run on fat, like the brain. The glycerol molecules also go to the liver and are turned into glucose.

The amount of glucose made from stored fat (glycerol) isn't enough to supply all the body's needs for glucose when you are running on fat (and thus getting negligible amounts of glucose from your diet), so another process, called gluconeogenesis, helps out. Gluconeogenesis turns protein into glucose. The body is remarkably adept at making all the glucose it needs; that's why there is no need for dietary glucose and why a carnivore diet is even possible.

The body stores roughly 1,200 to 2,000 calories of glycogen in the muscles and liver, but most of that glycogen is locked up in the muscles. Once glycogen is stored in the muscles, it can be used only by the muscles, and only in times of great need, such as during high-intensity workouts. If you go for a vigorous walk, though good for your health, you will not tap into your muscle glycogen. Glycogen is like your reserve fuel tank for times of fight-or-flight. If a lion started chasing you, you would need a burst of speed and energy. One study tested athletes who fully depleted muscle glycogen with high-intensity workouts of two hours or more to see how much glycogen was restored in their muscles when adding and not adding carbs. After about 24 hours, the athletes who added carbs after the workout had the same amount of glycogen in their muscles as those who didn't.[39] In other words, your body restores muscle glycogen even if you are eating no carbohydrates because it needs those reserves.

So really, the majority of the time, you are using liver glycogen for fuel, which for most people totals only about 400 calories' worth. That small amount gets depleted pretty quickly, and then your body has to shift to burning fat. That's why you see elevated blood ketones within

---

[39]J. S. Volek, D. J. Freidenreich, C. Saenz, L. J. Kunces, B. C. Creighton, J. M. Bartley, P. M. Davitt, et al, "Metabolic Characteristics of Keto-Adapted Ultra-Endurance Runners," *Metabolism* 65, no. 3 (2016): 100–10.

a day or two of starting a ketogenic diet, because most cells can run on ketones instead of glucose, reducing the need for glucose in the body. But there still is some need for glucose. Most parts of the brain love ketones, but certain parts, like the neurons, prefer glucose. That's where gluconeogenesis comes into play. It is primarily a demand-driven process that helps keep blood glucose levels from falling too low and replenishes muscle glycogen after an intense workout. Gluconeogenesis is occurring all the time to some extent. It ramps up when needed and slows down when more glucose is present. But dietary protein has little effect on gluconeogenesis.

You might be thinking, "I have a friend with type 1 diabetes who has to inject insulin for protein at about half the rate of carbohydrates, so doesn't that mean protein spikes blood sugar?" Type 1 diabetics don't make their own insulin, so they have to use exogenous, or external, insulin. All macronutrients require some insulin. Carbohydrates require the most, protein a moderate amount, and fat the least, as shown in the following chart.[40]

Insulin Needed to Process Macronutrients

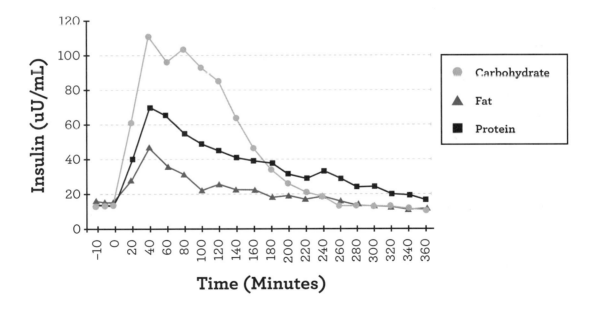

But the body is smart. It knows that it needs insulin to utilize protein in order to make muscle. It also knows that if you eat only protein and no carbs, that rise in insulin will cause blood glucose to drop. To prevent this, the body releases the hormone glucagon when you eat protein. Glucagon tells the liver to release some glucose in order to keep blood sugar levels from dropping too low. But a type 1 diabetic isn't making insulin, so all you see is glucagon

---

[40]K. E. Foster-Schubert, J. Overduin, C. F. Prudom, J. Liu, H. S. Callahan, B. D. Gaylinn, M. O. Thorner, and D. E. Cummings, "Acyl and Total Ghrelin Are Suppressed Strongly by Ingested Proteins, Weakly by Lipids, and Biphasically by Carbohydrates," *Journal of Clinical Endocrinology & Metabolism* 93, no. 5 (2008): 1971–9.

spilling glucose into the blood. This is why diabetics have to add insulin for protein—to enable the body to make use of that protein and prevent blood sugar from rising too much. This isn't a sign that gluconeogenesis is ramping up and converting a bunch of protein to glucose.

Hitting your protein goal every day ensures that your body has all the amino acids it needs to maintain your lean mass. What happens if you go over your protein goal? A couple of things can happen. First, your body can use more of that ingested protein to maintain glucose levels instead of using protein on the body (muscle or other lean mass). It can also use that protein to build more lean mass instead of just maintaining it. Processing protein takes a long time, and it's a very energy-intensive process. Digesting a large protein-heavy meal could trigger multiple cycles of protein synthesis over several hours.

The body processes dietary protein by breaking it down into amino acids. Once it has enough amino acids to start building lean mass, it triggers a process called muscle protein synthesis (MPS). The amount of amino acids needed to start protein synthesis varies by protein source, with whey protein requiring only about 27 grams and beef protein about 40 grams. Whole grain protein (gluten) never triggers protein synthesis because it doesn't contain the amino acid leucine. This is referred to as the leucine threshold. The amount of leucine needed to trigger protein synthesis varies from about 3.2 to 4.4 grams. When we are young, we need less leucine to trigger protein synthesis. As we get older, the leucine curve shifts, and we need more to trigger the same protein synthesis (called the leucine shift). That's why our requirement for protein increases as we age.

Once enough leucine is present, the body triggers MPS once. MPS is an energy-intensive process, so after the cycle is complete, the body rests for a bit. But this whole time, protein is being digested, and when the leucine threshold is reached again, the body triggers another cycle of MPS. You can have two or three cycles from one meal.

There is no reason to fear dietary protein. It is vital for maintaining your strength as you age, and it won't spike your blood sugar when you are carnivore.

DISPELLING THE MYTHS ABOUT MEAT

Myths about meat (or certain types of meat) causing cancer and harming the environment are common, so let's take a moment to expose the truth.

Does Meat Cause Cancer?

Many people believe that eating red meat, especially processed meats, leads to higher cancer risk and other health issues. They point to a few studies that they say support these claims. But, as is always the case with studies, the devil is in the details. Two important factors in evaluating a study are its funding and methods.

There have been many examples of studies that had suspicious funding and motives. In our book *Keto. The Complete Guide to Success on the Keto Diet,* we talk about the sugar industry's funding of studies to make saturated fat look like the enemy instead of sugar. The funding source is important to understand the study's motives.

The methods used are another important component. The double-blind randomized control trial (RCT) is the most trusted type of study. It aims to reduce bias by randomly allocating people to groups and evaluating the results without any bias in their allocation. *Double-blind* means that not even the researchers know which group is getting what, so they can't insert their own biases.

An observational study is much less controlled and therefore less accurate. Researchers simply observe people and their outcomes without trying to control anything. This typically includes a yearly nutrient analysis, which is a form participants fill out once a year that asks what they ate in the last *year!* That doesn't imply much accuracy. For this reason, researchers won't consider correlations below 200 to 300 percent to be relevant. That means the difference in outcomes (having disease or death) has to be 200 to 300 percent higher in one group than another for the study to be considered relevant and worth looking into further.

To date, unlike so many other risk factors (smoking, physical activity, and so on), there has not been an RCT looking at the effects of meat consumption on heart disease or heart health. Not one. And yet the public view is settled on the linkage between meat and heart disease, like it's a fact.

What studies are there that support the supposed link between meat consumption and heart disease or cancer? One of the biggest and most commonly pointed to is the China Study, which suggests that meat consumption is correlated to higher rates of cancer and heart disease. But the raw data from the epidemiological study (a type of observational study done on populations) tells a very different story than the authors of the study portray. This is another example of how a study can be manipulated—omitting and manipulating the data that doesn't fit your agenda.

First, the authors omitted data that contradicted their claims about meat's link to cancer and heart disease. The residents of the county of Tuoli in China ate 45 percent of their diet from fat and 134 grams of protein a day (almost twice the American average) and rarely ate vegetables or other plant foods. Yet, according to the study data, they were very healthy and had low rates of cancer and heart disease. In fact, they had lower rates of cancer and heart disease than most of the counties that were nearly vegan.[41]

Looking deeper at the study data reveals other striking evidence. One is the correlation of wheat intake to heart disease mortality. The data from this study actually shows a pretty strong correlation between higher wheat consumption and higher rates of heart disease deaths![42]

The Correlation of Wheat Consumption to Coronary Heart Disease Mortality

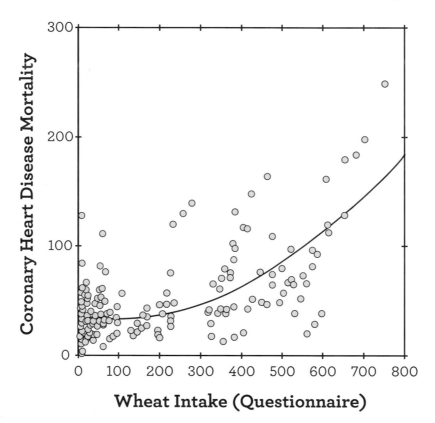

So was it the meat that caused higher cancer and heart disease, or was it the wheat? The study data points to people who eat more meat as having better health and those who eat more wheat as having worse health.

[41]Denise Minger, "The China Study: Fact or Fallacy?" accessed October 30, 2019, deniseminger.com/2010/07/07/the-china-study-fact-or-fallac/

[42]Denise Minger, "The China Study: Wheat and Heart Disease, Oh My," accessed October 30, 2019, deniseminger.com/2010/09/02/the-china-study-wheat-and-heart-disease-oh-my/#more-532

Many other observational studies purport to link meat consumption with cancer and heart disease, and even more are coming out. One published in 2019 reported a 20 percent increase in colorectal cancer in those subjects who ate more meat.[43] Yes, an observational study that has a 20 percent risk differential between the groups is being widely publicized. Remember, no serious researcher would consider it significant if it was less than 200 percent, ten times more than this study. But still it is reported as if it is fact. And did the group in the study that ate more meat also exercise less, smoke more, and have less-healthy lifestyles? Likely, but the study doesn't account for these factors. This is called "healthy user bias," and it is a major flaw in observational studies. Is someone who eats vegetarian generally more concerned about their health than someone who eats fast food every day? Vegetarians are likely to be more active, do yoga, and have many other lifestyle factors that skew the results. So not only is the 20 percent difference insignificant, but the healthy user bias in this type of study makes it virtually meaningless.

Then there are studies like the one titled "The Paradoxical Nature of Hunter-Gatherer Diets: Meat-Based, Yet Non-Atherogenic," which shows that even though hunter gathers ate primarily a meat-based diet, they were free of signs of heart disease.[44] There are many other contradictory studies and examples. The new dietary guidelines removed dietary saturated fat as a concern due to growing evidence that it doesn't affect heart disease risk.

We could fill a whole book dissecting other examples. The important takeaway is to always look at the latest study claiming that something causes cancer or heart disease with an eye on the details. What kind of study was it? How many subjects were included? Who funded the study? If it was an observational study, was the risk ratio above 200 percent? This will filter out the noise from the important data.

What About Nitrates/Nitrites and Processed Meats?

Nitrates and nitrites are another concern that comes up when talking about meat consumption, especially consumption of processed meats. It is said that the increased nitrates in processed meats lead to increased risk of cancer and heart disease. But are they really something to be concerned about?

First, let's look at where nitrates come from. You might be surprised to learn that 70 to 90 percent of nitrite exposure comes from your own saliva. And about 93 percent of dietary nitrites come from vegetables. That's right, you get most of your nitrates from vegetables. Here are some of the foods highest in nitrates.

---

[43]K. E. Bradburger, N. Murphy, and T. J. Key, "Diet and Colorectal Cancer in UK Biobank: A Prospective Study," *International Journal of Epidemiology* pii (2019): dyz064.

[44]L. Cordain, S. B. Eaton, J. B. Miller, N. Mann, and K. Hill, "The Paradoxical Natural of Hunter-Gatherer Diets: Meat-Based, Yet Non-Atherogenic," *European Journal of Clinical Nutrition* 56 (2002): S42–52.

Food	Nitrates Per Serving (ppm)
Arugula	4,677
Basil	2,292
Celery	1,103
Spinach	1,066
Hot dogs	10
Bacon	10

That's right, you can eat 460 hot dogs and get less nitrate than you would get from just one serving of arugula. Some argue that plants have "natural nitrates" that are somehow different. Nitrate is NO_3—one nitrogen atom and three oxygen atoms. Either it is NO_3 or it isn't a nitrate. There is no difference between the nitrates in processed meats and the nitrates in vegetables.

Nitrate we eat comes in contact with our saliva to create salivary nitrite, with 20 percent being converted to nitrite. The rest of the nitrate leaves through the urine within five hours of being eaten. Any small amount that is absorbed stays in the body for only about five minutes.[45] Some of the nitrite is converted to nitric oxide in the gut, which has been shown to have beneficial effects in the body.[46] So don't fear processed meats or nitrates in foods.

Does Beef Contribute to Climate Change?

Another common belief is that the methane gas emitted by cows (via their burps and farts) contributes to climate change and that we should eat less beef to help. This, like so many other popular beliefs (eat healthy whole grains, eat low-fat, etc.), is a result of a poor understanding of the larger picture. The truth is, properly raised ruminants such as cows that graze on grass can help remove carbon from the environment.

Grasses sequester, or store, lots of carbon. They take in carbon dioxide to grow. That is where the cows get their carbon: the grass. More cows eating grass means more carbon coming out of the atmosphere, into the plants and then into the cows. Here's how that breaks down. Cows can only "emit" carbon that they got from food. For every pound of carbon "emitted," the cow enabled about 3.2 pounds of carbon to be removed from the air and fixed in the plants' roots and the cow itself. Therefore, a cow helps remove carbon from the atmosphere.[47]

[45]N. G. Hord, Y. Tang, and N. S. Bryan, "Food Sources of Nitrates and Nitrites: The Physiologic Context for Potential Health Benefits," *American Journal of Clinical Nutrition* 90, no. 1 (2009): 1–10.

[46]D. L. Archer, "Evidence That Ingested Nitrate and Nitrite Are Beneficial to Health," *Journal of Food Protection* 65, no. 5 (2002): 872–5.

[47]Pete B., "Cattle 'Emissions,'" *Grass Based Health* blog, August 12, 2012, grassbasedhealth.blogspot.com/2012/08/cattle-emissions.html

Also, only about 4 percent of the Earth's surface can be used to grow crops, but 14 percent is suitable for rangeland.[48] That's almost four times as much land available for grazing animals than for crops. In addition, modern agriculture strips the topsoil of nutrients and depletes it of vegetation (roots, etc.). This means less carbon in the soil. Grazing cattle enrich the soil with nutrients and fertilizer (their feces). More grazing ruminants can help sequester a lot of carbon into the soil and the cows themselves. Studies have shown this as well. For example, the study "The Role of Ruminants in Reducing Agriculture's Carbon Footprint in North America" found that "to ensure long-term sustainability and ecological resilience of agroecosystems, agricultural production should be guided by policies and regenerative management protocols that include ruminant grazing."[49]

Even the data used to make cows look like the enemy reveals that about 9 percent of greenhouse gas emissions come from all of agriculture. Less than half of that is from animals, and cows make up only about 2 percent of all animal emissions in the U.S. So cows contribute 2 percent of greenhouse gas emissions and crops contribute 5 percent. But the cows are the problem when they supply a much more efficient source of protein and minerals that are more bioavailable to humans (see the sections "Bioavailability of Nutrients" and "Bioavailability of Proteins")? This doesn't account for all the carbon being sequestered in the soil from the grazing animals, as mentioned above.

For reference, healthcare contributes about 10 percent of all greenhouse gas emissions.[50] Could we reduce those emissions even more by getting people off of pharmaceuticals and requiring less healthcare?

The Takeaway

Fearing beef is not founded in good science. Taking some simple steps, such as buying properly raised beef, can ensure that you, and the Earth, experience no negative effects.

---

[48]D. C. Church, *The Ruminant Animal: Digestive Physiology and Nutrition* (Long Grove, IL: Waveland Press, 1993).

[49]W. R. Teague, S. Apfelbaum, R. Lal, U. P. Kreuter, J. Rowntree, C. A. Davies, R. Conser, et al, "The Role of Ruminants in Reducing Agriculture's Carbon Footprint in North America," *Journal of Soil and Water Conservation* 71, no. 2 (2016): 156–64.

[50]David Blumenthal and Shanoor Seervai, "To Be High-Performing, the U.S. Health System Will Need to Adapt to Climate Change," *To the Point* blog, the Commonwealth Fund, April 18, 2018, www.commonwealthfund.org/blog/2018/be-high-performing-us-health-system-will-need-adapt-climate-change?redirect_source=/publications/blog/2018/apr/health-system-and-climate-change

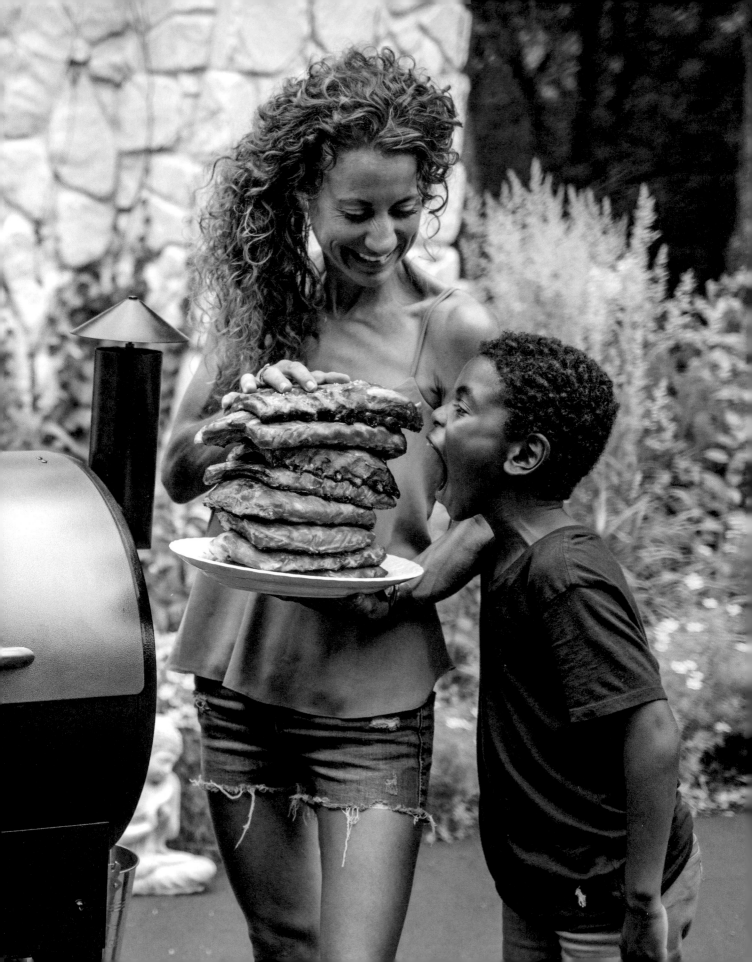

Chapter 2:

Implementing a Carnivore Diet

Now that you have some background in the science behind a carnivore diet, let's talk about how to start eating this way and what you can expect.

CARNIVORE LEVELS

Based on our experience and the research we have done, we have created four levels of carnivore to serve different needs.

Level 1: Beef, Beef Tallow, and Salt

This phase is about elimination and healing. You eat only beef products and salt. Here are the foods included in Level 1:

- All parts of the cow—muscle meat, organ meats, tallow, bone marrow

- Beef tallow for cooking

- Salt for seasoning

- Melted beef tallow as a sauce

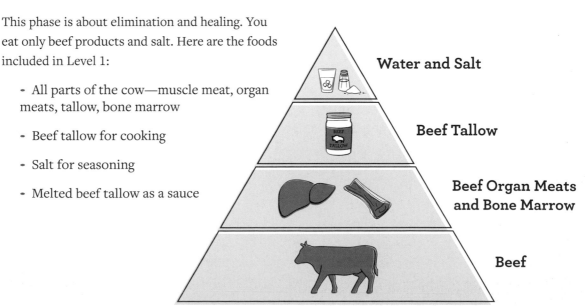

Water and Salt

Beef Tallow

Beef Organ Meats and Bone Marrow

Beef

Level 2: All Meats, All Animal Fats, and Salt

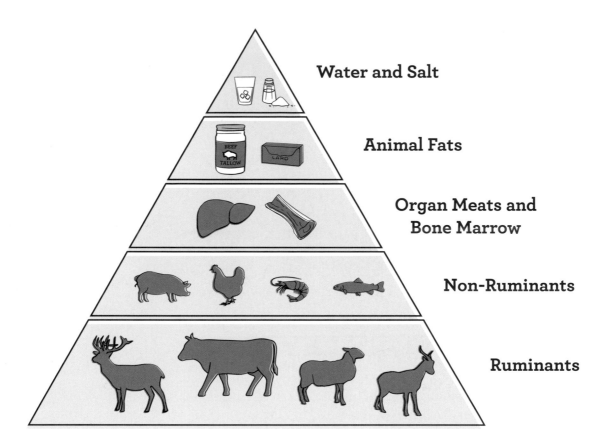

In this phase, you can eat all types of animal protein. Here are the foods included in Level 2:

- All parts of any animal—beef, pork, lamb, goat, venison, poultry, fish, seafood, etc.

- Beef tallow, lard, duck fat, and schmaltz for cooking

- Salt for seasoning

- Melted beef tallow, lard, duck fat, and schmaltz as a sauce

If you are coming to this level from Level 1, try adding one type of protein at a time (like pork) and give it a week to see how your body reacts. Also, every recipe from Level 1 can be used for Level 2.

Level 3: All Meats, All Animal Fats, Salt, Dairy, and Eggs

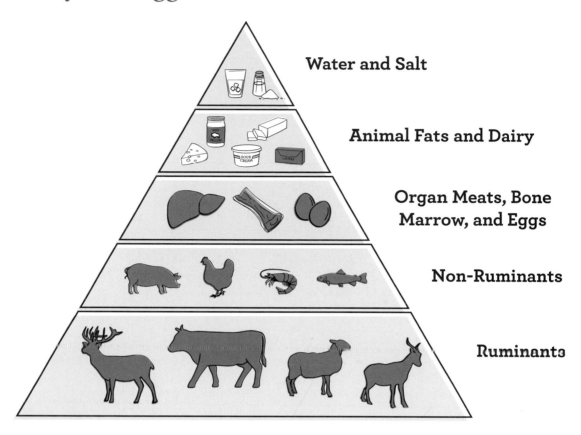

Water and Salt

Animal Fats and Dairy

Organ Meats, Bone Marrow, and Eggs

Non-Ruminants

Ruminants

Level 3 introduces eggs and dairy. Here are the foods included in Level 3:

- All parts of any animal—beef, pork, lamb, goat, venison, poultry, fish, seafood, etc.

- Eggs

- Low-sugar dairy products such as butter, cheese, sour cream, and heavy cream

- Beef tallow, lard, duck fat, schmaltz, butter, and ghee for cooking

- Salt for seasoning

- Sauces made with animal fats, eggs, and/or dairy, such as mayonnaise, hollandaise, and cheese sauce

Every recipe from Levels 1 and 2 can be used for Level 3.

Level 4: All Meats, All Animal Fats, Salt, Dairy, Eggs, Spices, and Some Low-Sugar Plant-Based Sauces

We would argue that Level 4 is not really carnivore, as it includes plants. This level introduces some low-sugar plant-based spices and sauces and is what some people call Zero-Carb Keto. This level can work well for those who are trying to lose weight and don't have chronic issues like Lyme or autoimmune disease. Here are the foods included in Level 4:

- All parts of any animal—beef, pork, lamb, goat, poultry, fish, seafood, etc.

- Eggs

- Low-sugar dairy products such as butter, cheese, sour cream, and heavy cream

- Beef tallow, lard, duck fat, and schmaltz for cooking

- Salt and low-sugar spices for seasoning

- Some low-sugar plant-based sauces and condiments, such as ranch dressing, hollandaise, cheese sauce, béarnaise, mayonnaise, and mustard

There are no plants included in the recipes in this book; that's what makes them carnivore. Adding lettuce, onions, tomato sauce, and spices (which come from plants) makes a meal keto, not carnivore. This approach may work well for some people and could be something you progress to with time, but all the recipes in this book are Level 1, 2, or 3. That said, if you find that you are not sensitive to certain spices and your main goal is weight loss, you can easily add your favorite spice or a little low-sugar sauce to these recipes.

"Carnivore Level 1, day 4!

I can honestly say my nighttime anxiety has improved! I have a 50/50 chance of getting eight hours of sleep at night or not sleeping at all. Ever since I had my son five years ago, I've had a lot of health problems and nighttime anxiety has been consistent. I almost feel postpartum! I'm constantly worried about the safety of my son. It's been running me ragged the past five years. I've tried cold therapy, wild yam cream, lavender oil, magnesium, meditation, you name it!

Last night was the easiest I've ever gone to sleep in the past five years. Basically, so far so good! I'm excited to see if it helps my severe pain!"

—Erin

Which Level Is Right for You?

Which level is best to start with depends on your goals; the two main categories are healing and weight loss. If you are doing carnivore to heal a leaky gut or to manage conditions like autoimmune disease or a mood disorder, follow the guidelines in the section "Carnivore Autoimmune Protocol (CAIP) for Healing." For weight loss and general health, you have more flexibility in how you implement the carnivore diet. The following section will help you get started.

CARNIVORE FOR WEIGHT LOSS

In general, if your goal is to lose weight—which really means losing body fat—it's a good idea to start with Level 1 or 2. These levels eliminate dairy and eggs, which can help with weight loss. Some people can enter at Level 3 and do fine, but Level 1 or 2 is typically a more effective starting point.

Learning how our bodies work helps us understand why carnivore is great for fat loss. In this section, we take a look at the key components of our biology and metabolisms that make a carnivore diet so powerful for weight loss.

Oxidative Priority

Oxidative priority is the order in which the body processes fuels coming in from the diet. At any moment, there isn't much fuel in the blood. Normal blood glucose is 85 mg/dL, which is about 4 grams of glucose, or 16 calories' worth. We know that very high blood glucose can be lethal, but an excess of any other fuel can be lethal as well. Alcohol, exogenous ketones, glucose (from carbohydrates), protein, and fat will all cause damage if allowed to build up in the blood.

To understand the power of oxidative priority, let's refer to a study titled "Changes in Macronutrient Balance During Over- and Underfeeding Assessed by 12-d Continuous Whole-Body Calorimetry."[51] This study examined where the fuels for the body came from in an overfed state versus an underfed state. In an overfed state, you are taking in more macronutrients than your body needs at that time. In an underfed state, you are taking in fewer macronutrients than your body needs, or nothing at all.

---

[51] S. A. Jebb, A. M. Prentice, G. R. Goldberg, P. R. Murgatroyd, A. E. Black, and W. A. Coward, "Changes in Macronutrient Balance During Over- and Underfeeding Assessed by 12-d Continuous Whole-Body Calorimetry," *American Journal of Clinical Nutrition* 64, no. 3 (1996): 259–66.

When you eat a large meal (500 to 1,000 calories, or maybe even more), your body has to deal with all those food coming in and do it quickly so that you don't die from hyperglycemia (high blood glucose), hypertriglyceridemia (high blood fat), or alcohol toxicity (if you have consumed alcohol). The body is smart; it deals with the different types of "meal inputs" you consume in reverse order of storage capacity, as shown in the following chart. This means the fuel that it has no capacity to store—alcohol—is burned off first.

Oxidative Priority

	Alcohol	Exogenous Ketones	Carbo-hydrate	Protein	Fat
Oxidative Priority Level	1	2	3	4	5
Storage System	None	Blood	Blood (glucose), glycogen	Limited (plasma AA)/tissue	Adipose (fat)
Storage Capacity (in Calories)	None	20	1,200–2,000	360–480	Unlimited
Postprandial (Blood)					
Diet-Induced Thermogenesis (4–6 Hours After Meal)	15%	3%	8%	25%	3%

The second priority is exogenous ketones, which are ketone supplements. The body doesn't like blood ketones to be too high and has almost no storage space for them, so it burns those off next. We don't recommend taking ketone supplements, by the way; on a carnivore diet, your body will make all the ketones it needs from your fat stores.

The third priority is carbohydrate because the body's storage capacity for it is relatively small. Carbohydrates are turned into glucose in the blood when digested. That glucose is either burned for fuel or stored in the muscles or liver in the form of glycogen. You can store around 1,200 to 2,000 calories of glycogen in your muscles and liver. The glycogen in the muscles is locked away to be used by the muscles only during very intense exercise; a brisk walk around the block or a typical workout will not tap into your muscle glycogen stores in any significant way. Most people are really only replenishing liver glycogen on a typical day, which is only about 320 to 400 calories' worth.

The fourth priority is protein, which is a little different. It is preferentially used to build lean mass (muscle, skin, and so on). The body is constantly turning over cells in the skin and other body parts, so it needs a steady supply of amino acids from complete protein sources to rebuild cells. Protein is used as a fuel only when no other fuels are present. If you were very lean and you ate only protein, you could run into problems as your body struggled to turn enough protein into fuel. This is known as rabbit starvation. Turning protein into fuel is an energy-intensive process (see the section "Thermic Effect of Food" on page 63), so the body does it only when it has no other option.

The last priority is fat, which is the easiest of the five fuels to store. Our bodies have a theoretically unlimited fat storage capacity. There are people who have millions of calories of stored fat. Therefore, the body deals with all the other fuels and stores the fat to deal with later.

What does this look like in a typical meal? Let's say you have a couple glasses of wine with a meal high in protein, carbohydrates, and fat. Because your body can't store the alcohol from the wine, it burns off as much of the alcohol as quickly as it can. While it is prioritizing the alcohol, your body stores the carbs and fat for later and sends the protein into muscle protein synthesis, which is the body's process for building and rebuilding lean mass. Therefore, the majority of the carbs and fat you consumed go into storage due to the alcohol that is present. This is why drinking alcohol greatly limits fat loss.

Energy Expenditure for Protein, Carbohydrates, and Fat

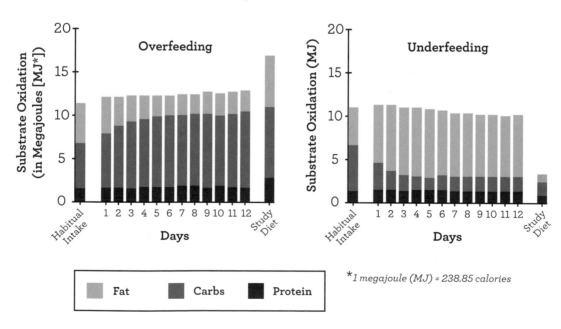

*1 megajoule (MJ) = 238.85 calories

There are a couple of striking things to note in the chart on the previous page, which is from the same study on oxidative priority. One is that in both overfed and underfed states, the energy expenditure for protein doesn't really change. This reflects the body's preference to use protein for building lean mass, not as a fuel. Then second thing that jumps out is the drastic change in fat being used for fuel between the underfed and overfed states. The body's requirement for energy doesn't really change, but when carbohydrates are present in an overfed state, very little fat is used for fuel. In an underfed state, where less carbohydrates are coming in from the diet, the body oxidizes, or burns, much more fat for fuel. Dietary carbohydrates are simply displacing fat burning because they take oxidative priority over fat.

Another interesting example of the power of oxidative priority is in alcoholics. Hemoglobin A1c (HbA1c or just A1c) is a measure of average blood glucose over the last three months or so. In healthy people, A1c should be below 5.4, ideally 5.0 or less. You are considered at risk for diabetes with A1c above 5.7 and considered diabetic with A1c above 6.5. If you have an A1c level of 5.0 (a good goal for overall health), you had average blood glucose of 97 mg/dL over that period. An alcoholic always has elevated blood alcohol levels, and alcohol is the number-one priority fuel. Therefore, the body stores all carbs and fat that come in when alcohol levels are elevated. The result is very low A1c in alcoholics, typically in the fours or even the threes, no matter what they eat. They can eat tons of sugar and carbohydrates and still have very low A1c. Now, we are not advocating becoming an alcoholic to get your A1c down, but it does demonstrate the power of oxidative priority.

"Okay, so this carnivore thing does have side effects...

I was up at o'dark thirty this morning. No big deal...got to work early and got lots accomplished. Thought burnout would happen, as usual, around noon. Nope, still chugging along. Okay, I will get drowsy about 3 p.m., and I can snuggle with the cat for a nap. Nope! Didn't happen. Instead, I met up with a neighbor and made plans to be walking buddies. 6 p.m....I can sit down now, right? Oh look, the WHOLE UPSTAIRS needs to be vacuumed. (Seriously, did someone slip me some drugs?) Hmmmm, that's done, let me weed and feed the yard. Now, here's the best part...the hose exploded! The only way to shut it off was to get absolutely baptized by it. Let's just say I can cross 'clean the front porch' off the summer to-do list. (And BTW hubby said, yeah I left that hose out in the sun too long, it was probably bad.) Hmmm... (I'm a teacher) report cards are due soon, oh what the heck, let me do all of them now before hubby gets home so we can have a nice evening. For goodness sake, what am I going to do tomorrow? I think I did my whole to-do list for the next year today..."

—Susan

Thermic Effect of Food

The thermic effect of food (TEF) is the amount of energy the body needs to expend in order to process a macronutrient. Each macronutrient has a different thermic effect, as shown in the following table.

Energy Source	TEF	Calories Consumed	Resulting Calories
Alcohol	15%	100	85
Exogenous ketones	3%	100	97
Protein	25%	100	75
Carbohydrates	8%	100	92
Fat	3%	100	97

Ketones and fat have the lowest thermic effect. The body needs only about 3 percent of the calories consumed to utilize fat in the body. Next are carbohydrates at 8 percent, then alcohol at 15 percent, and finally protein at 25 percent. Some forms of protein can even be 30 percent TEF. That means 30 percent of the calories consumed don't really count because the body has to burn that many calories just to process the protein. So eating 100 calories of protein results in only 70 to 75 calories in the body. This can help with fat loss.

How a Carnivore Diet Helps with Fat Loss

Looking at the biology makes it easy to see why carnivore can be so powerful for fat loss. By leveraging oxidative priority and the thermic effect of food, a carnivore diet primes the body to use fat as fuel. The fuel chart basically looks like this:

Weight-Loss Carnivore Diet

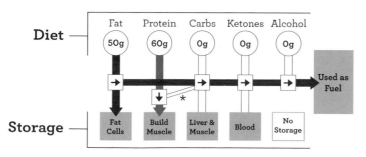

*Used for muscle building only as fuel when no other fuels are present

See mariamindbodyhealth.com/charts/ for more charts and explanation.

By eating carnivore, you are eliminating the fuels that can displace fat oxidation (the burning of fat for fuel)—no alcohol, no exogenous ketones, no carbohydrates. Protein goes toward maintaining lean mass and glucose levels. So you are left with fat as your fuel. The body can burn dietary fat and body fat equally well, so just upping or lowering your fat intake will result in fat loss or maintenance. (If you upped the fat enough, you could gain weight, too.) If weight loss is your goal, just adjust the fat down a bit so that your body uses more body fat for fuel. This is easy when eating carnivore: Simply select leaner proteins, like skinless chicken breasts, egg yolks, and loin. If you want to maintain your weight, select fattier meats, like brisket, rib-eye steak, and bacon.

What to Do if You Hit a Stall

If you are stalled, first try moving to a lower level. So, if you are at Level 3, move to Level 2 or 1 (which eliminate dairy, which can cause people to stall). Next, try adjusting to leaner cuts of meat. The charts in the section "Protein Sources" are sorted in order of lowest fat-to-protein ratio (per calorie) to highest. All you have to do is move up the chart for leaner cuts to help improve weight loss and down the chart to move toward maintenance.

Another strategy for breaking a stall or improving weight loss results is to do a protein-sparing modified fast (PSMF) day a couple days a week. This involves drastically cutting dietary fat to about 30 grams per day, which means choosing the leanest cuts of meat, like skinless chicken breast. PSMF can be a powerful tool for weight loss. It mimics many of the benefits of longer-term fasting (greater than 24 hours) without any loss of lean mass. For more information about PSMF, check out our website, keto-adapted.com.

What's Next After Reaching Your Fat Loss Goals?

If you have reached your weight target, what's next? We suggest one of two paths. First, you can stay carnivore if you like. It can be an easy lifestyle to maintain, with less preparation of meals and no counting of macronutrients. You eat foods that are rich in bioavailable nutrients. You can thrive on this diet for life. One note we would emphasize is that if you plan to make carnivore a long-term lifestyle, you should make sure you are eating organ meats like beef liver to ensure that you are getting all the nutrients your body needs.

Another option is to transition to a ketogenic lifestyle and slowly add back in some nutrient-dense low-carb vegetables, sauces, spices, and maybe even occasional treats like baked goods. We recommend reintroducing these foods one by one, giving it a few days to see how your body reacts and how well you tolerate that food. Remain mindful of potential issues with plants, and avoid frequent consumption of foods that are dense in antinutrients (see page 25). A cake or dessert made with almond flour is an occasional treat, not a daily food. Likewise, spinach and kale add color, flavor, and texture to a plate, but you don't want to drink a green smoothie that has a high concentration of oxalates (see page 26).

CARNIVORE AUTOIMMUNE PROTOCOL (CAIP) FOR HEALING

One of the biggest reasons for following a carnivore diet is to help manage chronic conditions that following a ketogenic diet may improve but not totally resolve. Those conditions include

- ADHD, autism, and obsessive-compulsive disorder (OCD)

- Alopecia

- Alzheimer's disease, dementia, and other brain health issues

- Anxiety and depression

- Arthritis and joint pain

- Asthma

- Autoimmune disorders

- Autoimmune thyroid (Hashimoto's)

- Bipolar disorder

- Crohn's disease, colitis, irritable bowel syndrome (IBS), acid reflux, and other gastrointestinal issues

- Eczema, psoriasis, acne, and other skin issues

- Epilepsy and seizures

- Fertility, polycystic ovary syndrome (PCOS), and menopause

- Fibromyalgia and other chronic pain

- Gout

- Graves' disease

- Inflammation

- Kidney stones and kidney disease

- Liver health

- Lyme disease

- Multiple sclerosis (MS)

- Parkinson's disease

- Sleep issues

- Type 2 diabetes and metabolic syndrome control

In clients with all of these conditions, we have seen symptoms greatly improve with a keto diet, and most of the time they realize even more relief when they go carnivore. Craig started eating primarily carnivore when he was diagnosed with Lyme disease in 2017. Although keto enabled him to function much better than a standard American diet ever would, going carnivore reduced his symptoms and pain significantly.

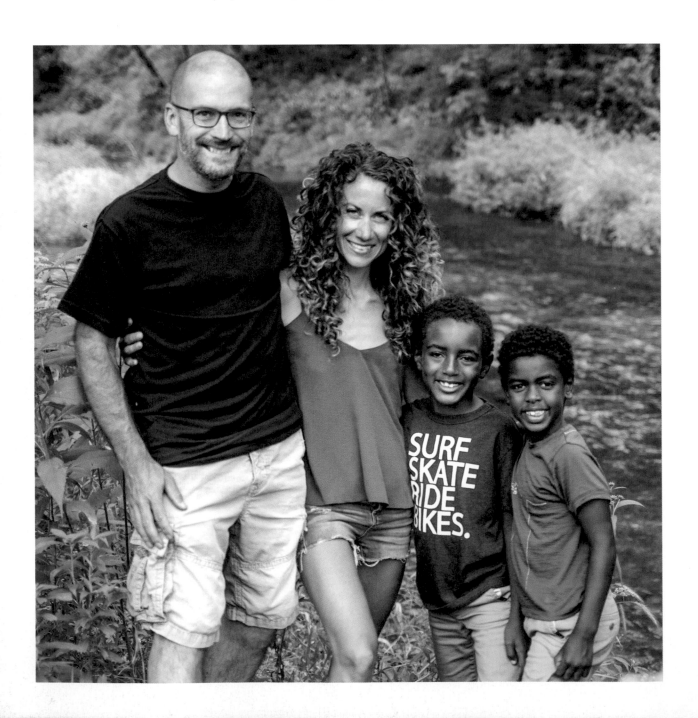

For about six years, I slowly developed increasing pain in my back. At first, I thought it was from an old football injury I sustained in high school that damaged a disk in my low back and had given me trouble on and off ever since. But this was different. It wasn't shooting pain; it was constant pain and stiffness. Over the years, it progressed to my upper back and then to my neck. I also started having migrating pain in my knees, ankles, and hips. I would wake up in the morning and feel like I had sprained my knee or ankle, sometimes both. The hip pain was the hardest, as it would be hard to walk that day.

About three years into this, I went to the doctor to get checked for Lyme disease. Given the knowledge I had about it, I felt that is what I had. My doctor ran the standard Western blot test, and it came back negative. I now know that test results in up to 70 percent false negatives. I went another two years of progressing pain not knowing what was wrong.

It got to the point where I couldn't stand up straight or turn my head. My 8-year-old son could throw a football farther than I could, and my energy was very low. Finally, Maria told me this wasn't normal, and I had to figure this out. I went to a functional doctor we know and got some blood tests done. My C-reactive protein (CRP) came back at 50. You want CRP to be ideally less than 1.0, and Maria and I get clients eating a ketogenic diet to below 1.0 all the time. I had been keto for almost ten years at that point. I knew something was really wrong. I was also anemic with a low red blood cell count (which is why I was low in energy) even though I ate lots of red meat. Our good friend and publisher, Erich, told me I needed to get a more accurate Lyme test from IGeneX, and when I did, I learned that I did in fact have Lyme.

This started me on a journey to try to reverse this disease. Being keto for all that time lessened the effects of the Lyme and the treatments. Most people with chronic Lyme are frequently bedridden during the first year of treatment. I was able to function fairly well, helping clients and homeschooling our boys. I went through all the standard treatments (nine months of three antibiotics, antiparasitic drugs, Cowden herbal protocol, and others) with little improvement in symptoms. I had cavitation surgery on two cavities where my wisdom teeth were and one root canal. I also got all my silver amalgam fillings removed, as my heavy metals were high as well.

Eventually, I decided to go full carnivore to see how it would affect my symptoms. Within a few weeks of going Level 1 and sometimes Level 2 carnivore, the migrating pain went away completely. I also started full-spectrum infrared sauna treatments to help detox from high mold and heavy metals.

I am still a work in progress. I am starting to regain mobility, my migrating pain is gone, my overall pain and stiffness in my neck and back are reduced. My energy has improved. I attribute almost all of it to the carnivore diet. Chronic Lyme can be a debilitating disease, but I believe that carnivore can help people get their life back.

—Craig Emmerich

If you are doing carnivore to manage any of these conditions, or if you are wondering whether a carnivore diet will help with other conditions, we suggest you try following the Carnivore Autoimmune Protocol (CAIP):

1. **Start at Level 1.** This means eating only beef and beef organ meets along with salt and water. This will act as the ultimate elimination diet, removing all the common allergens and sources of leaky gut and autoimmune food reactions. Give this level at least 30 days. Also, take a closer look at the topical products you use. Our skin absorbs everything that we apply to it, so try to use animal-based products (beef tallow is a great moisturizer) and avoid products containing plant ingredients like almond oil. And watch for chemicals in makeup and other beauty products that can trigger symptoms or interfere with your hormone balance (makeup can be very estrogenic). It can be helpful to make over your environment, too. That means removing scented candles, dryer sheets, or other sources of chemicals or estrogenic compounds. This includes plastics, so no plastic water bottles, no storing food in plastic, and absolutely no heating food in plastic, which can greatly increase the estrogenic effects. It also helps to get vitamin D3 levels into a good range (we recommend 45 to 85 ng/mL) by getting commonsense sun exposure of 20 to 30 minutes each day, with as much skin exposed as possible.

2. **After 30 days of Level 1, you can try transitioning to Level 2.** Eating beef nose to tail gives you all the nutrients your body needs, but many people need more variety, so adding other proteins can help. If you want to expand your diet, try adding one protein from Level 2, like chicken, for a week and see how your body responds. If some symptoms reoccur, then drop back to Level 1 for another week or so, and then try another protein, such as pork, and give that a week to see how your body handles it. This will allow you to pinpoint which foods trigger you.

3. **Once you have found the proteins that your body is comfortable with, you can try Level 3 by adding dairy or eggs.** Start by adding eggs for a week and see how your body reacts. If you don't see an escalation of symptoms, water retention, or other issues after a week of eating eggs, then you are safe to include eggs to your diet. Next, you can try adding dairy for a week and see how it affects you. If at any time you see symptoms creeping back in, drop back down to Level 2 until they subside. Stay at Level 2 for another month or so, and then try going back up to Level 3 again.

4. **If you want to expand your diet further, you can try adding spices or zero-carb sauces like ranch dressing or mustard.** If any of these plant foods trigger more symptoms, move down a level and eliminate them.

The CAIP is the ultimate elimination diet for rooting out the source of your health issues. We believe that the majority of problems people have today are related to food, and eliminating the food that is causing the issue or autoimmune reaction can result in healing and reversal of many conditions. The CAIP is a powerful tool for healing and alleviating symptoms from a wide range of diseases and issues.

For either the CAIP or just the carnivore diet in general, adjusting for weight loss, maintenance, or weight gain is easy. If you want to lose weight, just adjust the fat content of the meat accordingly. If you are at Level 1 and are getting some relief from symptoms but not losing weight like you want, try switching to leaner cuts of beef. Use the charts on pages 39 to 45 to pick proteins with lower fat-to-protein ratios. If you want to maintain or gain weight, go down the charts to select proteins with higher fat-to-protein ratios.

I have been following a Paleo and keto approach for nine years, and these supported me while dealing with autoimmune thyroid disease. About ten months ago, I came across the carnivore diet and read about how it was helping so many people, so I decided to give it a chance for 30 days.

Within 24 hours of cutting vegetables out of my diet, I felt like a new person.

There was no more bloating, and over time my digestion dramatically improved. I lost all my sugar cravings for keto treats and started craving red meat every meal. After a few months, my doctor reduced my thyroid medication and my antibodies went down to the lowest levels ever.

Also, I lost 20 stubborn pounds and my body composition improved. My mood is more solid and my energy is improved. Now I sleep like a rock, and I am never hungry between meals. I plan to stay on carnivore for the long term and am excited about even more healing progress.

—Caitlin Weeks, @grassfedgirl

WHAT TO EXPECT WHEN TRANSITIONING TO CARNIVORE

Whether you're coming from a high-carb standard American diet or a ketogenic diet, going carnivore will involve a transition period. Here's some information about what to expect.

Transitioning from a Standard American Diet to a Carnivore Diet

When transitioning from a standard American diet (that is, a high-carb diet) to carnivore, you will experience a phase of adaptation. This is the same adaptation phase that people see when transitioning to a ketogenic diet, with some possible added issues.

Your body needs to deplete itself of glucose and then start the process of becoming efficient at burning fat as its primary fuel. The depletion of glucose takes only one to two days, and after a couple of days, your blood ketones will rise. But your body won't be good at burning fat as its primary fuel yet; that can take four to six weeks or even longer. During this time, you may experience "keto flu" symptoms such as low energy, brain fog, and possibly even "keto rash," which is likely due to oxalate dumping (see page 71). Focusing on a couple of things will help ease the transition.

Electrolytes

Many keto flu symptoms are just signs of dehydration—the low energy, brain fog, and sore or heavy legs. When you cut carbohydrates from your diet, your body retains less water. You may see a large drop in weight in the first week of going carnivore (10 pounds in some cases) that is the result of your body releasing retained water. This is generally a good thing, but it also requires you to be diligent about your electrolyte intake, because along with the retained water goes a lot of electrolytes.

You must be much more mindful about adding salt to your food when eating carnivore, especially when you are coming from a higher-carb diet. For one, you get a lot of sodium without even knowing it from processed foods, fast food, and drinks. For example, at McDonald's, a milkshake has more even sodium than an order of fries. When you switch to carnivore, the meat doesn't come with sodium, so you have to add it.

A good goal for sodium intake is 4 to 5 grams per day, or about 2½ teaspoons of fine sea salt. But everyone is different, so you must find what works best for your body. We advise that you lean toward the higher end of this range because studies have shown that getting more than enough salt is less risky than getting too little salt. Some people find that they feel best with 10 grams of sodium a day. Add salt to your food and even a bit to your drinks until you find the level at which your body feels best.

Digestion

If you weren't eating a lot of animal protein prior to going carnivore, there may be an adjustment period for your body to process the added proteins. Vegetarians experience this when they add meat back into their diets. Their bodies stopped making the enzymes required to digest meat, so when they reintroduce it suddenly, they can feel ill. In these cases, it helps to take hydrochloric acid (HCl) with pepsin and digestive enzymes to support digestion until your body adjusts and is making enough enzymes on its own.

If you are experiencing digestive issues such as bloating, try taking an HCl with pepsin capsule with the first bite of food, then maybe one or two more capsules during your meal if your symptoms don't subside. At the end of the meal, take a digestive enzyme supplement with ox bile in it. Over time, you are likely to find that you can use less, and eventually, once your body has adjusted, you can stop taking the supplements altogether. Typically, your body will be making enough of its own enzymes in a couple of weeks.

Oxalate Dumping

Another possible "side effect" when going carnivore is oxalate dumping, which can cause skin rash or irritation. As we discussed on page 26, oxalates are nasty crystals that can cause all kinds of problems in the body. When you remove plants with oxalates from your diet, your body goes to work getting rid of those that have accumulated. This is hard work and can lead to some discomfort. Oxalates commonly collect in the mouth, teeth, salivary glands, jaw, sinuses, and face. You may even get a stye, which is really just oxalates being pushed out of your body through your eyelid.

Removing oxalates from the body can be a long process. Oxalate dumping issues can show up a year or more after you start eating carnivore. You could feel great for a year or two of eating this way and then suddenly feel pain in your hips, joints, or back. The pain might persist for a couple weeks, and then you will feel fine again. Hang in there and let your body detox.

If you do get a stye or other oxalate-dumping skin irritation, one great solution is to apply coconut oil to the affected area. The coconut oil will help unclog it and allow the oxalates to be expelled from your body. A tallow-based moisturizer is a carnivore alternative.

Transitioning from Keto to Carnivore

If you are already eating a ketogenic diet, then your body has made the switch to burning fat as its primary fuel (that is, you are keto adapted). Transitioning to carnivore should be fairly easy because you don't have to go through the keto adaptation phase. You may experience slight digestive issues from the added meat. After a couple of weeks, your body should adjust.

Electrolytes

When coming from a keto diet, you won't get the keto flu types of issues that stem from hydration. Electrolytes are still important, however. You may notice a more manageable electrolyte balance in your body and possibly less need for sodium. If you weren't getting a lot of potassium in your keto diet (many of the foods that are high in potassium are also high in carbs), you may have needed more sodium to feel your best. The body likes sodium and potassium to be in balance, so when potassium is lower, it leaches sodium until the two are in balance, which might require you to add salt to your diet to compensate. Animal proteins are very high in potassium, so when you eat carnivore, you are likely getting more potassium. Many people find that on a carnivore diet, they get enough sodium just from salting their meat to taste.

Digestion

As noted earlier, if you weren't eating a lot of animal protein prior to going carnivore, there may be an adjustment period for your body to process the added proteins. It may be helpful to take HCl with pepsin and digestive enzymes to support digestion until your body adapts. (Refer to page 71 for details.)

Oxalate Dumping

If you are coming from a keto diet, you won't get keto flu issues with dehydration or other problems. But oxalate dumping issues can show up a year or more after you switch to carnivore. Refer to page 71 for more on this "side effect."

Measuring Success

So many people rely on the scale to measure their success with a diet, but the number on the scale can be really deceiving. Your body can hold on to water, lose water due to dehydration, or put on muscle while losing fat. Water weight alone can move the scale several pounds in one day. Many factors can make your weight stall or even increase, but when you focus on the right thing—body recomposition—you realize that they aren't a problem.

Body recomposition, which means reducing stored body fat while maintaining or increasing muscle, which makes you stronger, should be your main goal when following a carnivore diet. But body composition is not always easy to measure, and the scale isn't going to show your progress.

Let's look at an example. The man in the photos at the top of the next page is Dr. Ted Naiman. The photo on the left shows Dr. Naiman after years of eating vegetarian. The photo on the right shows him after following an animal protein-focused keto diet.

What is striking about these photos, other than the obvious improvements in body composition, is that Dr. Naiman weighs the same in both photos. This is a great example of how the scale can be an enemy of real progress.

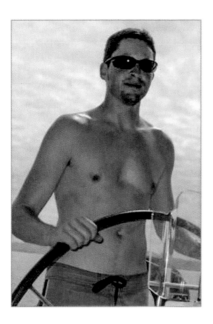 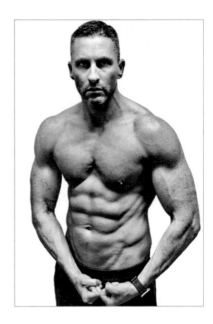

Take Measurements

So how do you measure success on a carnivore diet? One way is to take measurements. Measure your body in several places to see changes in inches. Muscle takes up less space than fat, so you will see inches go down while the number on the scale stays the same. Here are some key measurements you can take to track your progress:

- **Bust:** Measure around the chest right at the nipple line, but don't pull the tape too tight.

- **Chest:** Measure just under your bust.

- **Waist:** Measure ½ inch above your belly button or around the smallest part of your waist.

- **Hips:** Measure around the widest part of your hips.

- **Thighs:** Measure around the widest part of each thigh.

- **Calves:** Measure around the biggest part of each calf.

- **Upper arm:** Measure around the largest part of each arm above the elbow.

You can take these measurements once a week or once a month and track them in an app or just write them down. Seeing the numbers of inches decrease will show you progress that the scale might not.

See How Your Clothes Fit

Another way to track your progress is to go by how your clothes fit. If the scale hasn't moved but the waistband of your favorite pants is looser, or a shirt isn't as tight, that is a good sign that things are going in the right direction. Another great visual tool is to take a before photo in the bathroom mirror. Then take more photos to see how your body looks as you progress. Many times, you can see visual improvements in your body composition that might not show up on the scale.

Body Fat Scan

The most accurate way to gauge body recomposition and progress is with a body fat analysis. But we will warn you: many of the methods for test body fat numbers are not very accurate and are skewed by hydration level, especially impedance measurements (like those you get from a bathroom scale). One of the more accurate measurements is a DEXA body scan, where an X-ray scan is taken of your body and lean mass can be separated from body fat. It isn't a perfect method, as hydration levels can still affect it somewhat, but it does give you a pretty good idea of how much lean mass (muscle, organs, bones) you have compared to body fat. Seeing body fat go down while lean mass stays the same or goes up shows that you are making good progress in body recomposition.

CARNIVORE SUPPLEMENTS

A carnivore diet provides all the vitamins and minerals your body needs to function properly, but if you have a chronic deficiency or a hormone imbalance, supplements can help get things into balance quicker.

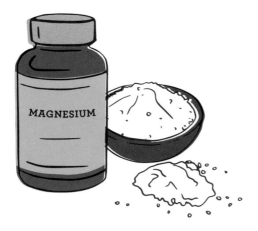

Collagen

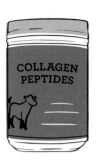

We suggest that everyone supplement with collagen because it has many health benefits:

- Helps with skin elasticity and aging; when losing a lot of weight, it can help the skin shrink, reducing wrinkles and cellulite

- Helps strengthen hair and reduce hair loss

- Improves joint health

- Builds bone strength

- Contains 18 amino acids that help muscle and ligament repair and recovery

- Contains glycine, which helps with immune system health and digestion

Collagen contains amino acids (mainly glycine) that you don't get from muscle meat. You can get it by eating the connective tissue of the animal, and there is some collagen in bone broth as well. But not a lot of people like eating those tough sinewy parts, so we suggest that everyone supplement with a scoop of quality collagen powder each day for everyone, regardless of diet.

Other Safe Supplements

Most vitamin and mineral supplements are safe if needed. Taking minerals like magnesium, potassium, selenium, and/or zinc and/or vitamins like B, C, D3, and K2 to help with imbalances or symptoms is generally okay.

The only supplements you really need when eating carnivore, however, are magnesium and salt. Magnesium glycinate, the most absorbable form, is good for everyone regardless of diet. The majority of us are deficient in magnesium because it is filtered out of our drinking water, so a daily supplement can be beneficial. Magnesium is needed for over 300 biochemical reactions in the body. It helps maintain nerve and muscle function and supports immune health, steady heartbeat, strong bones, and much more. The body needs sodium to retain water. When eating a whole-food, meat-based diet, you don't get all the sodium that is added to processed foods, so you have to add it yourself. Salt your food to taste, and if you get leg cramps, fatigue, or other symptoms of dehydration, add more salt.

Avoiding Plant-Based Supplements

When you are carnivore, you want to watch which supplements you take to eliminate plant sources. Here two supplements we often recommend, along with carnivore alternatives. Make sure to avoid tinctures or supplements that contain herbs, including ginger, kelp, resveratrol, and turmeric. These have high concentrations of oxalates, which you want to avoid (see page 26), especially when following the CAIP.

Common Plant-Based Supplement Alternatives

Supplement	Carnivore Alternative	What It's Good For
Evening primrose oil	Emu oil	Low progesterone Sleep issues
Kelp	Iodine drops	Thyroid issues

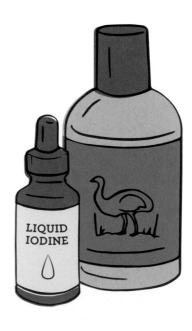

"Today is Day 31 carnivore. I can't believe it! Truly life transforming in every way! For the first 30 days I had butter and ghee but no other dairy, and I'm still having black coffee in the morning. I'm going to tackle the coffee in September. Given my crazy work schedule this summer I'm not ready to go there yet. Even still, cutting back to just mostly red meat and the occasional seafood or chicken has had profound effects on my life. Here are some of the benefits I wanted to share:

1. SLEEP: Sleep is crazy good! Very deep and I dream every night. I fall asleep easily and if I wake up in the middle of the night to use the bathroom I go right back to sleep.

2. MOOD + ENERGY: I have the best mood I've ever had. Always upbeat and energetic and it's helping me to be my best in all areas of my life (spouse, mother of two teenage daughters, friend, employee with lots of responsibilities, etc.).

3. WEIGHT LOSS: It is now effortless. When I went carnivore, I had come off a major carb binger. It was not pretty. It was at that moment that I vowed it was time to try something really different. I was keto, but it wasn't fully working for me. I had gained some serious water weight with my setback. Today I'm down 21.2 pounds from Day 1. Wow!

4. CRAVINGS: What's that? If it's not a juicy steak or bacon I have zero interest in it. Total freedom from self-sabotage!

5. INFLAMMATION: Completely gone. I have extensive osteoarthritis in both knees, but they don't hurt at all! They don't fully function properly, but I have zero pain. Same with my shoulder that went through MAJOR surgery 2.5 years ago. Never take anything for joint pain.

6. MIGRAINES: Completely gone.

Carnivore has helped me to become the best version of myself and to finally see that my goals that have felt so elusive for the past few years will become a reality soon. I'm just 15 pounds away from my goal weight. Wow! I'm 50 but I feel like I have the energy of a 25-year-old. It is truly fantastic! I strongly encourage anyone who's on the fence about it but is struggling to give it a go.

Thank you, Maria and Craig, for all you do to support all of us and spread the word. I can't wait for your new book!"

—Julia

STORING MEATS

Eating a carnivore diet means buying a lot of animal proteins. Buying in bulk will help keep the costs down. Each type of animal protein has a different storage time in the fridge or freezer. Whether it is cooked or raw matters, too. Here is a guide for storing common proteins.

	FRIDGE 39°F or colder	FREEZE 0°F
Chicken	RAW: 1–2 days COOKED: 3–4 days	RAW: 9–12 months COOKED: 4–6 months
Cow / Pig	STEAKS: 3–5 days CHOPS: 3–5 days BACON: 1 week SAUSAGE: 1–2 days SOUPS: 3–4 days STOCK: 3–4 days STEWS: 3–4 days	STEAKS: 6-12 months CHOPS: 4–6 months BACON: 1 month SAUSAGE: 1–2 months SOUPS: 4 months STOCK: 4–6 months STEWS: 4–6 months
Fish	RAW FISH: 1–2 days COOKED FISH: 3–4 days SEAFOOD: 1–2 days	RAW FISH: 2-6 months COOKED FISH: 4–6 months SEAFOOD: 3–6 months

TOP GADGETS

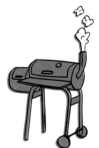

These kitchen gadgets helped us fall in love with eating carnivore:

- **Smoker:** A smoker is great for adding flavor to meats, which helps change things up when you eat only meat.

- **Sous vide machine:** With a sous vide machine, it is easy to get a perfect cook on your meats. Just make sure to avoid plastic bags, which can leach compounds into your food; use a silicone bag instead.

- **Air fryer:** An air fryer is useful for cooking steak or getting a good sear on meats. It is also handy in the summer so you don't heat up the kitchen too much.

- **Quality meat thermometer:** Getting the right internal temperature on your meats ensures that they are perfectly cooked to your desired doneness, and to a safe level.

SMOKING FOODS WITHOUT A SMOKER

Smoking can add a lot of flavor to meats. Having a smoker (we have a Treager) is great for simplifying the smoking process—just turn it on and fill it with wood pellets and it does the rest. But if buying a smoker isn't an option for you, you can smoke meats without a smoker.

First, you need wood chips. You can use hickory, applewood, or pecan wood. Soak the chips in enough water to cover them for at least four hours to ensure that the moisture penetrates the wood. This important step will cause the chips to smoke instead of catching on fire.

ON THE GRILL

If using a grill to smoke meats or eggs, you will need to make an aluminum foil bag for your soaked wood chips. Simply place the chips on a sheet of foil, place another sheet of foil on top, and twist the ends into a bag shape. Then poke a few holes in the top to let the smoke escape.

If using a charcoal grill, put the coals under the foil bag, not under the meat. You want indirect heat to avoid overcooking the meat. If using a gas grill, just turn on the burners on one side (under the foil bag) and put the meat on the other side. Adjust the heat as needed to maintain a temperature of 225°F to 275°F. Then just follow your chosen recipe for the cook time.

IN THE OVEN

You can also use your oven to smoke meats. You will need a roasting pan that has a raised rack that will keep the meat from touching the soaked wood chips as it cooks. Line the bottom of the pan with aluminum foil, add a layer of soaked wood chips, and then put the rack on top. Place the meat on the rack, cover the top of the pan with foil, and seal completely. Low and slow heat is still important, so cook the meat at 225°F to 275°F.

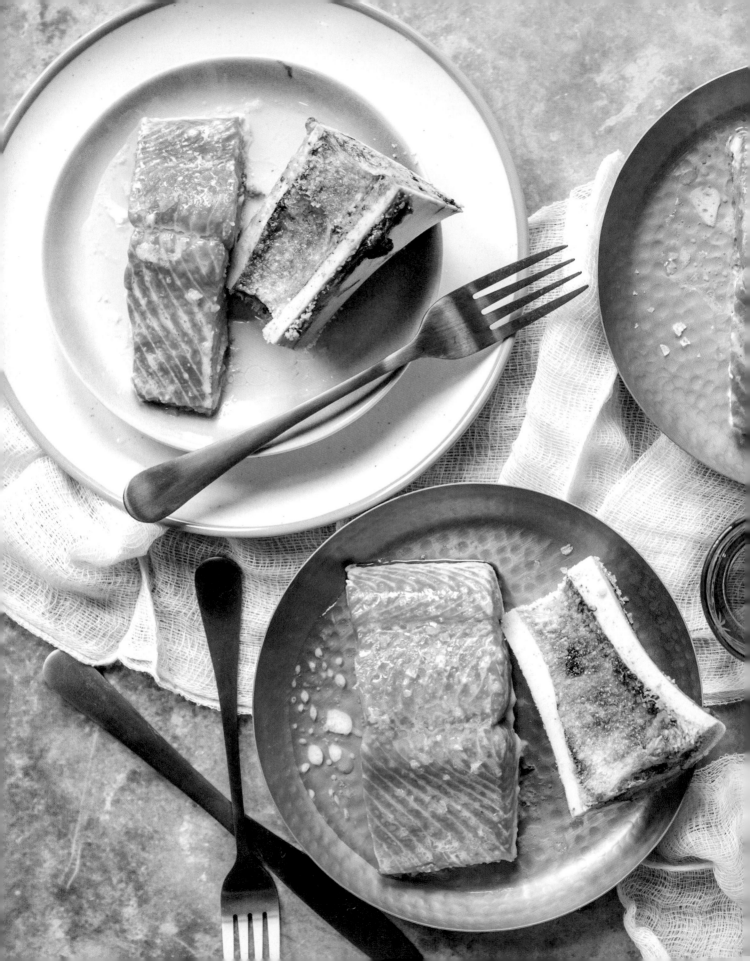

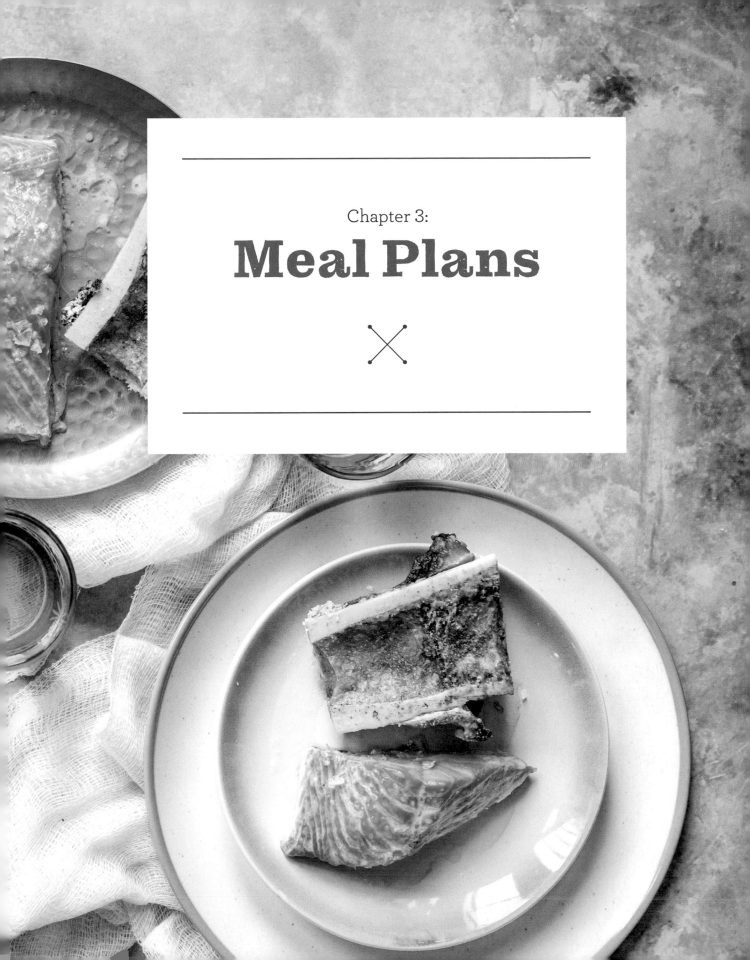

Chapter 3:

Meal Plans

Carnivore Weight Loss Meal Plan

Week 1 Menu

(#) = number of servings

	Breakfast	Snack	Dinner	Nutrient Per Serving	
DAY 1	Salmon French Eggs (2) 102	Chicken Wings (4) 164	Bacon-Wrapped Pork Chops (4) 254	Calories	1,169
				Fat	86g
				Protein	90g
				Carbs	1g
DAY 2	Bon Vie Scrambler (4) 104		Scotch Eggs (4) 252	Calories	1,123
				Fat	85g
				Protein	107g
				Carbs	2g
DAY 3	Ham Hocks and Fried Eggs (4) 106	Chicken Wings leftovers	Bacon-Wrapped Pork Chops leftovers	Calories	1,167
				Fat	87g
				Protein	90g
				Carbs	0g
DAY 4	Bon Vie Scrambler leftovers		Scotch Eggs leftovers	Calories	1,123
				Fat	85g
				Protein	107g
				Carbs	2g
DAY 5	Ham Hocks and Fried Eggs leftovers		Prosciutto-Wrapped Stuffed Chicken (4) 274	Calories	1,146
				Fat	76g
				Protein	108g
				Carbs	0g
DAY 6	Pork Fried Eggs (1) 112		Crispy Chicken Legs (2) 276	Calories	1,101
				Fat	76g
				Protein	95g
				Carbs	3g
DAY 7	Steak and Eggs (2) 122		Prosciutto-Wrapped Stuffed Chicken leftovers	Calories	925
				Fat	51g
				Protein	108g
				Carbs	0g

Week 1 Grocery List

Note: *In each week's grocery list, we have included enough food to feed two people, which means doubling the recipes that serve one. When a recipe gives more than one option for an ingredient, only the first option is included here. Refer to the recipes for dairy-free and other alternatives.*

Proteins

Bacon, 8 thin slices

Chicken breast halves, boneless, skinless, 4 (8 ounces each)

Chicken legs, 4

Chicken wings or drummies, 1 pound

Filet mignons, 2 (4 ounces each)

Ground pork, 2¾ pounds

Ham hocks, smoked, 4 (10 ounces each)

Pork chops, boneless, 4 (about ¾ inch thick)

Prosciutto, 16 thin slices

Smoked salmon, 4 ounces

Seasonings

Fine sea salt

Also purchase the ingredients for Easy Carnivore Hollandaise (page 314) if you plan to serve it with the dishes in this week's plan.

Dairy and Eggs

Brie, 8 ounces

Cheddar cheese, 1 ounce

Mascarpone, 2 tablespoons

Parmesan cheese, powdered, ½ cup

Eggs, large, 33

Fats

Butter, unsalted, 1 teaspoon

Duck fat, for greasing the air fryer (if needed)

Lard, ¼ cup + 1 teaspoon

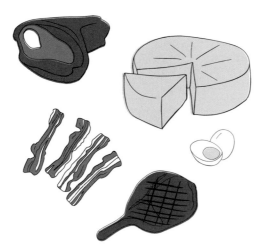

Week 2 Menu

	Breakfast	Snack	Dinner	Nutrient Per Serving	
DAY 1	Ham 'n' Cheese Frittata (2) 124		Reverse Sear Long-Bone (2) 182	Calories	1,273
				Fat	95g
				Protein	102g
				Carbs	6g
DAY 2	Carnivore Omelet (1) 126		Bacon-Wrapped Shrimp (2) 296	Calories	1,174
				Fat	85g
				Protein	94g
				Carbs	3g
DAY 3	Ham 'n' Cheese Frittata (2) 124		Reverse Sear Long-Bone (2) 182	Calories	1,273
				Fat	95g
				Protein	102g
				Carbs	6g
DAY 4	Breakfast Pie (4) 118	Meat Lollipops (12) 138	Carnivore Shabu Shabu (4) 184	Calories	1,281
				Fat	106g
				Protein	78g
				Carbs	2g
DAY 5	Breakfast Pie *leftovers*	Meat Lollipops *leftovers*	Slow Cooker Shredded Chicken with Cheddar and Bacon (4) 284	Calories	1,318
				Fat	100g
				Protein	102g
				Carbs	3g
DAY 6	Carnivore Omelet (1) 126		Carnivore Shabu Shabu *leftovers*	Calories	1,271
				Fat	100g
				Protein	83g
				Carbs	3g
DAY 7	Carnivore Eggs Benedict (1) 120		Slow Cooker Shredded Chicken with Cheddar and Bacon *leftovers*	Calories	1,131
				Fat	85g
				Protein	86g
				Carbs	3g

Week 2 Grocery List

Dairy and Eggs

Blue cheese, crumbled, 4 ounces

Cheddar cheese, 11 ounces

Heavy cream, ½ cup

Eggs, large, 30 (make sure to save some shells for making Carnivore Bone Broth)

Fats

Butter, unsalted, ¾ cup (1½ sticks)

Lard, ½ cup

Proteins

Bacon, 30 thin slices (be sure to save the fat for making Bacon Hollandaise)

Beef bones, 4

Beef chuck roast, boneless, 1 pound

Beef tenderloin, 1 pound

Canadian bacon, 4 slices

Chicken breast halves or thighs, boneless, skinless, 4 (6 ounces each)

Ground beef, 1 pound

Ground pork, 2 pounds

Ham, 4 ounces

Ham, cubed, 4 cups

Leftover bones and skin from 1 pastured chicken

Shrimp, large, raw, 12

Steaks, rib-eye, bone-in, 2 (1¼ pounds each)

Seasonings

Fine sea salt

Special Equipment

Chopsticks

Small skewers or toothpicks

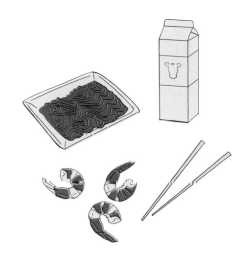

Week 3 Menu

(#) = number of servings

	Breakfast	Snack	Dinner	Nutrient Per Serving	
DAY 1	Breakfast Kabobs (4) 108	Easy Baked Chicken Livers (4) 282	Slow-Roasted Salmon with Bone Marrow (4) 294	Calories Fat Protein Carbs	999 70g 87g 1g
DAY 2	Breakfast Patties (6) 116		Salisbury Steak (2) 186	Calories Fat Protein Carbs	792 66g 60g 0g
DAY 3	Breakfast Kabobs *leftovers*	Easy Baked Chicken Livers *leftovers*	Slow-Roasted Salmon with Bone Marrow *leftovers*	Calories Fat Protein Carbs	999 70g 87g 1g
DAY 4	Breakfast Patties *leftovers*		Brisket (8) 190	Calories Fat Protein Carbs	1,208 95g 96g 0g
DAY 5	Breakfast Patties *leftovers*		Brisket *leftovers*	Calories Fat Protein Carbs	1,208 95g 96g 0g
DAY 6	Steak and Eggs (2) 122		Brisket *leftovers*	Calories Fat Protein Carbs	1,020 71g 87g 0g
DAY 7	Scotch Eggs (4) 252		Bacon-Wrapped Juicy Lucy (4) 198	Calories Fat Protein Carbs	1,291 95g 120g 1g

Week 3 Grocery List

Dairy and Eggs

Blue cheese crumbles, for serving (optional, for Salisbury Steak)

Provolone or Muenster cheese, 4 slices

Eggs, large, 10 (make sure to save some shells for making Carnivore Bone Broth)

Fats

Lard, ¼ cup plus 1 teaspoon

Tallow, ¾ cup

Proteins

Bacon, 16 thin slices (make sure to save the fat for making Easy Carnivore Hollandaise)

Beef bones, 4

Beef brisket, 4 pounds

Chicken livers, 1 pound

Filet mignons, 2 (4 ounces each)

Ground beef, 1½ pounds

Ground pork, 4 pounds

Ham steak, smoked, boneless, 1 (8 ounces)

Marrow bones, 4 large

Pork breakfast sausage links, precooked, 4

Prosciutto, 8 thin slices

Salmon fillet, skinless, 1 (2 pounds)

Seasonings

Fine sea salt

Flaked sea salt

Smoked sea salt (if making homemade, see page 310)

Special Equipment

Metal or wooden skewers (4 inches long), 8

Also purchase the ingredients for Easy Carnivore Hollandaise (page 314) and Bacon Mayonnaise (page 318) if you plan to serve it with the dishes in this week's plan.

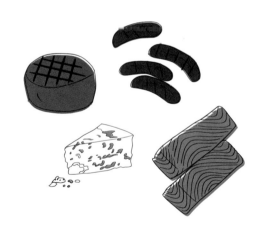

Week 4 Menu

(#) = number of servings

	Breakfast	Snack	Dinner	Nutrient Per Serving	
DAY 1	Bacon-Wrapped Filet Mignons (2) 202		Brick Chicken (6) 264	Calories	852
				Fat	53g
				Protein	90g
				Carbs	0g
DAY 2	Egg-cellent Meatloaf Cupcakes (4) 204	Bacon Burger Lover's Deviled Eggs (12) 146	Chicken Cordon Bleu Roulade (4) 280	Calories	984
				Fat	67g
				Protein	90g
				Carbs	1g
DAY 3	Carnivore Eggs Benedict (1) 120		Brick Chicken leftovers	Calories	1,122
				Fat	80g
				Protein	95g
				Carbs	2g
DAY 4	Egg-cellent Meatloaf Cupcakes leftovers	Bacon Burger Lover's Deviled Eggs leftovers	Chicken Cordon Bleu Roulade leftovers	Calories	984
				Fat	67g
				Protein	90g
				Carbs	1g
DAY 5	Carnivore Eggs Benedict (1) 120		Brick Chicken leftovers	Calories	1,122
				Fat	80g
				Protein	95g
				Carbs	2g
DAY 6	Ham 'n' Cheese Frittata (2) 124	Bacon Burger Lover's Deviled Eggs leftovers	Air-Fried T-Bone Steaks with Smoked Butter (2) 212	Calories	1,220
				Fat	92g
				Protein	85g
				Carbs	6g
DAY 7	Carnivore Omelet (1) 126		Basted Top Sirloin (1) 210	Calories	1,254
				Fat	96g
				Protein	87g
				Carbs	3g

Week 4 Grocery List

Condiments

Fish sauce, 1 teaspoon (optional, for deviled eggs)

Dairy and Eggs

Cheddar cheese, 4 ounces

Provolone cheese, 4 thin slices

Eggs, large, 34

Fats

Butter, unsalted, 1 cup (2 sticks)

Ghee, 3 tablespoons

Lard, 6 tablespoons

Tallow, 1 tablespoon

Proteins

Bacon, 14 thin slices (make sure to save the fat for making Bacon Mayonnaise and Easy Carnivore Hollandaise)

Canadian bacon, 8 slices

Chicken breast halves, boneless, skinless, 4 (4 ounces each)

Chicken, whole, 1 (3 pounds)

Deli ham, 4 thin slices

Filet mignons, 2 (4 ounces each)

Ground beef, 1¾ pounds

Ground pork, 2 pounds

Ham, 7 ounces

Steaks, T-bone, 2 (8 ounces each)

Steaks, top sirloin, 2 (8 ounces each)

Seasonings

Fine sea salt

Smoked sea salt (if making homemade, see page 310)

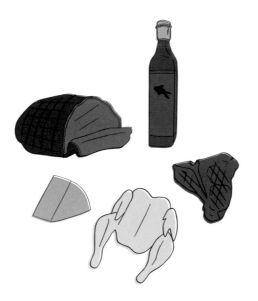

Carnivore Autoimmune Protocol Level 1 Meal Plan

Week 1 Menu

(#) = number of servings

	Breakfast	Snack	Dinner	Nutrient Per Serving	
DAY 1	Breakfast Patties (6)		Basted Top Sirloin (1)	Calories	999
				Fat	83g
				Protein	73g
				Carbs	0g
DAY 2	Beef Pemmican (8)	Short Rib Terrine (8)	Bacon-Wrapped Filet Mignons (2)	Calories	1,575
				Fat	134g
				Protein	82g
				Carbs	0g
DAY 3	Breakfast Patties	Short Rib Terrine	Roast Beef (8)	Calories	1,437
				Fat	121g
				Protein	94g
				Carbs	0g
DAY 4	Breakfast Patties	Short Rib Terrine	Roast Beef	Calories	1,437
				Fat	121g
				Protein	94g
				Carbs	0g
DAY 5	Beef Pemmican	Short Rib Terrine	Roast Beef	Calories	1,659
				Fat	142g
				Protein	84g
				Carbs	0g
DAY 6	Grilled Sweetbreads (4)		Reverse Sear Long-Bone (2)	Calories	1,340
				Fat	107g
				Protein	106g
				Carbs	0g
DAY 7	Grilled Sweetbreads		Grilled Porterhouse (2)	Calories	1,029
				Fat	76g
				Protein	91g
				Carbs	0g

Week 1 Grocery List

Fats

Beef tallow, 2¾ cups

Proteins

Beef bacon, 2 thin slices

Beef bones, 4

Beef roasts, boneless, 2 (2 pounds each)

Beef short ribs, 8 pounds

Filet mignons, 2 (4 ounces each)

Ground beef, 2 pounds

Steak, porterhouse, 1 (1¼ pounds)

Steak, rib-eye, bone-in, 1 (1¼ pounds)

Steaks, top sirloin, 2 (8 ounces each)

Sweetbreads, 1 pound

Seasonings

Fine sea salt

Special Equipment

Smoker and wood chips

Metal or wooden skewers, 8 inches long, 4

This meal plan focuses on Carnivore Level 1 recipes. Omit any Level 3 ingredients, such as Easy Carnivore Hollandaise or Salt-Cured Egg Yolks. (They are not included in the shopping lists.) Butter can be replaced with tallow.

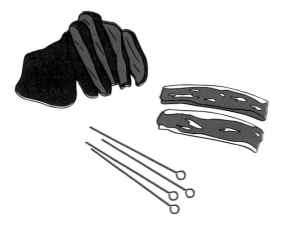

Week 2 Menu

	Breakfast	Dinner	Nutrient Per Serving	
DAY 1	Smoked Beef Roast (12) `240`	Smoked Short Ribs (8) `242`	Calories	1,067
			Fat	83g
			Protein	75g
			Carbs	0g
DAY 2	Smoked Beef Roast `leftovers`	Smoked Short Ribs `leftovers`	Calories	1,067
			Fat	83g
			Protein	75g
			Carbs	0g
DAY 3	Smoked Beef Roast `leftovers`	Smoked Short Ribs `leftovers`	Calories	1,067
			Fat	83g
			Protein	75g
			Carbs	0g
DAY 4	Smoked Beef Roast `leftovers`	Smoked Short Ribs `leftovers`	Calories	1,067
			Fat	83g
			Protein	75g
			Carbs	0g
DAY 5	Smoked Beef Roast `leftovers`	Grilled Porterhouse (2) `222`	Calories	1,107
			Fat	74g
			Protein	104g
			Carbs	0g
DAY 6	Beef Heart Steak (2) `244`	Beef Tongue (4) `216`	Calories	1,021
			Fat	75g
			Protein	107g
			Carbs	0g
DAY 7	Air-Fried T-Bone Steaks with Smoked Butter (2) (replace butter with tallow) `212`	Beef Tongue `leftovers`	Calories	1,192
			Fat	104g
			Protein	88g
			Carbs	0g

Week 2 Grocery List

Fats

Beef tallow, 6 tablespoons

Proteins

Beef bones, 4

Beef heart slices, 2 (8 ounces each)

Beef roast, boneless, 5 pounds

Beef short ribs, 8 pounds

Beef tongue, 2 pounds

Steak, porterhouse, 1 (1¼ pounds)

Steaks, T-bone, 2 (8 ounces each)

Seasonings

Fine sea salt

Smoked sea salt (if making homemade, see page 310)

Special Equipment

Smoker and wood chips

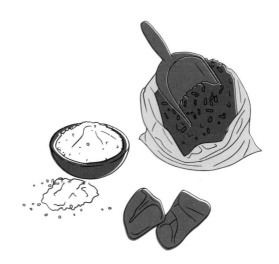

Week 3 Menu

(#) = number of servings

	Breakfast	Dinner	Nutrient Per Serving	
DAY 1	Basted Top Sirloin (1)	Brisket (8)	Calories	1,349
			Fat	106g
			Protein	91g
			Carbs	0g
DAY 2	Slow Cooker Short Ribs (omit Brown Butter) (16)	Brisket	Calories	1,358
			Fat	112g
			Protein	82g
			Carbs	0g
DAY 3	Slow Cooker Short Ribs	Brisket	Calories	1,358
			Fat	112g
			Protein	82g
			Carbs	0g
DAY 4	Slow Cooker Short Ribs	Brisket	Calories	1,358
			Fat	112g
			Protein	82g
			Carbs	0g
DAY 5	Slow Cooker Short Ribs	Reverse Sear Long-Bone (2)	Calories	1,490
			Fat	125g
			Protein	95g
			Carbs	0g
DAY 6	Salisbury Steak (2)	Air-Fried T-Bone Steaks with Smoked Butter (2) (replace butter with tallow)	Calories	1,043
			Fat	84g
			Protein	65g
			Carbs	0g
DAY 7	Reverse Sear Long-Bone (2)	Air-Fried T-Bone Steaks with Smoked Butter (2) (replace butter with tallow)	Calories	1,591
			Fat	126g
			Protein	114g
			Carbs	0g

Week 3 Grocery List

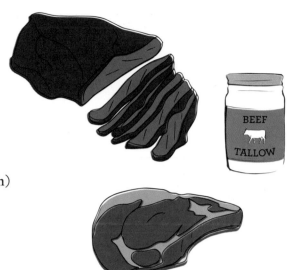

Fats
Beef tallow, 1½ cups

Proteins
Beef bones, 4

Beef brisket, 4 pounds

Beef short ribs, bone-in, 8 pounds

Ground beef, 8 ounces

Steaks, rib-eye, bone-in, 2 (1¼ pounds each)

Steaks, T-bone, 4 (8 ounces each)

Steaks, top sirloin, 2 (8 ounces each)

Seasonings
Fine sea salt

Smoked sea salt (if making homemade, see page 310)

Week 4 Menu

(#) = number of servings

		Breakfast	Snack	Dinner	Nutrient Per Serving	
DAY 1		Grilled Porterhouse (2) 222		Roast Beef (8) 206	Calories	921
					Fat	62g
					Protein	84g
					Carbs	0g
DAY 2		Carnivore Shabu Shabu (4) 184	Grilled Sweetbreads (4) 234	Roast Beef leftovers	Calories	1,337
					Fat	107g
					Protein	95g
					Carbs	0g
DAY 3		Oxtail (8) 230	Grilled Sweetbreads leftovers	Roast Beef leftovers	Calories	1,110
					Fat	81g
					Protein	96g
					Carbs	0g
DAY 4		Grilled Porterhouse (2) 222		Roast Beef leftovers	Calories	921
					Fat	62g
					Protein	84g
					Carbs	0g
DAY 5		Carnivore Shabu Shabu leftovers		Reverse Sear Long-Bone (2) 182	Calories	1,498
					Fat	123g
					Protein	100g
					Carbs	0g
DAY 6		Oxtail leftovers		Reverse Sear Long-Bone (2) 182	Calories	1,271
					Fat	97g
					Protein	101g
					Carbs	0g
DAY 7		Oxtail leftovers		Reverse Sear Long-Bone (2) 182	Calories	1,271
					Fat	97g
					Protein	101g
					Carbs	0g

Week 4 Grocery List

Fats

Beef tallow, 1¼ cups

Proteins

Beef bones, 4

Beef chuck roast, boneless, 1 pound

Beef roast, boneless, 1 (2 pounds)

Oxtails, 2 pounds

Steaks, porterhouse, 2 (1¼ pounds each)

Steaks, rib-eye, bone-in, 3 (1¼ pounds each)

Sweetbreads, 1 pound

Seasonings

Fine sea salt

Special Equipment

Chopsticks

Metal or wooden skewers (8 inches long), 4

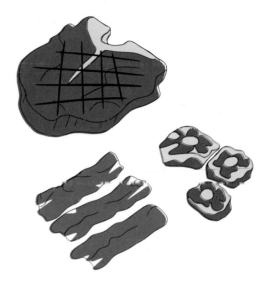

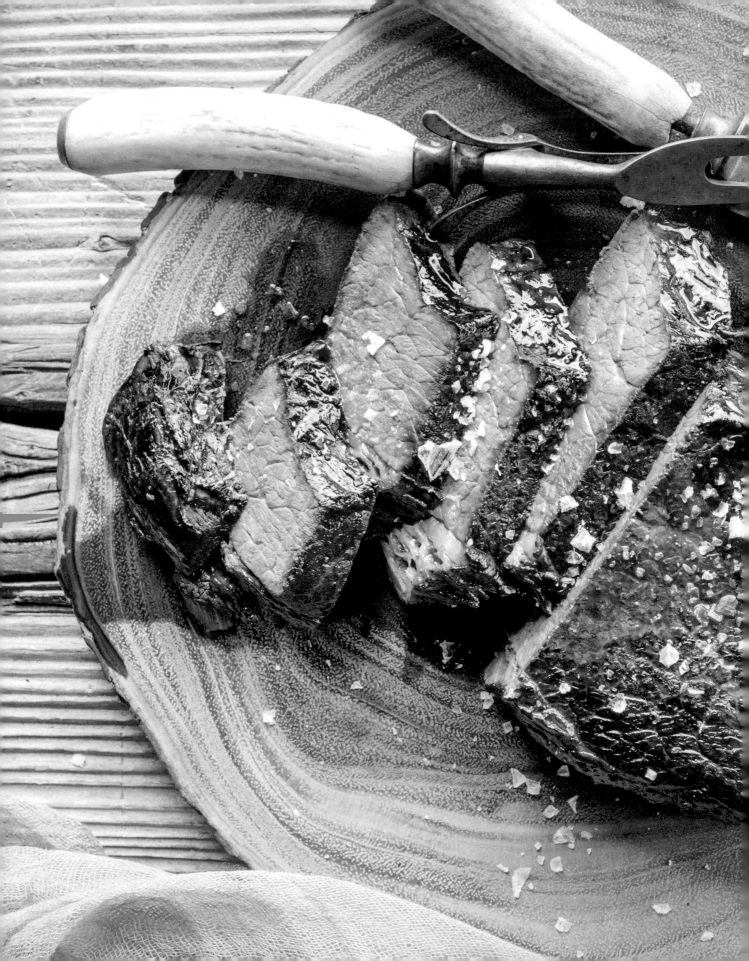

Chapter 4:

Recipes

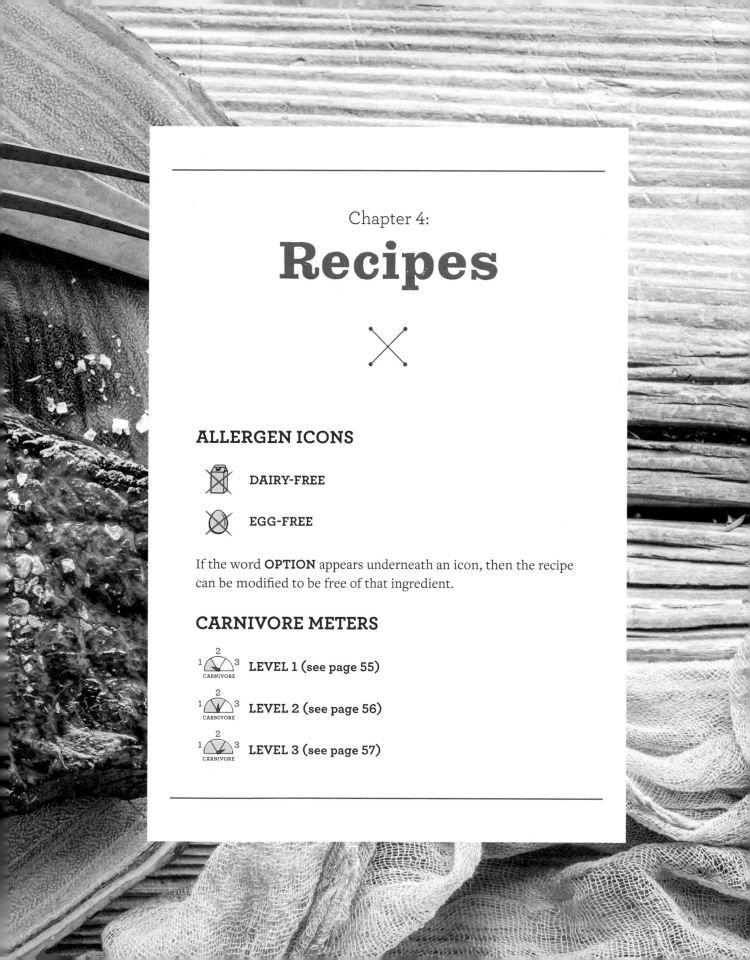

ALLERGEN ICONS

DAIRY-FREE

EGG-FREE

If the word **OPTION** appears underneath an icon, then the recipe can be modified to be free of that ingredient.

CARNIVORE METERS

LEVEL 1 (see page 55)

LEVEL 2 (see page 56)

LEVEL 3 (see page 57)

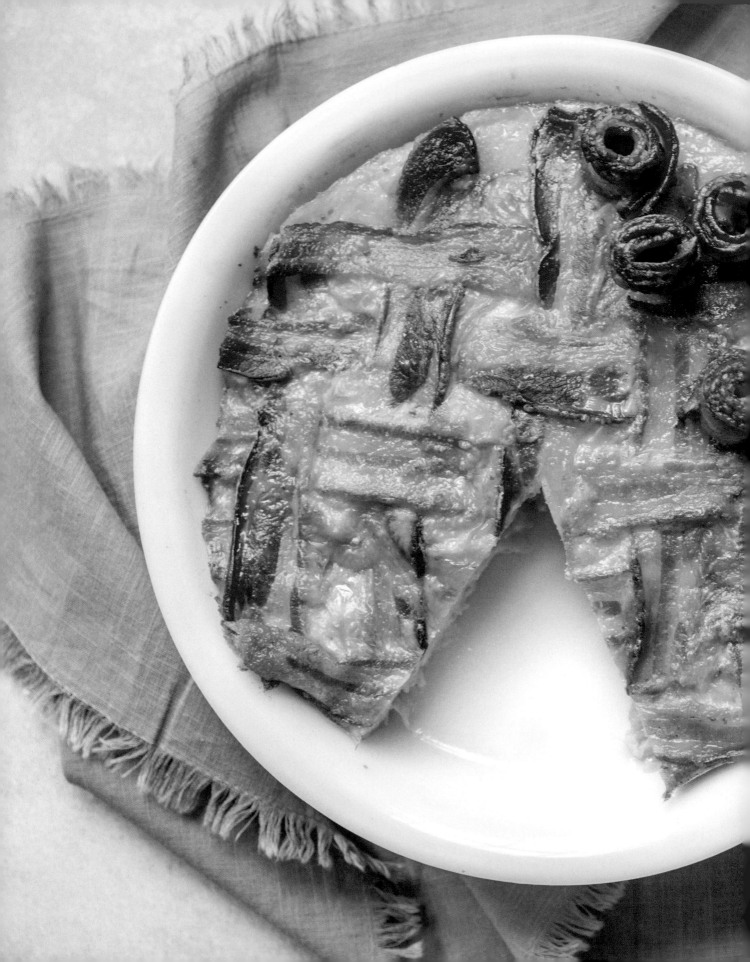

BREAKFAST

SALMON FRENCH EGGS

Yield: 2 servings
Prep Time: 5 minutes   **Cook Time:** 7 minutes

French eggs are very creamy, soft scrambled eggs. This breakfast is one of my favorite meals, and I have eaten it many times in Paris with a view of the Eiffel Tower!

2 tablespoons lard or unsalted butter

6 large eggs

½ teaspoon fine sea salt

4 ounces smoked salmon, chopped into small pieces

2 tablespoons mascarpone, room temperature

1. Melt the lard in a small saucepan over medium-low heat.

2. In a large bowl, whisk the eggs with the salt.

3. Pour the eggs into the saucepan and cook, whisking constantly, until the eggs are soft scrambled. Remove from the heat.

4. Add the smoked salmon and mascarpone and stir to combine with the eggs. Best served immediately.

Per Serving:

Calories: 464   Fat: 36 g   Protein: 30 g   Carbs: 1 g

1 2 3 CARNIVORE

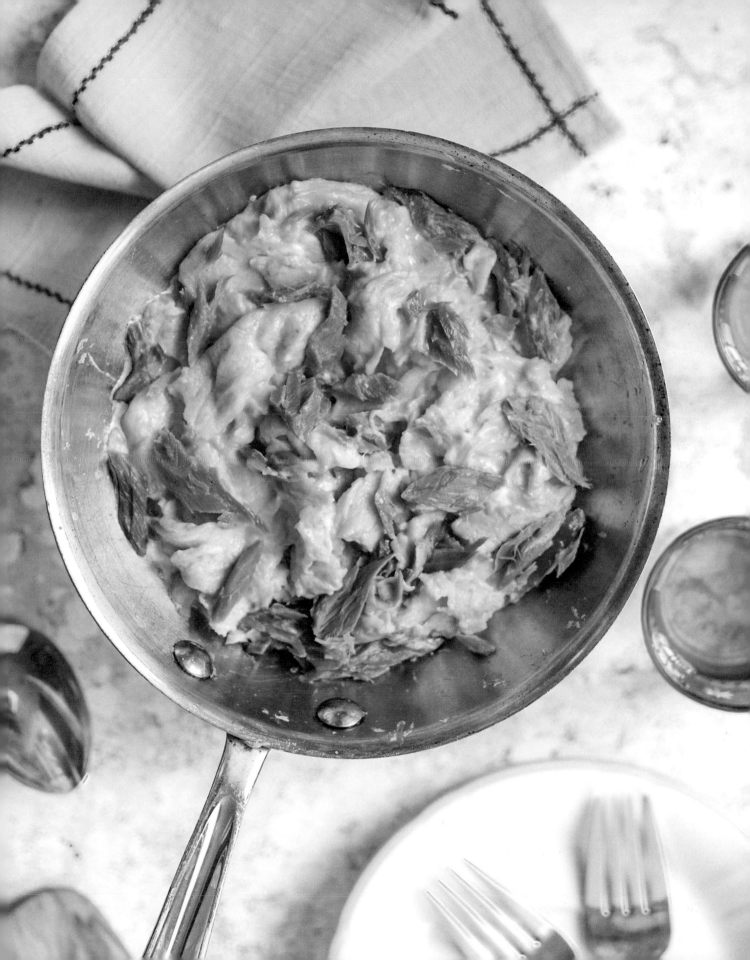

BON VIE SCRAMBLER

Yield: 4 servings
Prep Time: 4 minutes   **Cook Time:** 7 minutes

I often get asked what my kids eat since they are totally keto. On Saturdays, we love to go to a quaint breakfast restaurant in St. Paul, Minnesota, called Bon Vie, which means "good life" in French. My boys love to order the Bon Vie Scrambler with a side of sausages. You simply must try this kid-friendly breakfast—which is an excellent carnivore meal!

1 teaspoon unsalted butter or lard

8 ounces ground pork or ground beef

1 teaspoon fine sea salt

8 large eggs, lightly beaten

1 ounce cheddar cheese, shredded (about ¼ cup)

1. Melt the butter in a large skillet over medium heat.

2. Add the ground pork and season with the salt. Cook, crumbling the meat with a spatula to break up the clumps, until the meat is no longer pink, about 4 minutes.

3. Add the beaten eggs and use a whisk to scramble slightly. Cook until the eggs are set, about 3 minutes.

4. Add the cheese and mix well to combine. Remove from the heat and serve.

5. Store in an airtight container in the refrigerator for up to 4 days. To reheat, place a little butter or lard in a skillet over medium heat and stir frequently for 2 minutes, or until heated through.

Per Serving:

Calories: 330   Fat: 25g   Protein: 29g   Carbs: 1g

2
1 3
CARNIVORE

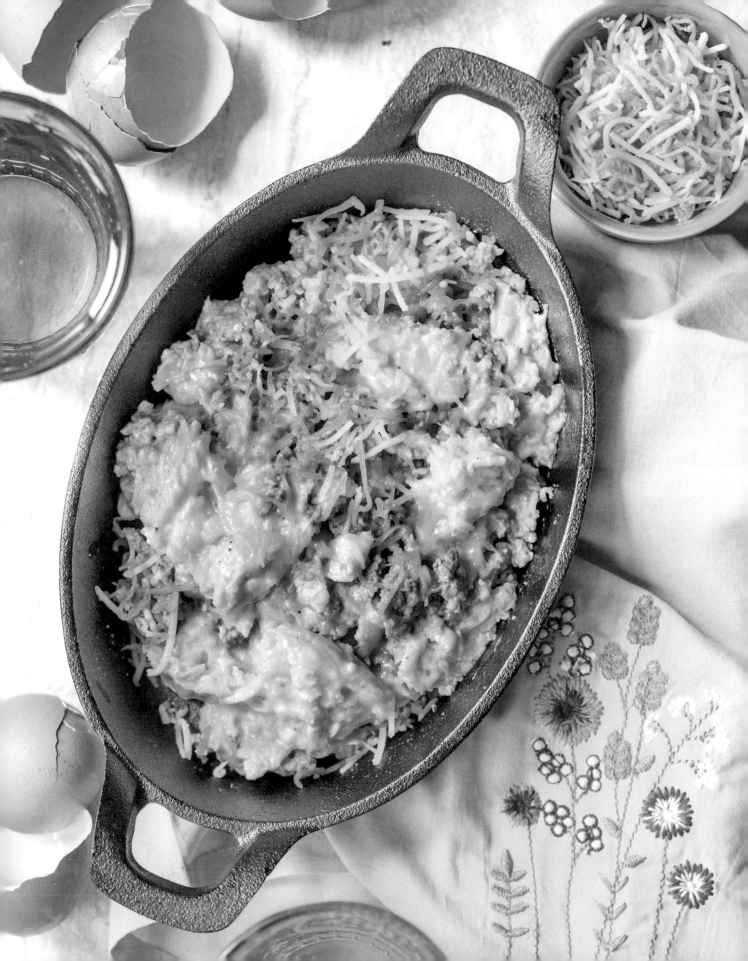

HAM HOCKS AND FRIED EGGS

Yield: 4 servings
Prep Time: 5 minutes   **Cook Time:** 10 minutes

4 (10-ounce) smoked ham hocks

1 tablespoon lard or tallow (page 312)

4 large eggs

¼ teaspoon fine sea salt

½ cup Easy Carnivore Hollandaise (page 314), for serving (optional)

1. Preheat the oven to 425°F.

2. Place the ham hocks on a rimmed baking sheet. Bake for 10 minutes, or until the skin gets crispy.

3. Meanwhile, fry the eggs: Heat the lard in a large cast-iron skillet over low heat. Crack the eggs side by side into the skillet. Season with the salt. Cover the pan with a lid and fry until the egg whites are cooked through but the yolks are still runny, about 4 minutes. Remove the eggs from the pan.

4. Place a ham hock along with a fried egg on a plate. Top with 2 tablespoons of hollandaise, if using. Best served immediately. (*Note:* Smoked ham hocks can be served cold, too.)

Per Serving (with hollandaise):

Calories: 462   Fat: 37 g   Protein: 30 g   Carbs: 0.4 g

1 2 3
CARNIVORE

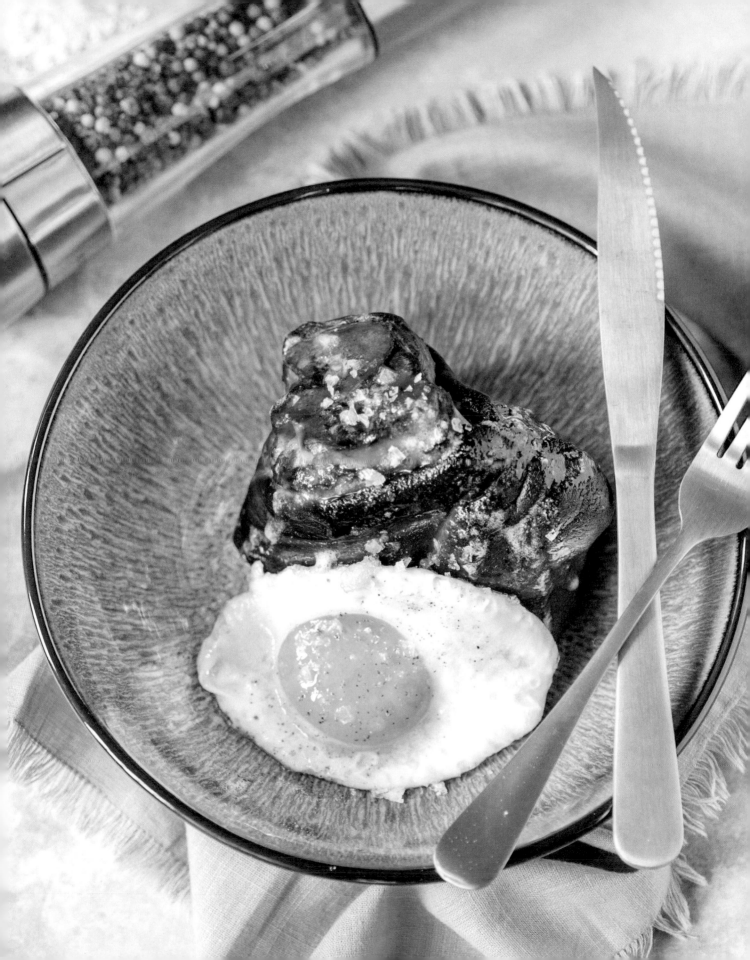

BREAKFAST KABOBS

Yield: 4 servings
Prep Time: 10 minutes   **Cook Time:** 8 minutes

Eating off a stick is so much fun! My kids love this playful and delicious breakfast.

8 thick slices pork or beef bacon

4 precooked pork breakfast sausage links, cut into 1-inch pieces

1 (8-ounce) fully cooked smoked boneless ham steak, ¾ inch thick, cut into 1-inch pieces

Special Equipment:
8 (4-inch) metal or wooden skewers

1. If using wooden skewers, soak them in water for 10 minutes. Preheat a grill to medium-high heat.

2. Thread 1 piece of bacon onto a skewer, starting about ½ inch from one end of the bacon. Thread on a piece of sausage, then weave the bacon around the sausage and thread the bacon onto the skewer again. Place a slice of ham on the skewer and weave the bacon around the ham, then thread the bacon onto the skewer again. Repeat with another slice of sausage and another slice of ham, weaving the bacon around the sausage and ham. Repeat with the remaining skewers.

3. Place the skewers on the hot grill and grill for 6 to 8 minutes, flipping after 3 minutes, until the bacon is slightly crisp and cooked to your liking. Remove from the grill and serve.

4. Store in an airtight container in the refrigerator for up to 4 days or in the freezer for up to a month. To reheat, place on a rimmed baking sheet in a preheated 350°F oven for 5 minutes, or until heated through.

Per Serving:

Calories: 295   Fat: 23 g   Protein: 22 g   Carbs: 1 g

1 2 3
CARNIVORE

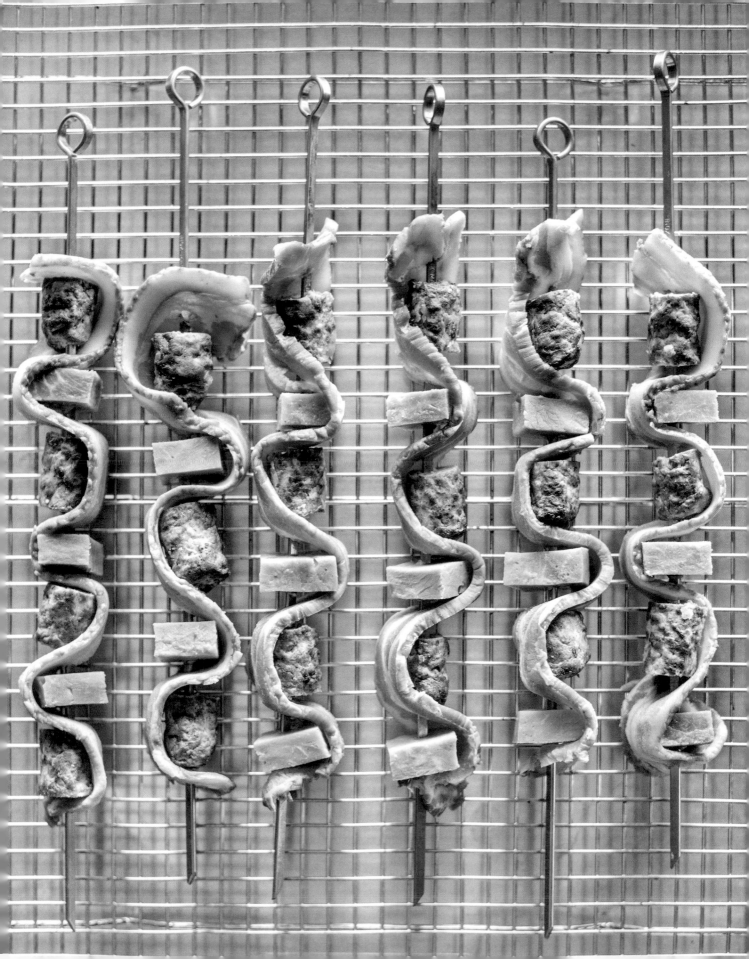

BACON KNOTS

Yield: 12 knots (2 per serving)
Prep Time: 5 minutes   **Cook Time:** 10 minutes

Serve these knots for breakfast or dip them in Smoky Chicken Salad (page 150), Tuna Salad (page 152), Smoky Salmon Salad (page 154), or Egg Salad (page 156).

12 slices pork or beef bacon

1. Preheat the oven to 400°F. Line a rimmed baking sheet with parchment paper.

2. Tie a slice of bacon in a very loose knot. Place on the lined baking sheet and fan the ends out so that the knots cook evenly. Repeat with the remaining bacon slices.

3. Bake for 10 minutes, or until cooked to your liking.

4. Store in an airtight container in the refrigerator for up to 4 days. To reheat, place on a rimmed baking sheet in a preheated 400°F oven for 2 minutes, or until heated through.

Per Serving:

Calories: 140   Fat: 12 g   Protein: 8 g   Carbs: 0 g

1 2 3 CARNIVORE   1 2 3 IF USING BEEF BACON

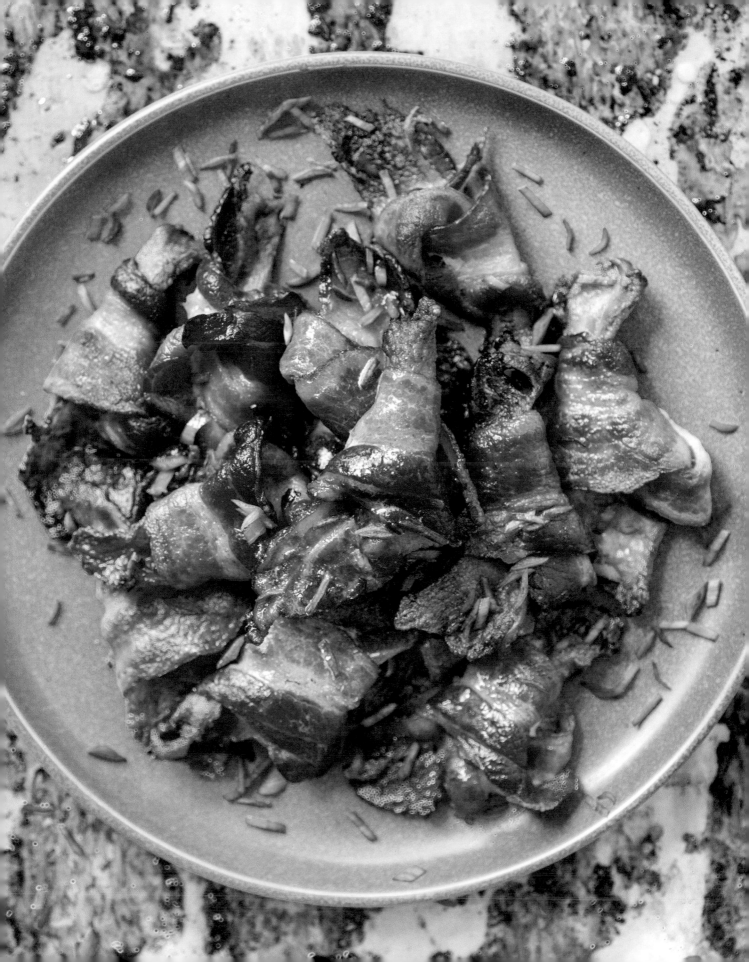

PORK FRIED EGGS

Yield: 1 serving
Prep Time: 4 minutes   **Cook Time:** 10 minutes

I often make this breakfast dish for my family. I used to use chorizo, but now I use ground pork to eliminate the undesired spices and fillers often found in chorizo for maximum healing. As shown in the photo, I sometimes garnish the dish with pink or purple salt to add a pretty color.

1½ teaspoons lard or tallow (page 312)

2 ounces ground pork

2 large eggs

¼ teaspoon fine sea salt

1. Heat the lard in a cast-iron skillet over medium heat. Add the ground pork and cook, crumbling the meat with a spatula to break up the clumps, until cooked through, about 4 minutes. Remove the pork from the skillet, leaving the drippings in the pan.

2. Reduce the heat to medium-low and crack the eggs side by side into the skillet. Sprinkle the eggs with the salt. Cook just until the whites are set and the yolks are runny.

3. Transfer the eggs to a plate, then top with the pork and serve.

Per Serving:

Calories: 464   Fat: 38 g   Protein: 27 g   Carbs: 2 g

CARNIVORE

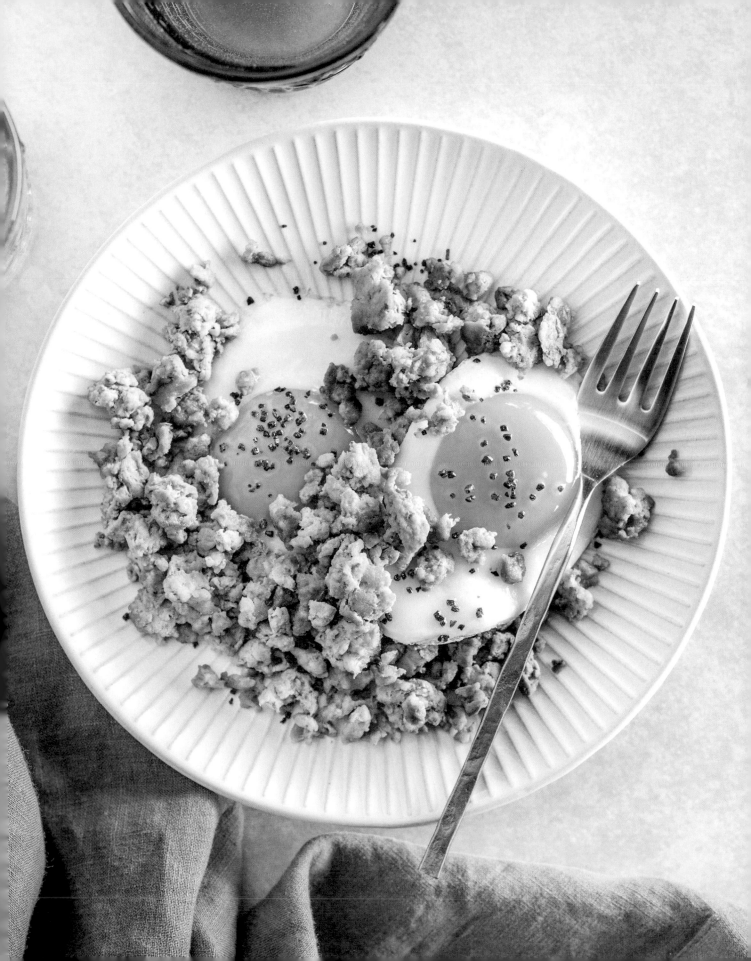

BACON CHEESEBURGER SCRAMBLED EGGS

Yield: 1 serving
Prep Time: 4 minutes   **Cook Time:** 13 minutes

I adore bacon cheeseburgers, and I love scrambled eggs. I married the two and made the most delicious carnivore breakfast. You must try it!

1 slice pork or beef bacon, diced

2 ounces ground beef

¼ teaspoon fine sea salt, divided

2 large eggs, beaten

2 ounces sharp cheddar cheese, shredded (about ½ cup)

1. Heat a cast-iron skillet over medium heat. Place the bacon in the pan and cook, stirring occasionally, until the bacon is cooked to your liking. Remove the bacon from the skillet, leaving the drippings in the pan. Set the bacon aside.

2. Add the ground beef to the skillet, season with ⅛ teaspoon of the salt, and cook, crumbling the meat with a spatula to break up the clumps, for 4 minutes, or until cooked through.

3. Reduce the heat to medium-low. Pour the beaten eggs into the skillet and cook for about 4 minutes, stirring often to scramble. Just before the eggs are set, sprinkle them with the remaining ⅛ teaspoon of salt. Stir well.

4. Sprinkle the cheese on top of the beef and egg mixture. Once the cheese is melted, transfer to a serving plate and top with the reserved bacon.

Per Serving:

Calories: 460   Fat: 35 g   Protein: 34 g   Carbs: 2 g

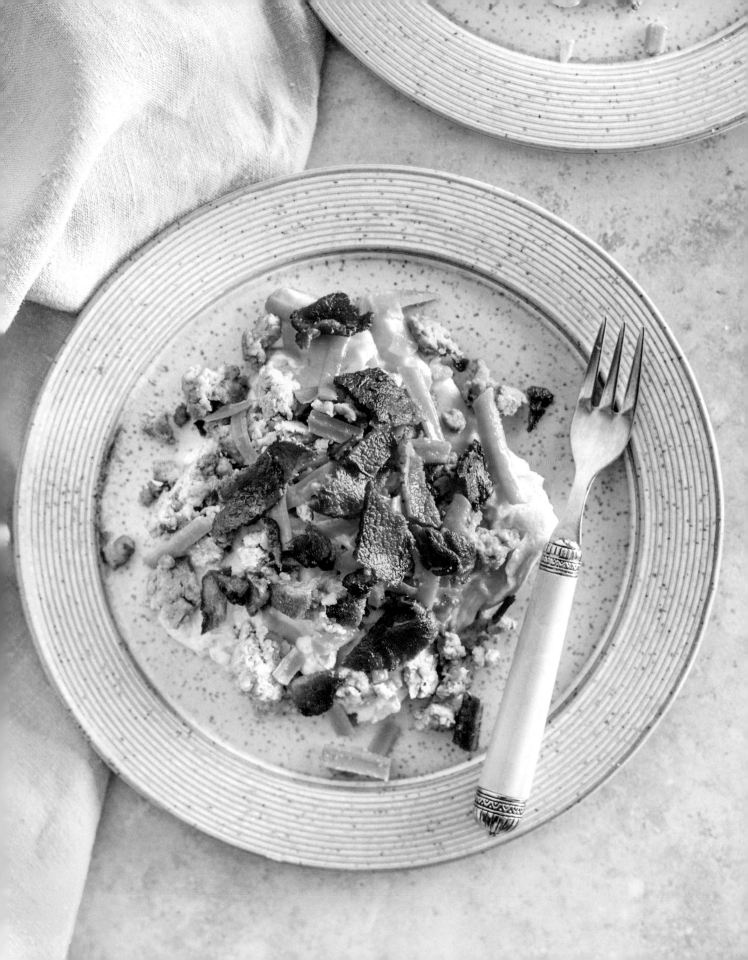

BREAKFAST PATTIES

Yield: 12 patties (2 per serving)
Prep Time: 8 minutes   **Cook Time:** 8 minutes per batch

I like to make a triple batch of these patties every month and store them in the refrigerator or freezer for easy breakfasts. The uncooked patties will keep in the fridge for up to 5 days or in the freezer for up to 6 months.

2 pounds ground pork or ground beef

2 teaspoons fine sea salt

2 tablespoons lard or tallow (page 312)

1. Place the ground pork and salt in a large bowl. Using your hands, mix well to work the salt into the meat, then form the mixture into twelve 3-inch patties.

2. Heat the lard in a cast-iron skillet over medium-high heat. Once hot, add the patties, working in batches if needed to avoid overcrowding the skillet. Cook for 4 minutes, then flip the patties over and cook for 4 minutes on the other side, or until the patties are no longer pink inside.

3. Store the cooked patties in an airtight container in the refrigerator for up to 5 days or in the freezer for up to 6 months. To reheat, place on a greased cast-iron skillet over medium heat for a few minutes on each side, until warmed through.

Per Serving:

Calories: 429   Fat: 36 g   Protein: 39 g   Carbs: 0 g

CARNIVORE   IF USING BEEF AND TALLOW

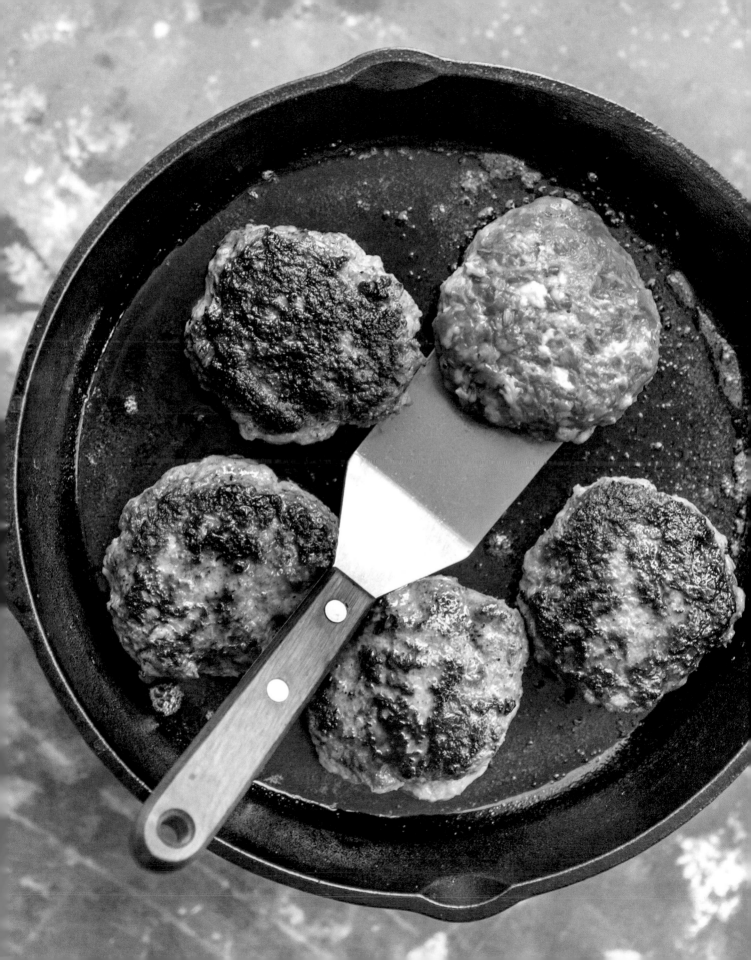

BREAKFAST PIE

Yield: 4 servings
Prep Time: 5 minutes   **Cook Time:** 28 minutes

As a busy mom, I understand that not everyone wants or has the time to spend hours in the kitchen. However, I do know that everyone loves tasty food. I have worked and worked to create recipes that will make the carnivore lifestyle easier for you! This lovely breakfast pie is not only super easy but also tastes amazing.

3 ounces sharp cheddar cheese, shredded (about ¾ cup), divided

8 large eggs

1 teaspoon fine sea salt

6 thin slices pork or beef bacon

1. Preheat the oven to 400°F.

2. Sprinkle ½ cup of the cheese evenly in a 9-inch pie pan. Bake for 3 minutes, or until melted.

3. Meanwhile, place the remaining ¼ cup of cheese in a medium bowl. Add the eggs and salt and whisk well to combine. Pour the eggs over the melted cheese in the pie pan.

4. Lay the bacon slices in a weave pattern over the eggs. Bake for 22 to 25 minutes, or until the eggs are set and the bacon is crisp.

5. Store in airtight container in the refrigerator for up to 5 days. To reheat, place a slice in a preheated 350°F oven for a few minutes, until warmed through.

Per Serving:

Calories: 336   Fat: 26 g   Protein: 24 g   Carbs: 2 g

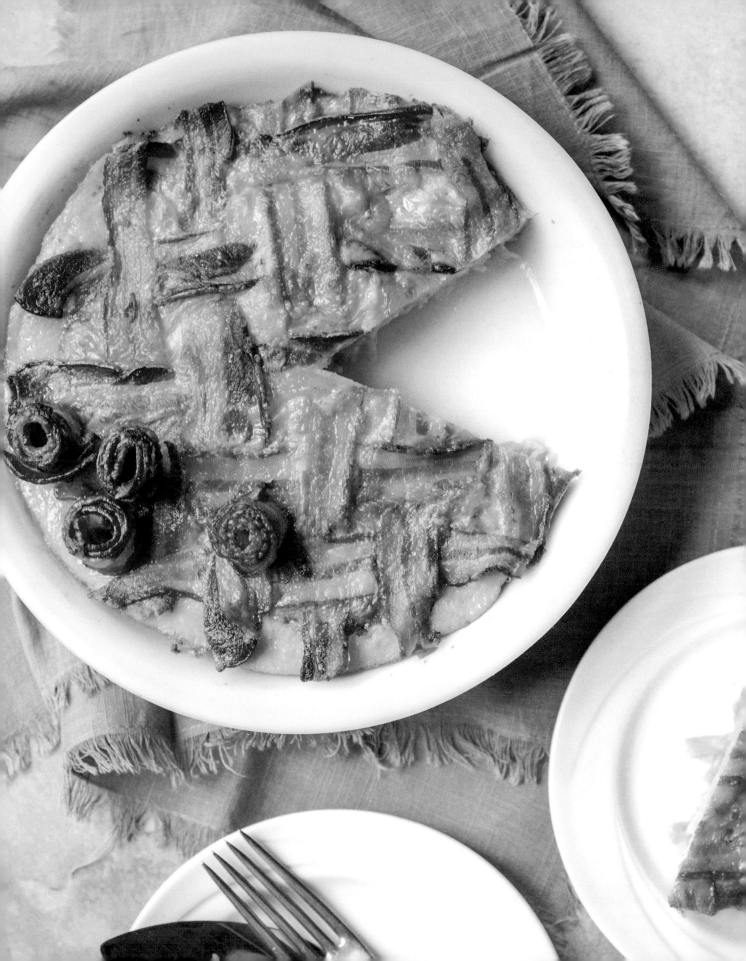

CARNIVORE EGGS BENEDICT

Yield: 1 serving   **Prep Time:** 5 minutes (not including time to make hollandaise)
Cook Time: 13 minutes

When making poached eggs, adding vinegar to the cooking water helps the whites coagulate. However, since vinegar isn't carnivore, you do not have to use it when poaching the eggs for this dish. Make sure that your eggs are fresh, because fresh eggs have a thicker albumen that won't disperse when placed in the poaching water. As eggs age, the albumen gets thinner and waterier, which causes the whites to fall apart in the hot water. Test eggs for freshness by placing them in a container of cold water—fresh eggs will sink, while older eggs will float.

1 tablespoon lard or tallow (page 312)

2 uncooked Breakfast Patties (page 116)

2 slices Canadian bacon

2 large eggs

2½ tablespoons Easy Carnivore Hollandaise (page 314)

1. Heat the lard in a cast-iron skillet over medium-high heat. Once hot, add the patties and cook for 4 minutes, then flip the patties over and cook for 4 minutes on the other side, or until the patties are no longer pink inside. Remove the patties to a serving plate, leaving the drippings in the skillet.

2. Add the Canadian bacon to the skillet and cook for 1 minute, then flip over and cook for another minute, or until heated through.

3. Poach the eggs: Fill a large saucepan with about 4 inches of water. Bring to a simmer. Swirl the water in one direction with a spoon and gently crack the eggs into the swirling water. Poach the eggs until the whites are just cooked but the yolks are still soft and runny, about 3 minutes.

4. To serve, top each patty with a slice of Canadian bacon, a poached egg, and a drizzle of hollandaise.

Per Serving:

Calories: 507   Fat: 40 g   Protein: 32 g   Carbs: 2 g

2
1 3
CARNIVORE

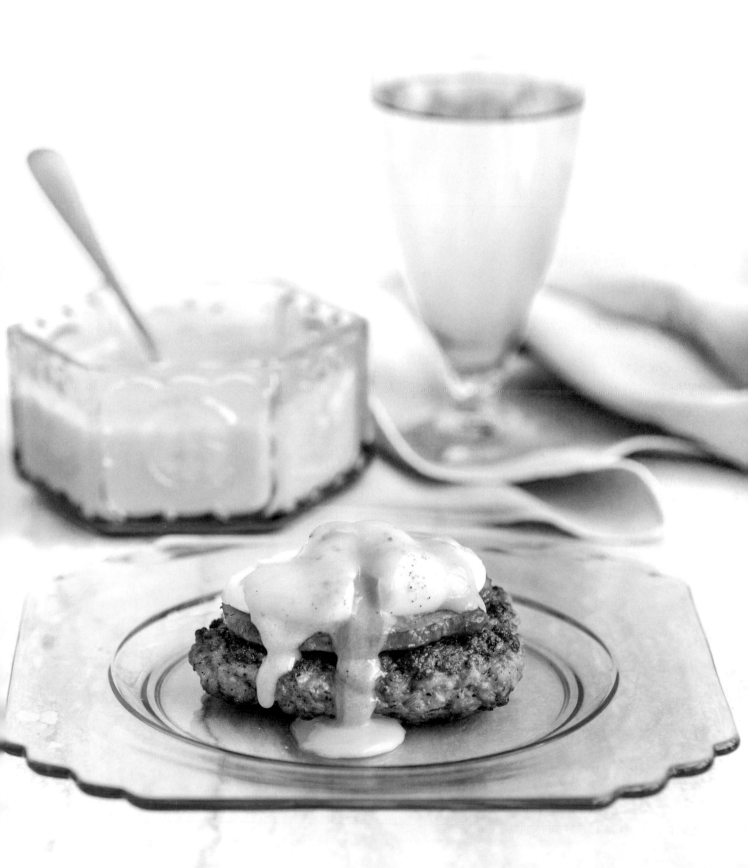

STEAK AND EGGS

Yield: 2 servings   **Prep Time:** 5 minutes, plus 25 minutes for steak to come to room temperature and rest   **Cook Time:** 10 minutes

What's not to love about steak and eggs? This is a great recipe for breakfast or any time of the day! If you're particularly ravenous, add a slice or two of crispy bacon.

2 (4-ounce) filet mignons, about 1¼ inches thick

2 teaspoons fine sea salt, divided

1 teaspoon lard or tallow (page 312)

2 large eggs

2 tablespoons Easy Carnivore Hollandaise (page 314), for serving (optional)

1. Set the filets out to rest at room temperature for 15 minutes before cooking to ensure even cooking.

2. Preheat the oven or an air fryer to 400°F. Pat the filets dry, then season well on both sides with 1½ teaspoons of the salt.

3. Place the filets on a rimmed baking sheet or directly in the air fryer basket and cook for 10 minutes for rare filets, or until done to your liking (see the chart on page 180). Allow to rest for 10 minutes before serving.

4. Meanwhile, fry the eggs: Heat the lard in a cast-iron skillet over low heat. Crack the eggs into the pan. Season with the remaining ½ teaspoon of salt. Cover the pan with a lid and fry until the whites are cooked through but the yolks are still runny, about 4 minutes. Remove the eggs from the pan.

5. Slice the steaks and place on two plates. Add a fried egg to each plate and top with a tablespoon of hollandaise, if desired. Best served fresh.

Per Serving (with hollandaise):

Calories: 241   Fat: 12 g   Protein: 20 g   Carbs: 0.4 g

2
1 3
CARNIVORE

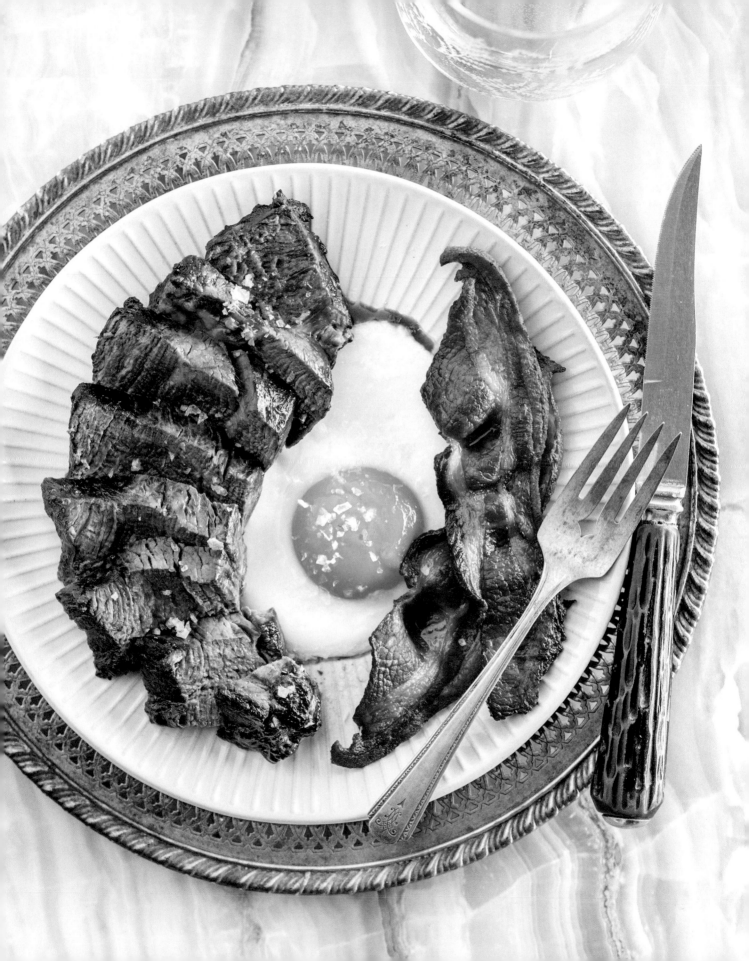

HAM 'N' CHEESE FRITTATA

Yield: 2 servings
Prep Time: 5 minutes   **Cook Time:** 24 minutes

Making a frittata is an easy way to enjoy a lovely breakfast. I often toss a frittata in the oven and then get ready for the day. When I return to the kitchen, my eggs are ready to eat.

1 cup cubed ham (about 5 ounces)

4 large eggs, lightly beaten

2 ounces cheddar cheese, shredded (about ½ cup)

½ teaspoon fine sea salt

1. Preheat the oven or an air fryer to 350°F. Lightly grease a 6-inch round cake pan.

2. In a medium bowl, combine the ham, beaten eggs, cheese, and salt. Pour the egg mixture into the prepared cake pan. Cook for 20 to 24 minutes, or until the eggs are set. Best served fresh.

Per Serving:

Calories: 428   Fat: 31 g   Protein: 35 g   Carbs: 3 g

CARNIVORE

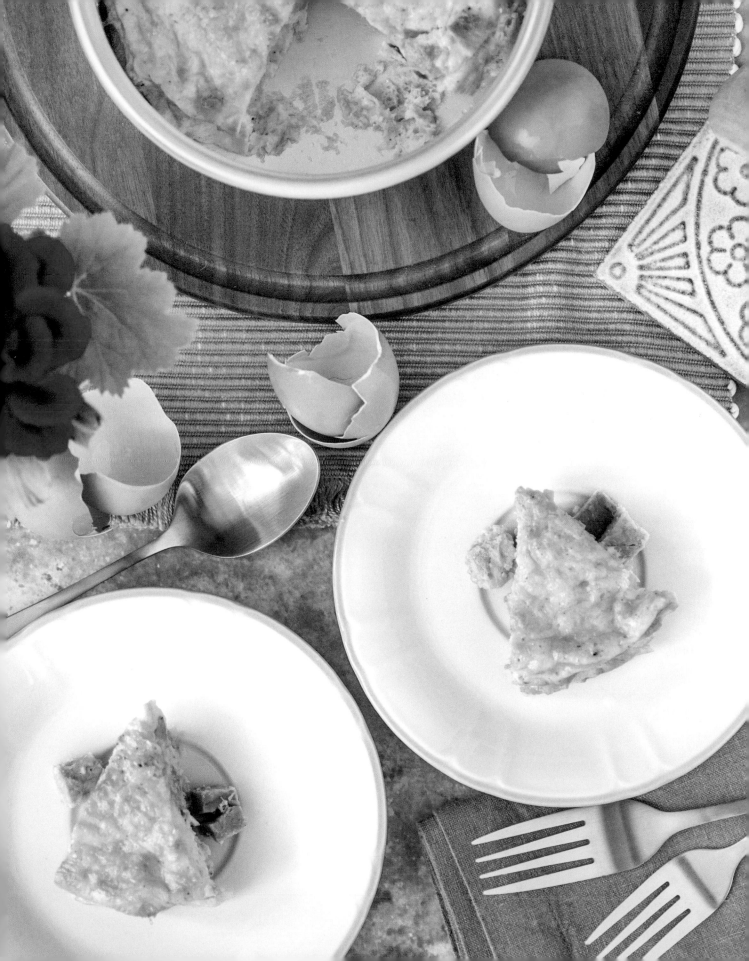

CARNIVORE OMELET

YIELD: 1 serving
PREP TIME: 3 minutes   **COOK TIME:** 5 minutes

I love omelets, and this omelet is filled with protein to make it a very hearty breakfast!

2 large eggs

1 tablespoon water

¼ teaspoon fine sea salt, divided

1 tablespoon unsalted butter or tallow (page 312)

4 ounces ground beef

1 ounce ham, cubed

1 ounce cheddar cheese, shredded (about ¼ cup)

1. Crack the eggs into a small bowl. Add the water and ⅛ teaspoon of the salt and whisk with a fork.

2. Heat a small skillet over medium-high heat. Once hot, melt the butter in the pan, then add the ground beef. Cook, crumbling the meat with a spatula to break up the clumps, until no longer pink, about 3 minutes. Season the beef with the remaining ⅛ teaspoon of salt.

3. Reduce the heat to medium-low. Pour the whisked eggs into the cooked beef and swirl the pan. For a few seconds, gently stir the eggs with a spatula (as if you were making scrambled eggs), then swirl the pan to make a nice round shape with the eggs.

4. Continue cooking for about 1 minute. The eggs will be set on the bottom but slightly liquid on top.

5. Remove the pan from the heat. Add the ham and cheese to the center of the omelet. Fold the omelet in half to cover the fillings and transfer to a plate.

Per Serving:

Calories: 716   Fat: 53 g   Protein: 54 g   Carbs: 3 g

2
1 3
CARNIVORE

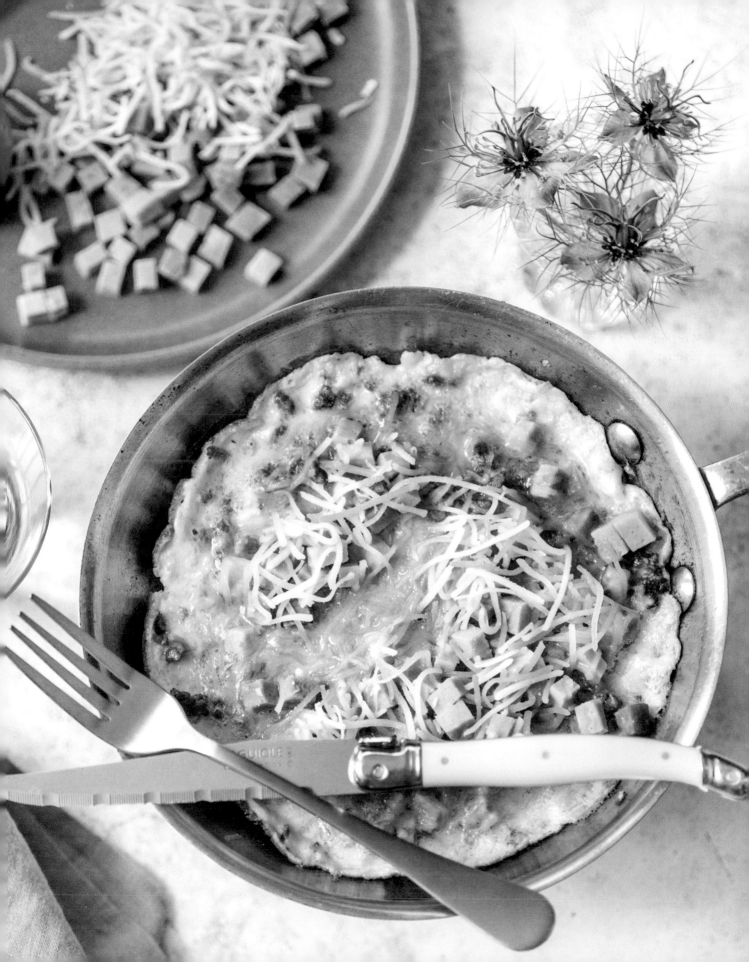

CARNIVORE WAFFLE

Yield: 1 serving
Prep Time: 5 minutes   **Cook Time:** 3 minutes

Why does everything seem to taste better in a waffle shape? I like to make extra Carnivore Waffles and store them in the fridge so my boys can heat them up for easy breakfasts.

4 ounces ground beef

2 large eggs

½ teaspoon fine sea salt

2½ tablespoons Easy Carnivore Hollandaise (page 314) (optional)

Special Equipment:
Waffle iron

1. Preheat a waffle iron. Place the beef, eggs, and salt in a small bowl and combine well using your hands.

2. Place the waffle "batter" in the center of the waffle iron and close the lid. Cook for 2 to 3 minutes, or until the waffle is golden brown and cooked through. Remove and place on a plate. Serve with hollandaise, if desired.

Per Serving (with hollandaise):

Calories: 628   Fat: 53 g   Protein: 34 g   Carbs: 1 g

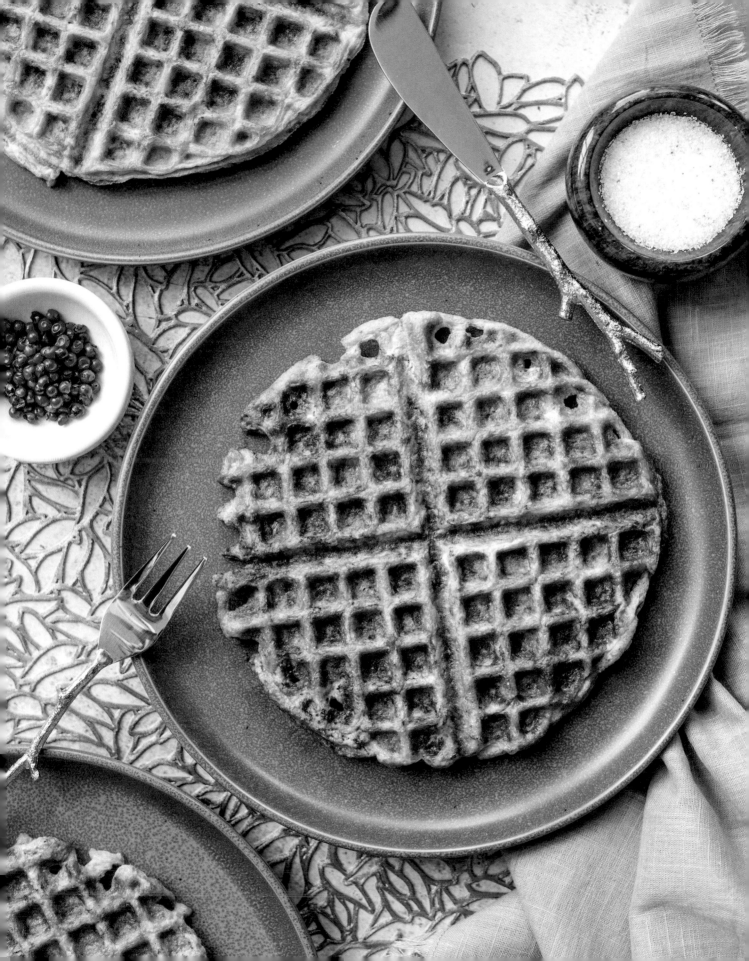

CARNIVORE EGG CUPS

Yield: 6 egg cups (3 per serving)
Prep Time: 5 minutes   **Cook Time:** 12 minutes

OPTION

Lard or tallow (page 312), for the pan

6 slices deli roast beef

6 slices cheddar cheese (omit for dairy-free)

6 large eggs

½ teaspoon fine sea salt

6 tablespoons Easy Carnivore Hollandaise (page 314), for serving (optional)

1. Preheat the oven to 400°F. Grease a 6-well muffin pan.

2. Place 1 slice of roast beef into each well. Place a slice of cheese into each beef-lined cup. Then break an egg into each beef cup.

3. Sprinkle the eggs with the salt.

4. Bake for 12 minutes, or until the egg whites are set but the yolks are still a bit runny.

5. Serve with hollandaise, if desired.

6. Store in an airtight container in the refrigerator for up to 4 days. To reheat, place cups in a muffin pan and into a preheated 350°F oven for 5 minutes, or until heated through.

Per Serving (with hollandaise):

Calories: 641   Fat: 52 g   Protein: 38 g   Carbs: 1 g

1   2   3
CARNIVORE

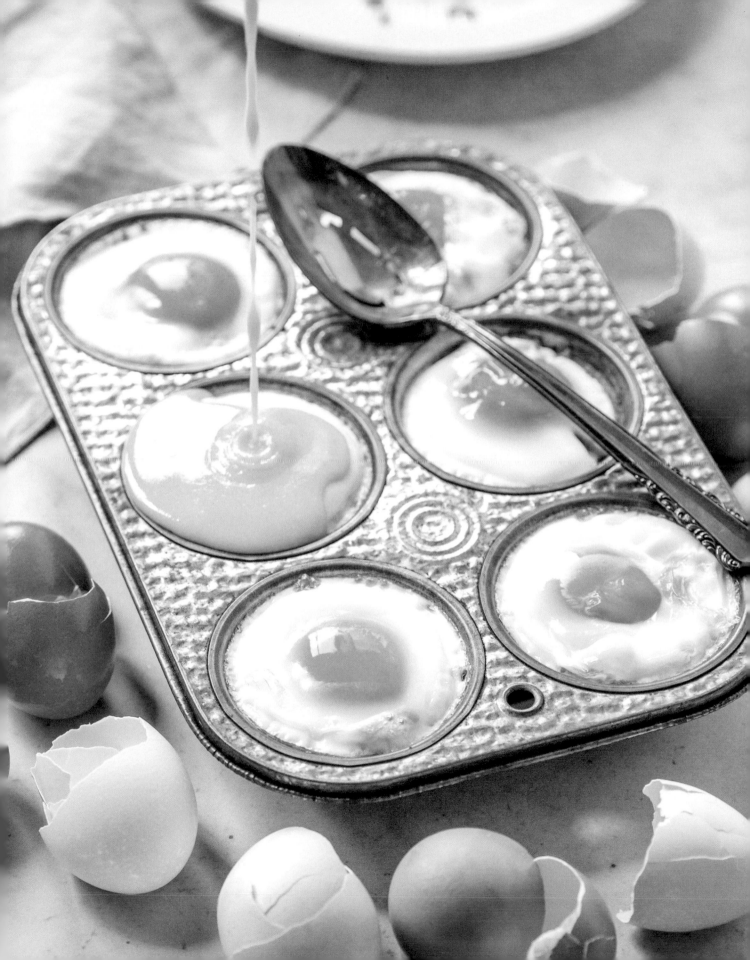

BREAKFAST MEATBALLS

OPTION

Yield: 12 meatballs (2 per serving)
Prep Time: 8 minutes, plus 5 minutes to rest   **Cook Time:** 20 minutes

1 pound ground beef

1 pound ground pork

4 ounces ham, finely chopped

2 teaspoons fine sea salt

1 teaspoon fresh ground black pepper

Easy Carnivore Hollandaise (page 314), for serving (optional)

1. Preheat the oven to 375°F.

2. Place the ground beef, ground pork, diced ham, salt, and pepper in a large bowl. Using your hands, mix well to evenly combine the ingredients. Form the mixture into twelve 1½-inch meatballs.

3. Arrange the meatballs in a single layer on a rimmed baking sheet. Bake for 15 to 20 minutes, turning occasionally, until evenly browned and cooked through. Remove from the oven and allow to rest for 5 minutes. Serve with hollandaise, if desired.

4. Store in an airtight container in the refrigerator for up to 5 days or in the freezer for up to a month. To reheat, place on a rimmed baking sheet in a preheated 350°F oven for about 3 minutes, until heated through.

Per Serving (without hollandaise):

Calories: 303   Fat: 23 g   Protein: 28 g   Carbs: 0.2 g

1 ⌄ 3   1 ⌄ 3
CARNIVORE   WITH HOLLANDAISE

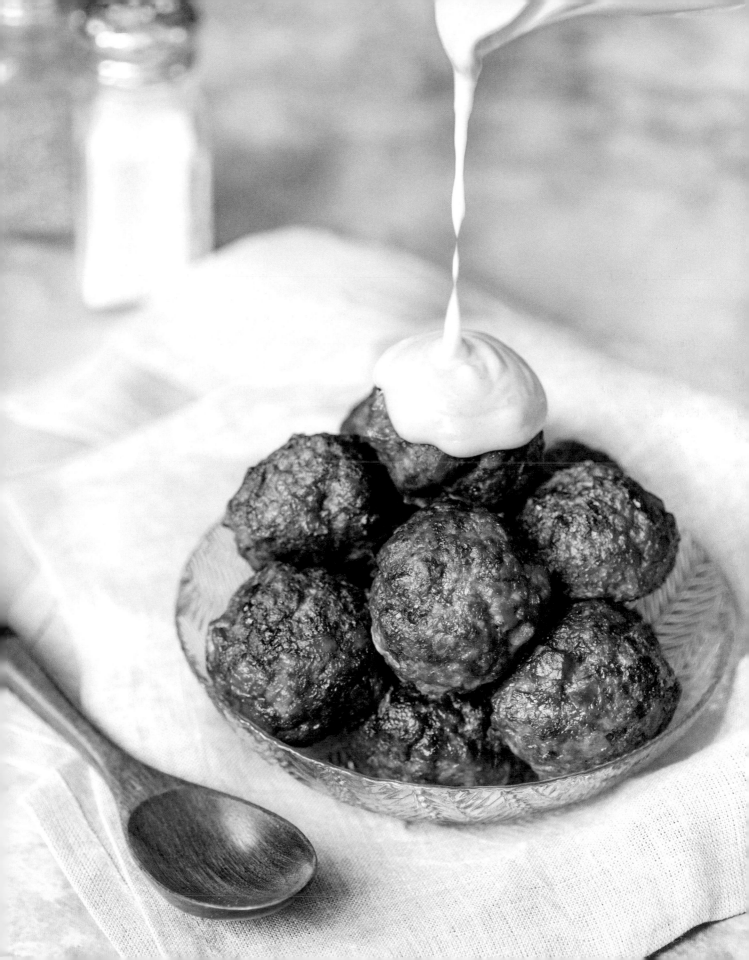

BREAKFAST BURGERS

Yield: 4 servings
Prep Time: 8 minutes   **Cook Time:** 18 minutes

4 slices pork or beef bacon

1 pound ground beef

1 teaspoon fine sea salt

4 large eggs

8 tablespoons Easy Carnivore Hollandaise (page 314)

1. Place the bacon in a cast-iron skillet over medium-high heat and cook for 4 minutes per side for crispy bacon. Remove the bacon from the skillet and set aside, leaving the drippings in the skillet.

2. While the bacon is cooking, divide the ground beef into 4 equal portions and form each portion into a ½-inch-thick patty (about 3½ inches in diameter). Season the patties well on both sides with the salt.

3. Place the seasoned patties in the cast-iron skillet over medium-high heat. Fry the patties for 3 minutes per side for medium-done burgers, or cook longer if you prefer more well-done burgers.

4. Remove the burgers from the skillet, leaving the grease in the skillet, and set aside on a warm plate. Crack the eggs into the skillet and cook over medium heat for 4 minutes, or until whites are set and yolks are still runny.

5. To serve, place the patties on four plates and top each burger with a fried egg, a slice of bacon, and 2 tablespoons of hollandaise.

6. Store in an airtight container in the refrigerator for up to 4 days. To reheat, place in a lightly greased skillet over medium heat for about 3 minutes, or until heated through.

Per Serving:

Calories: 592   Fat: 47 g   Protein: 39 g   Carbs: 0.4 g

1 2 3
CARNIVORE

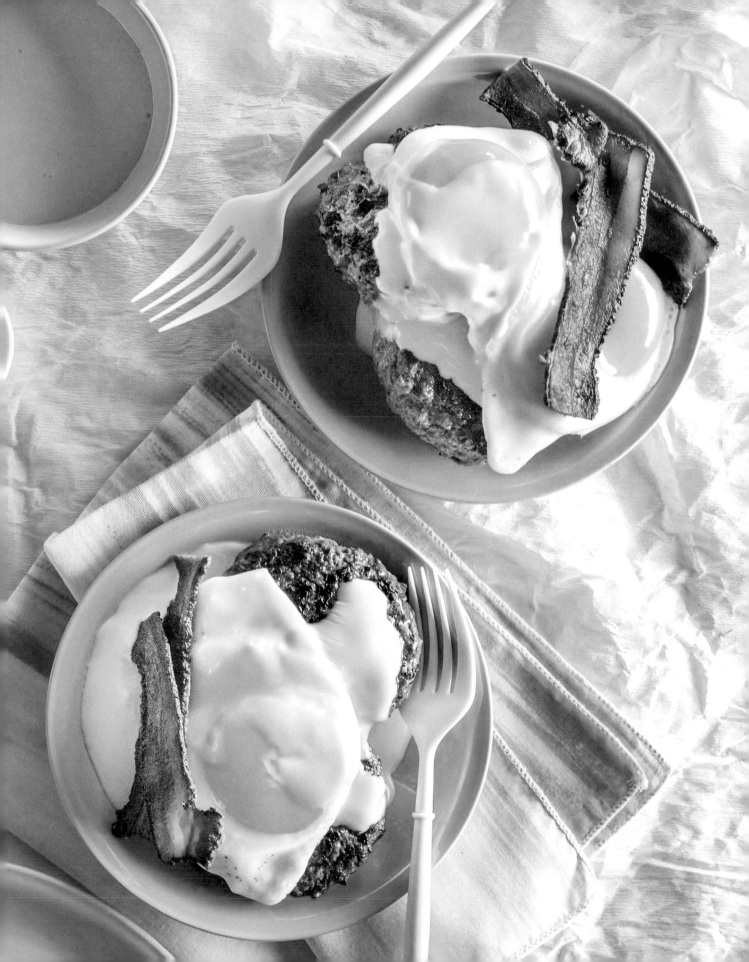

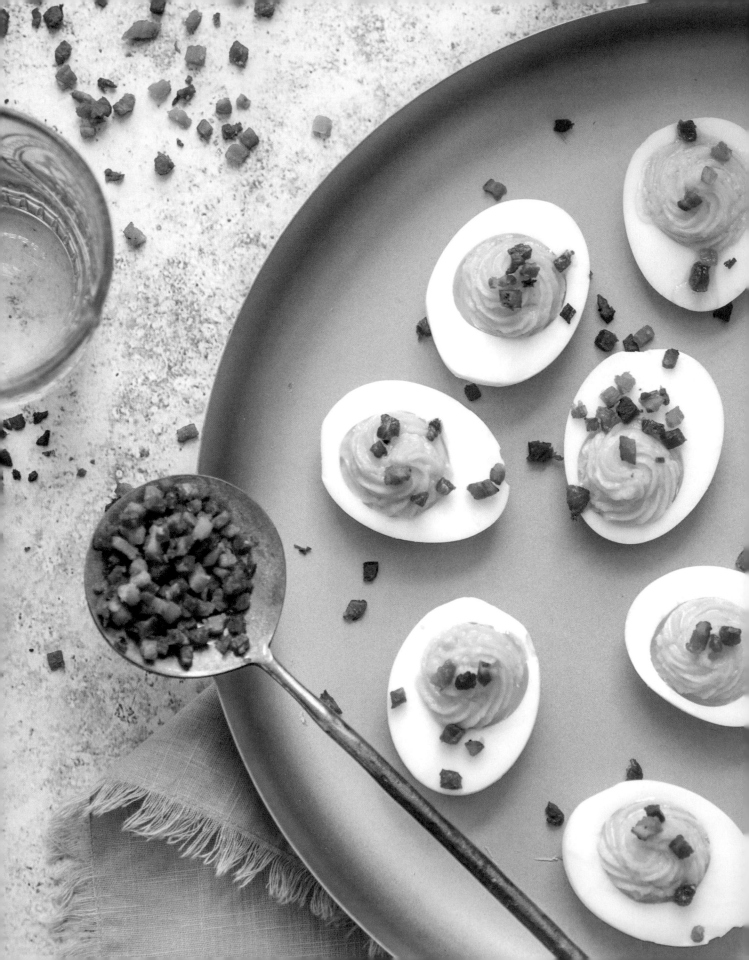

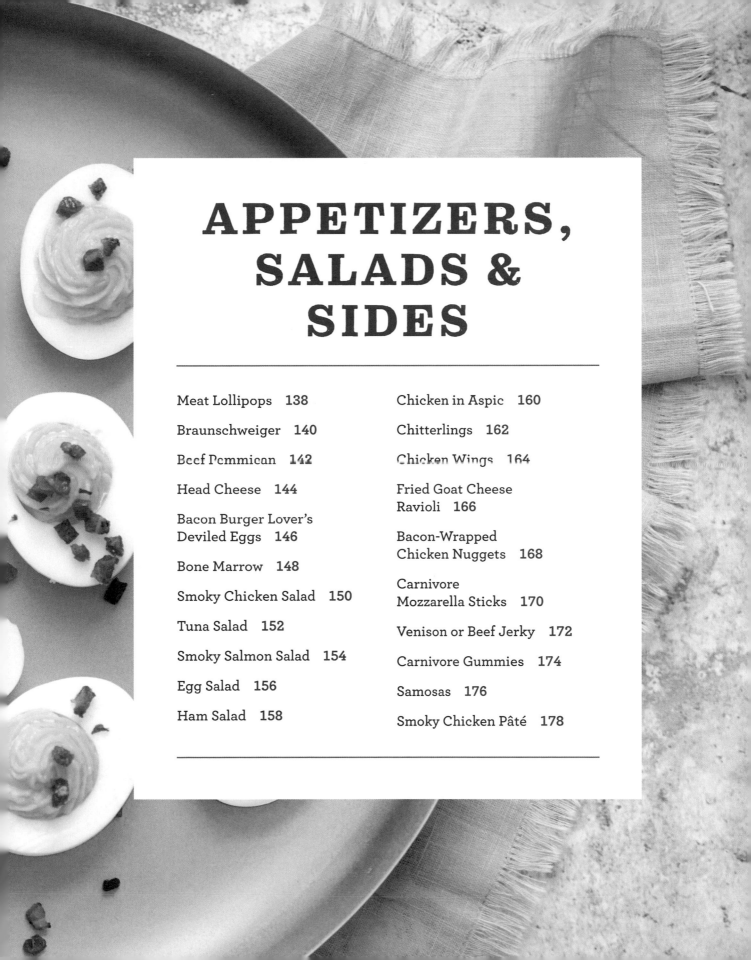

APPETIZERS, SALADS & SIDES

MEAT LOLLIPOPS

Yield: 24 lollipops (2 per serving)
Prep Time: 6 minutes   **Cook Time:** 17 minutes

This is a great appetizer to serve at a dinner party. Even the non-carnivores will be asking for more!

2 tablespoons lard or unsalted butter

1 pound beef tenderloin, cut into 24 (1½-inch) cubes

1 teaspoon fine sea salt

4 ounces crumbled blue cheese (about 1 cup)

Special Equipment:
24 small metal or wooden skewers or toothpicks

1. Preheat the oven to 350°F.

2. Heat the lard in a large skillet over medium-high heat. While it's heating, season the beef cubes with the salt. Once the lard is hot, add the beef and sauté until browned on all sides, about 3 minutes. (The meat will not be fully cooked at this point.)

3. Transfer the beef to an 8-inch square baking dish. Top each cube with 2 teaspoons of blue cheese.

4. Bake for about 8 minutes for medium-done beef, or until the meat is cooked to your desired doneness (see the chart on page 180). Remove to a serving plate and insert a skewer or toothpick into each cube for meat lollipops! Best served immediately.

Per Serving:

Calories: 358   Fat: 29 g   Protein: 24 g   Carbs: 0 g

2
1 3
CARNIVORE

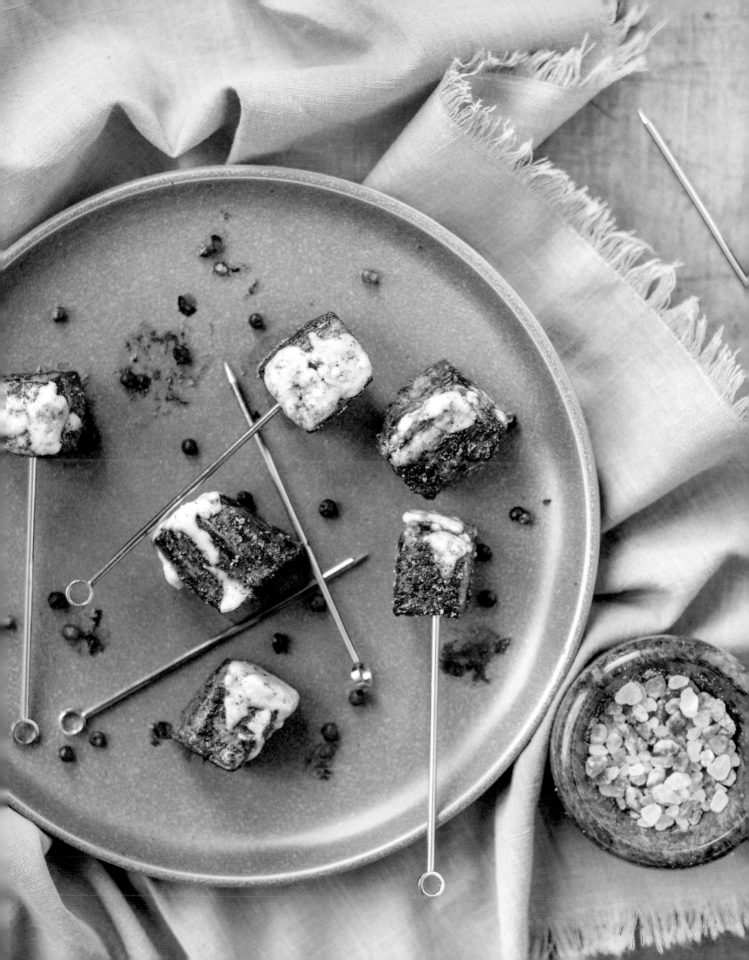

BRAUNSCHWEIGER

Yield: 8 servings
Prep Time: 10 minutes   **Cook Time:** 2 hours, plus 1 to 2 days to set

I grew up eating Braunschweige, a delicious liver pâté. We always ate it on crackers, but now I put it on top of a burger patty for a creamy bite. It also tastes great with pork rinds.

1¼ pounds pork or beef liver

12 ounces pork back fat

8 ounces boneless pork shoulder or beef tongue

1 tablespoon fine sea salt or smoked sea salt, store-bought or homemade (page 310)

1. Preheat the oven to 300°F.

2. Cut the pork liver, back fat, and shoulder into 1-inch cubes. Place in a food processor or blender with the salt and purée until smooth.

3. Spoon the pork purée into a pullman loaf pan or 9 by 5-inch loaf pan and cover tightly with aluminum foil. Pour an inch of boiling water into a roasting pan and set the loaf pan inside the roasting pan.

4. Bake for 2 hours, or until the sausage is thoroughly cooked but not browned and the internal temperature in the center of the loaf reaches 160°F.

5. Remove the loaf pan from the roasting pan and let the sausage cool completely in the pan. Refrigerate for 1 to 2 days, or until loaf is set, before slicing. Serve chilled.

6. Store in an airtight container in the refrigerator for up to 6 days.

Per Serving:

Calories: 433   Fat: 36 g   Protein: 23 g   Carbs: 2 g

CARNIVORE

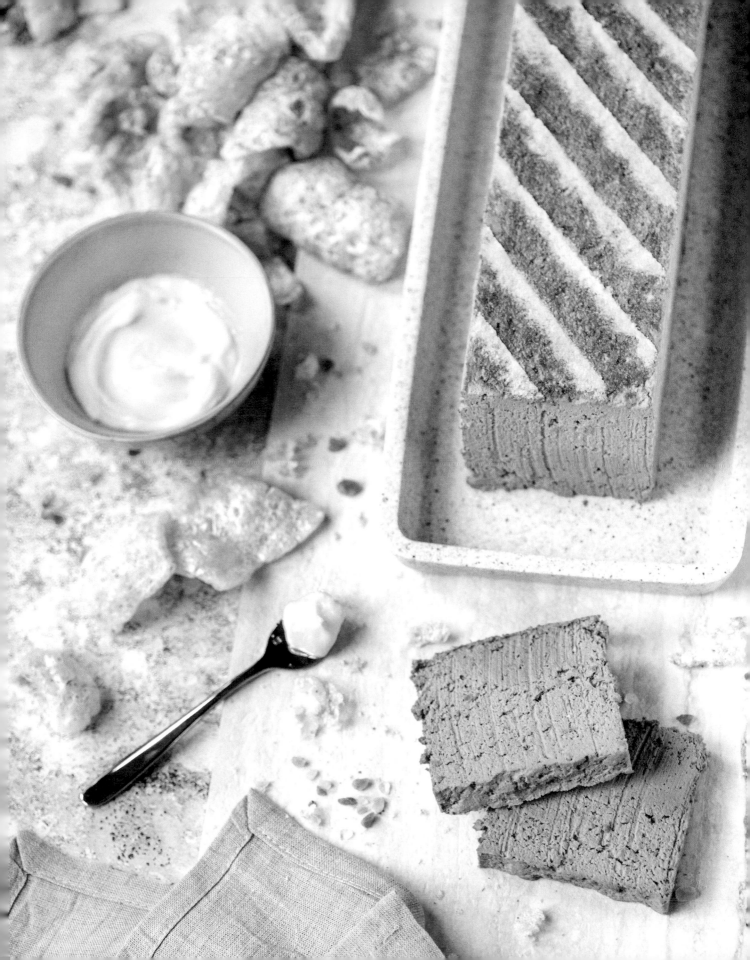

BEEF PEMMICAN

Yield: 8 servings
Prep Time: 5 minutes   **Cook Time:** 14 to 15 hours

Pemmican is a fantastic food to pack on long hiking trips when you have no access to refrigeration. I first discovered pemmican when I was a rock-climbing guide. We used to joke about the French Voyageurs from many years ago who would trade furs and goods in that area and eat pemmican that they stored in their "tukes" (hats).

1 (2-pound) boneless beef roast, cut into thin strips

1 tablespoon fine sea salt

1⅓ cups tallow (page 312), melted

1. Preheat the oven or dehydrator to 250°F.

2. Lay the strips of beef on 2 rimmed baking sheets or in the dehydrator basket. Season with the salt.

3. Bake for 14 to 15 hours, or until the beef is crispy and completely dehydrated.

4. Place the dehydrated beef in a blender or food processor and pulse until finely chopped. Add the tallow and pulse until well combined.

5. Remove the meat mixture from the blender and roll into eight 1½-inch balls.

6. Wrap the balls in parchment paper and store on the counter or in the pantry. The pemmican will keep for up to 3 weeks since the beef is completely dehydrated, or it can be stored in an airtight container in the freezer for up to 3 months.

Per Serving:

Calories: 651   Fat: 57 g   Protein: 29 g   Carbs: 0 g

1 — 2 — 3
CARNIVORE

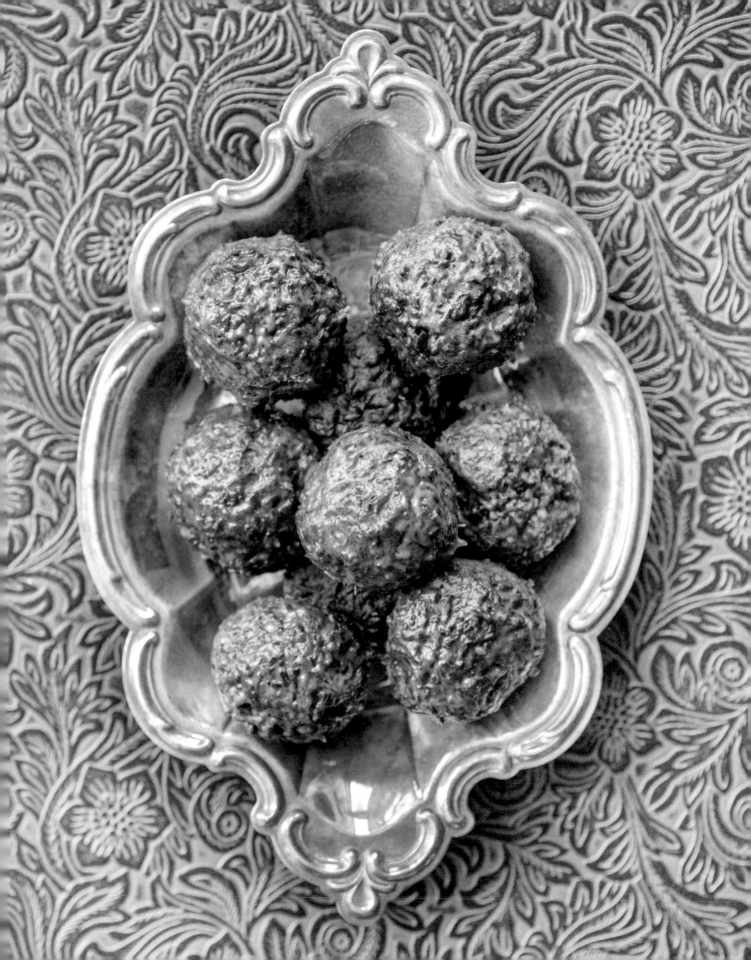

HEAD CHEESE

Yield: 12 servings
Prep Time: 3 minutes, plus time to chill overnight   **Cook Time:** 29 hours

Head cheese is delicious, and it is usually made with meaty bits of the head. I use ham hocks and veal shanks in this recipe because it is often hard to find quality sources of head.

6 fresh ham hocks

2 pounds veal shanks

2 teaspoons fine sea salt

¼ cup Carnivore Beef Bone Broth (page 308)

Special Equipment:
4 mini loaf pans

1. Place the ham hocks, veal shanks, and salt in a large, deep pot and cover entirely with water. Bring to a boil over medium-high heat, then reduce the heat to a low simmer. Simmer for 5 hours, or until the meat is fork-tender. Rearrange the meat every 30 to 45 minutes so it doesn't stick to the bottom of the pot. Add more boiling water if needed to keep the meat submerged.

2. Remove the meat from the pot and place on a rimmed baking sheet to cool. Strain the cooking liquid into another medium pot to remove any small bones.

3. Line the mini loaf pans with parchment paper.

4. Once the ham hocks and veal shanks are cool, remove the meat from the bones and cut the meat, skin, and soft gristle into tiny pieces. Add the pieces to the strained cooking liquid in the pot. Bring to a boil over medium-high heat, then reduce the heat to a very low simmer. Taste and add more salt, if needed. Simmer until the mixture has the consistency of Jell-O, 18 to 24 hours. Test the mixture occasionally to see if it will set by pouring a small amount into a bowl and placing it in the freezer for 20 to 30 minutes. Add the broth and remove the pot from the heat.

5. Spoon the mixture evenly into the lined mini loaf pans, filling the pans no more than three-quarters full. Allow to set at room temperature for 30 minutes or until cool, then refrigerate overnight.

6. Unmold the loaves onto parchment paper and double-wrap each loaf in aluminum foil. Refrigerate until ready to serve. Just before serving, cut each loaf into 12 slices.

7. Store in an airtight container in the refrigerator for up to 4 days.

Per Serving:

Calories: 183   Fat: 9 g   Protein: 23 g   Carbs: 0 g

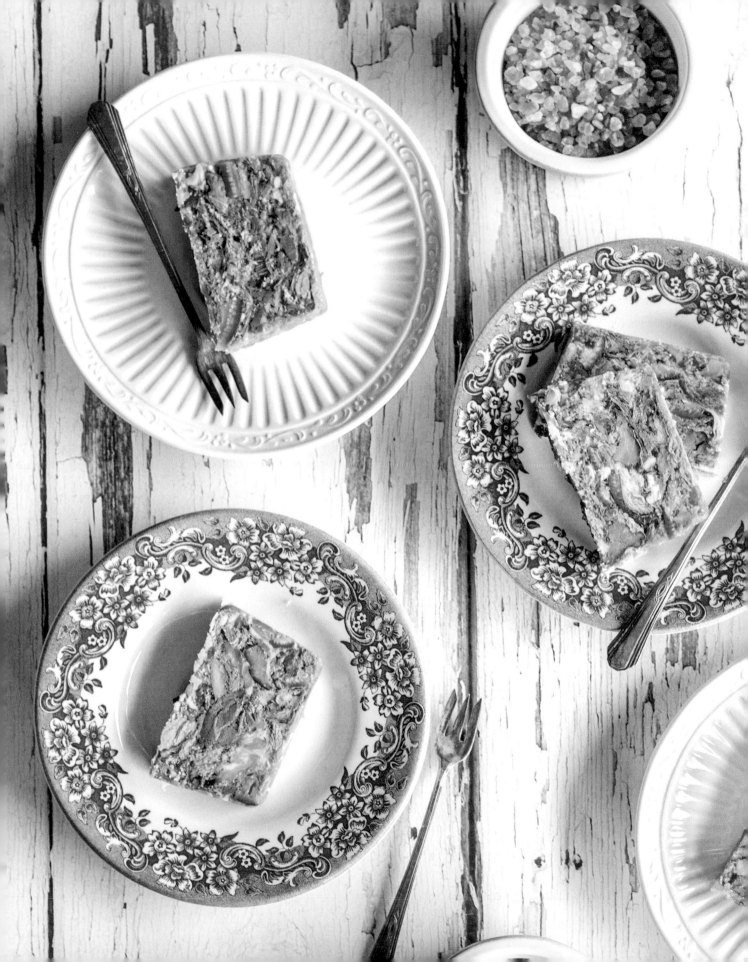

BACON BURGER LOVER'S DEVILED EGGS

Yield: 12 servings
Prep Time: 5 minutes   **Cook Time:** 15 minutes

I make these deviled eggs often for our family adventures and store them in my backpacking cooler. The fish sauce is optional, but it gives the eggs an extra boost of umami.

12 large eggs

4 slices pork or beef bacon, finely diced

4 ounces ground beef

½ cup Bacon Mayonnaise (page 318)

1 teaspoon fish sauce (optional)

1 teaspoon fine sea salt

1. Place the eggs in a large saucepan and cover with cold water. Bring to a boil over medium-high heat, then cover the pan and remove it from the heat. Allow the eggs to cook in the hot water for 11 minutes.

2. Meanwhile, cook the bacon. Heat a cast-iron skillet over high heat. Place the diced bacon in the hot skillet and cook, stirring often with a wooden spoon, for 4 minutes, or until cooked to your liking. Remove the bacon from the skillet, leaving the drippings in the pan, and place the bacon on a paper towel–lined plate to drain.

3. Place the ground beef in the skillet with the bacon drippings and cook over medium heat, crumbling the meat with a wooden spoon to break up the clumps, until the beef is browned and cooked through, 3 to 4 minutes. Remove the pan from the heat and set aside.

4. After the eggs have cooked, drain the water and rinse the eggs under very cold running water for a minute or two to stop the cooking. Peel the boiled eggs and cut them in half lengthwise.

5. Carefully remove the egg yolks and place them in a medium bowl. Mash the yolks with a fork until they have the texture of very fine crumbles. Add the mayonnaise, fish sauce (if using), and salt and mix with the fork until evenly combined. Add the cooked beef and stir gently to combine.

6. Fill the egg white halves with the yolk mixture. Garnish with the bacon and serve.

7. Store in an airtight container in the refrigerator for up to 3 days.

Per Serving:

Calories: 178   Fat: 15 g   Protein: 9 g   Carbs: 0.4 g

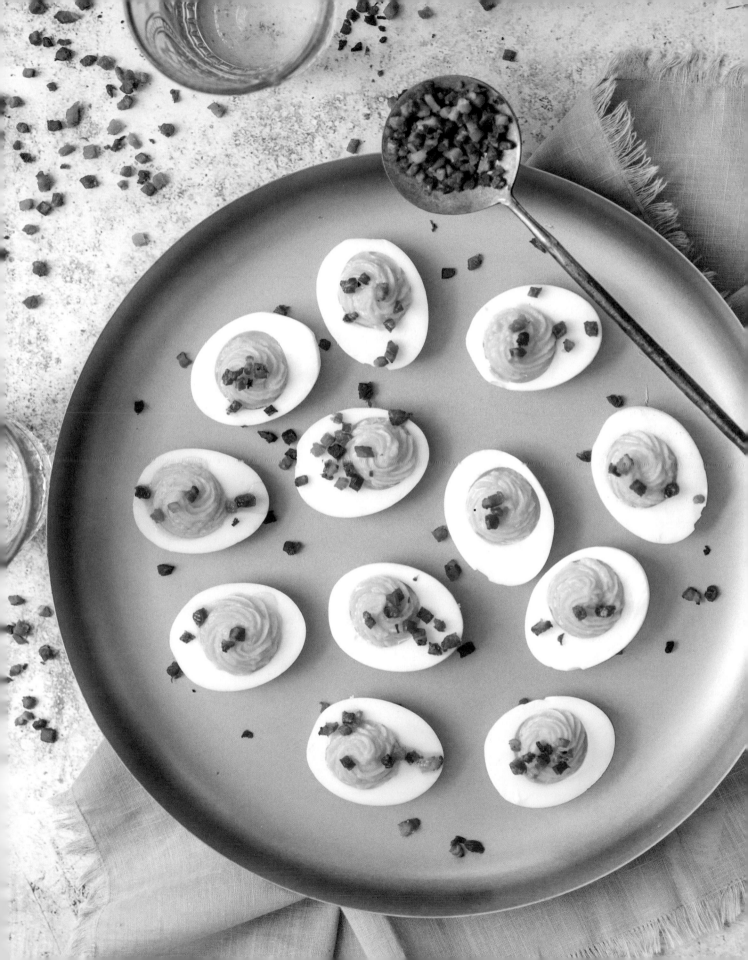

BONE MARROW

Yield: 2 servings
Prep Time: 3 minutes   **Cook Time:** 25 minutes

I know this dish may sound a little crazy, but let me list the reasons why you should consider bone marrow:

- *Marrow is made of osteoblasts, which form bone cells using minerals and are responsible for bone rebuilding.*

- *Marrow is also made of adipocytes (fat cells) and fibroblasts that form connective tissue.*

- *It is one of the only natural sources of vitamin K. Unlike K1, which is a blood clotter, K2 has been shown to help reverse artery calcification, reverse Alzheimer's disease, and boost fertility. It also has anti-aging properties as well as many other healing properties.*

- *Bone marrow is one of the best and densest sources of fat-soluble vitamins.*

- *It's a great high-fat, moderate-protein source for a carnivore or keto diet.*

- *The taste and creaminess are incredible! You can enjoy it right from the bone, use it to top a burger or steak, or add it to scrambled eggs or roasted salmon. My boys love it on salmon.*

6 marrow bones

Fine sea salt (optional)

1. Preheat the oven to 450°F. Rinse, drain, and pat the bones dry.

2. Place the bones in a roasting pan. If they are cut lengthwise, place them cut side up. If they are cut crosswise, place them standing up.

3. Roast for 15 to 25 minutes, until the marrow in the center has puffed slightly and is warm. (The exact timing will depend on the diameter of the bones; if they are 2 inches in diameter, it will take closer to 15 minutes.) To test for doneness, insert a metal skewer into the center of a bone; there should be no resistance when it is inserted, and some of the marrow will start to drip out.

4. Season with salt, if desired. Eat immediately.

Per Serving:

Calories: 630   Fat: 67 g   Protein: 6 g   Carbs: 0 g

1 — 2 — 3
CARNIVORE

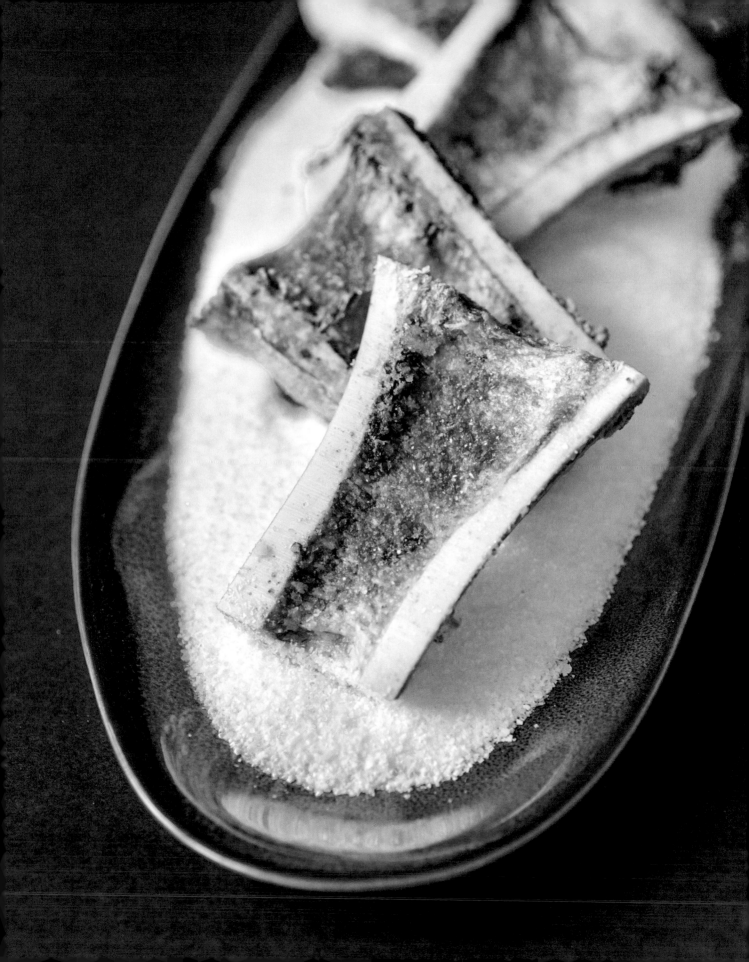

SMOKY CHICKEN SALAD

OPTION

Yield: 6 servings
Prep Time: 4 minutes, plus 2 hours to chill   **Cook Time:** 10 minutes

2 tablespoons lard or unsalted butter

1 pound boneless, skinless chicken thighs

1 teaspoon smoked sea salt, store-bought or homemade (page 310), divided

¾ cup Bacon Mayonnaise (page 318)

1. Heat the lard in a large cast-iron skillet over medium-high heat. Season the chicken on all sides with the salt. Once the lard is hot, add the chicken and cook for 5 minutes, then flip and cook for another 5 minutes, or until the chicken is cooked through and no longer pink inside. A meat thermometer inserted into the middle of a thigh should read 165°F. Remove the chicken from the skillet and let cool slightly.

2. Once the chicken is cool enough to handle, cut it into bite-sized pieces. Place the chicken in a large mixing bowl. Add the mayonnaise and toss to evenly coat. Refrigerate for 2 hours to allow the flavors to meld.

3. Serve chilled. Store in an airtight container in the refrigerator for up to 4 days.

Per Serving:

Calories: 350   Fat: 29 g   Protein: 21 g   Carbs: 0 g

2
1 / 3
CARNIVORE

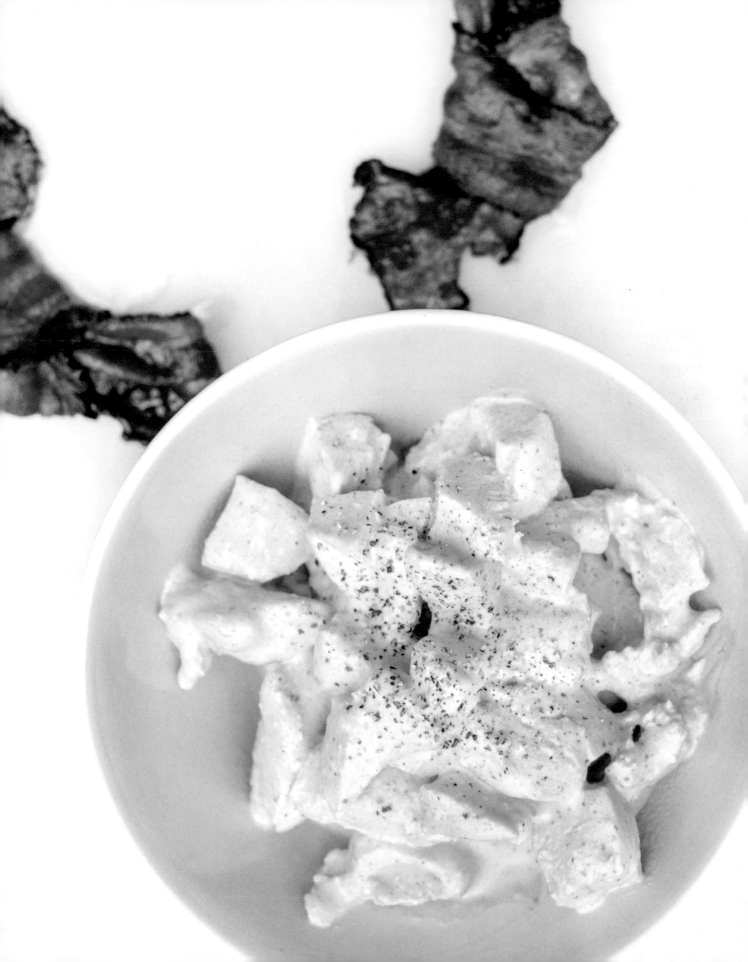

TUNA SALAD

Yield: 6 servings
Prep Time: 4 minutes, plus 2 hours to chill   **Cook Time:** —

This tuna salad tastes great with pork rinds or Bacon Knots (page 110).

4 (5-ounce) cans tuna, drained (we prefer Wild Planet brand)

¾ cup Bacon Mayonnaise (page 318)

½ teaspoon fine sea salt

1. Place the drained tuna in a large mixing bowl. Add the mayonnaise and toss to evenly coat. Season with the salt. Refrigerate for 2 hours to allow the flavors to meld.

2. Serve chilled. Store in an airtight container in the refrigerator for up to 4 days.

Per Serving:

Calories: 290   Fat: 21 g   Protein: 24 g   Carbs: 0 g

2
1   3
CARNIVORE

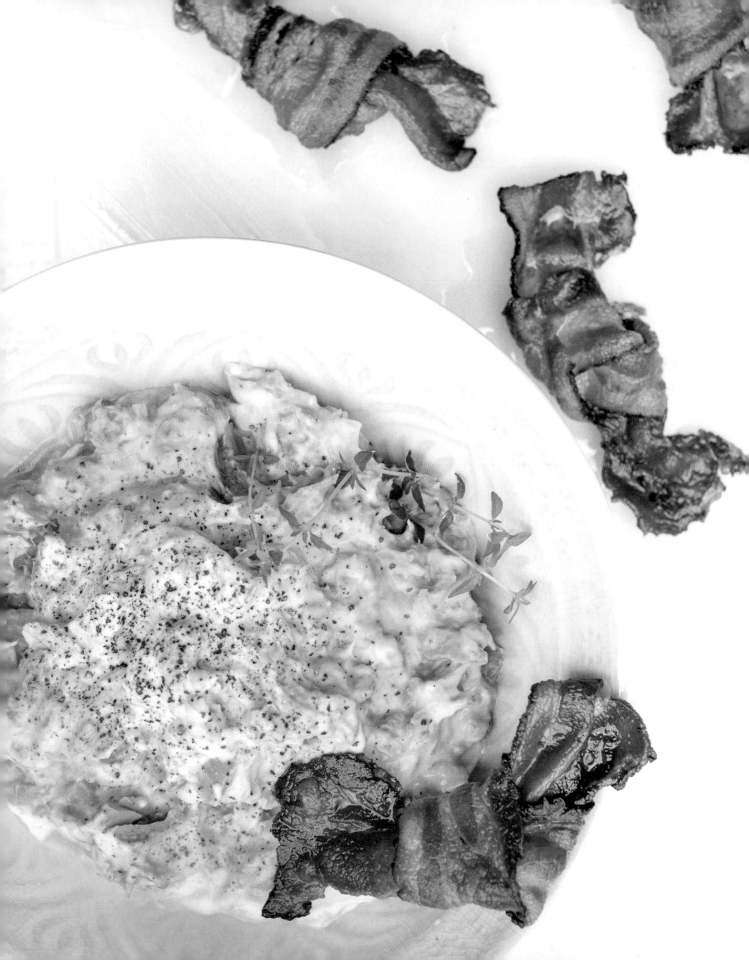

SMOKY SALMON SALAD

Yield: 6 servings
Prep Time: 4 minutes, plus 2 hours to chill   **Cook Time:** —

Try serving this salmon salad on with Bacon Knots (page 110).

4 (5-ounce) cans salmon, drained

¾ cup Bacon Mayonnaise (page 318)

½ teaspoon smoked sea salt, store-bought or homemade (page 310)

1. Place the drained salmon in a large mixing bowl. Add the mayonnaise and toss to evenly coat. Season with the salt. Refrigerate for 2 hours to allow the flavors to meld.

2. Serve chilled. Store in an airtight container in the refrigerator for up to 4 days.

Per Serving:

Calories: 330   Fat: 27 g   Protein: 23 g   Carbs: 0 g

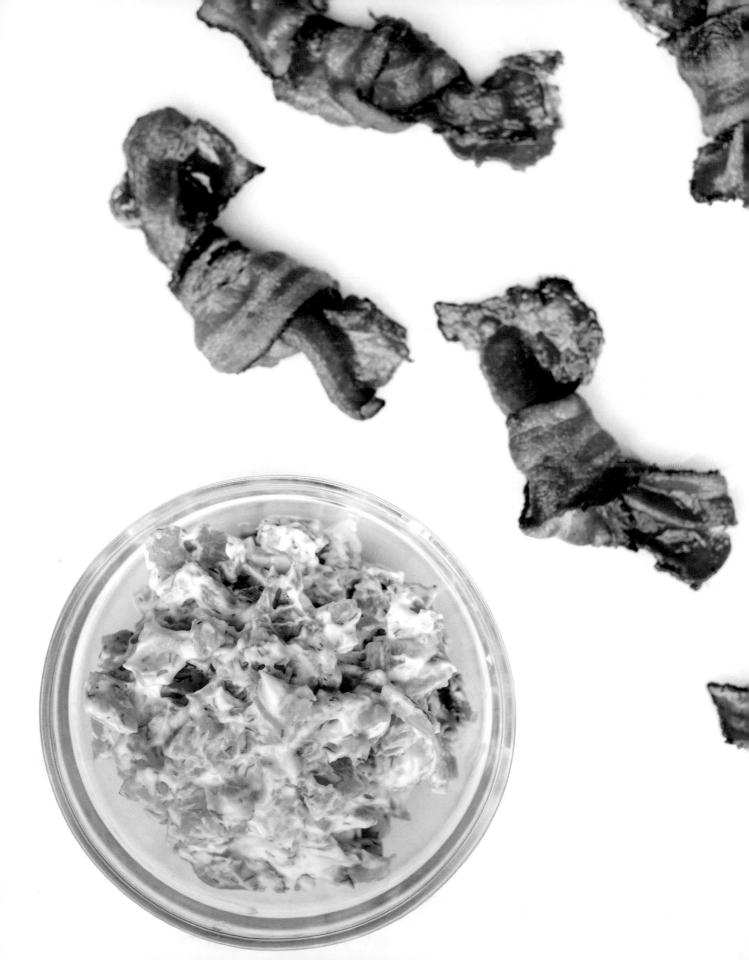

EGG SALAD

Yield: 4 servings
Prep Time: 5 minutes, plus 2 hours to chill   **Cook Time:** 11 minutes

8 large eggs

½ cup Bacon Mayonnaise (page 318)

¼ teaspoon fish sauce

½ teaspoon fine sea salt

1. Place the eggs in a medium saucepan and cover with cold water. Bring to a boil over medium-high heat, then immediately cover the pan and remove from the heat. Allow the eggs to cook in the hot water for 11 minutes.

2. Drain the water and rinse the eggs under very cold running water for a minute or two to stop the cooking. Peel and chop the eggs.

3. Place the chopped eggs, mayonnaise, fish sauce, and salt in a large bowl. Mash well with a fork or wooden spoon. Refrigerate for 2 hours to allow the flavors to meld.

4. Serve chilled. Store in an airtight container in the refrigerator for up to 4 days.

Per Serving:

Calories: 328   Fat: 30 g   Protein: 13 g   Carbs: 1 g

2
1 ◢◣ 3
CARNIVORE

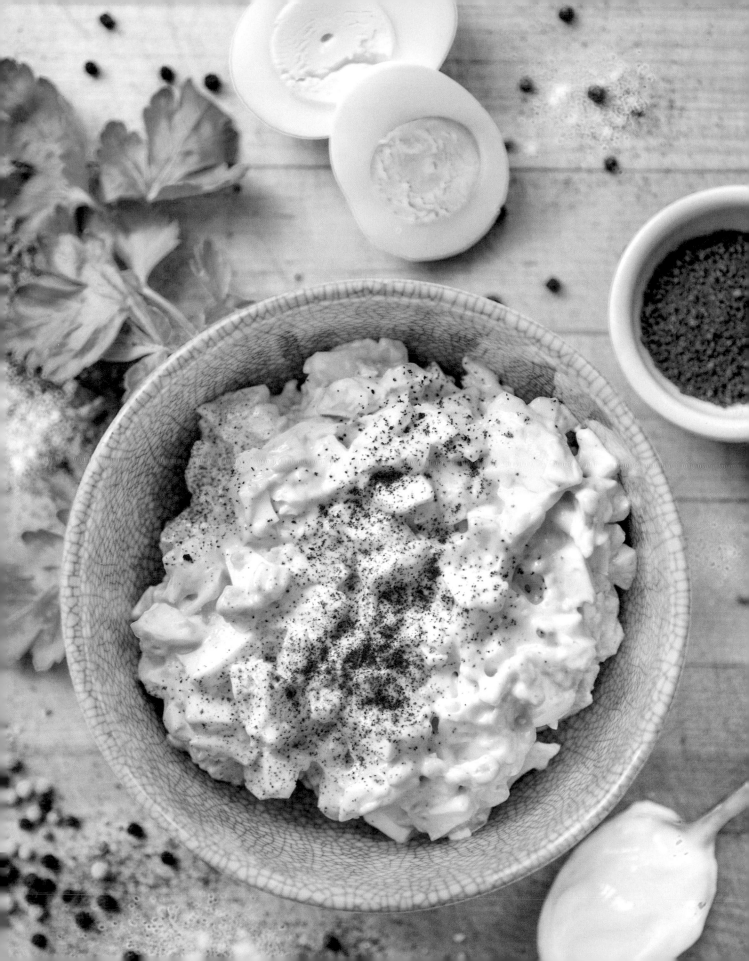

HAM SALAD

Yield: 4 servings
Prep Time: 5 minutes, plus 2 hours to chill   **Cook Time:** —

8 ounces fully cooked ham, roughly chopped

½ cup Bacon Mayonnaise (page 318)

½ teaspoon fine sea salt

1. Place the chopped ham in a food processor and pulse until you have very small pieces.

2. Transfer the ham to a large bowl and add the mayonnaise and salt. Mash well with a fork or wooden spoon. Refrigerate for 2 hours to allow the flavors to meld.

3. Serve chilled. Store in an airtight container in the refrigerator for up to 4 days.

Per Serving:

Calories: 343   Fat: 32 g   Protein: 12 g   Carbs: 0 g

1 2 3
CARNIVORE

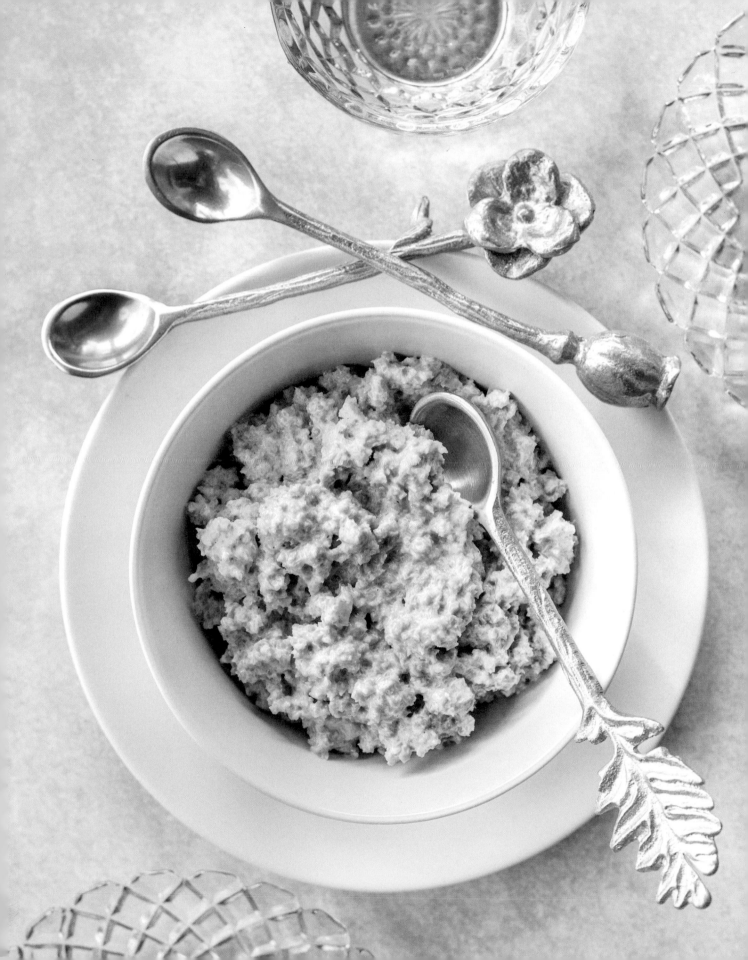

CHICKEN IN ASPIC

Yield: 12 servings
Prep Time: 7 minutes, plus at least 8 hours to chill   **Cook Time:** 1½ hours

Aspic is a delicious dish made with gelatin and meat, like a savory Jell-O. It is a true carnivore's dessert!

1 whole free-range chicken

1 tablespoon fine sea salt

3 tablespoons unflavored grass-fed gelatin

½ cup cold water

Special Equipment:
9-inch silicone Bundt mold

1. Place the chicken in a large stockpot and cover with water. Add the salt. Bring to a boil over medium-high heat, then reduce the heat to low. Simmer, uncovered, for 1½ hours. Skim the fat and foam that have risen to the surface.

2. Once the chicken is cooked through and no longer pink inside, carefully remove the chicken from the pot and place it on a cutting board. Allow to cool. Reserve the stock in the pot.

3. Once the chicken is cool enough to handle, remove the skin and bones. Use your hands to shred the meat. Place the shredded chicken in a 9-inch silicone Bundt mold.

4. Measure out 6 cups of stock from the pot and strain it into a large bowl. In a small bowl, whisk together the gelatin and cold water until the gelatin is dissolved. Then add the gelatin mixture to the stock and stir to combine.

5. Pour the stock mixture over the shredded chicken in the mold and place in the fridge overnight or for at least 8 hours, until the gelatin is set. Remove from the mold onto a decorative platter and serve.

6. Store in an airtight container in the refrigerator for up to 4 days.

Per Serving:

Calories: 281   Fat: 11 g   Protein: 43 g   Carbs: 0 g

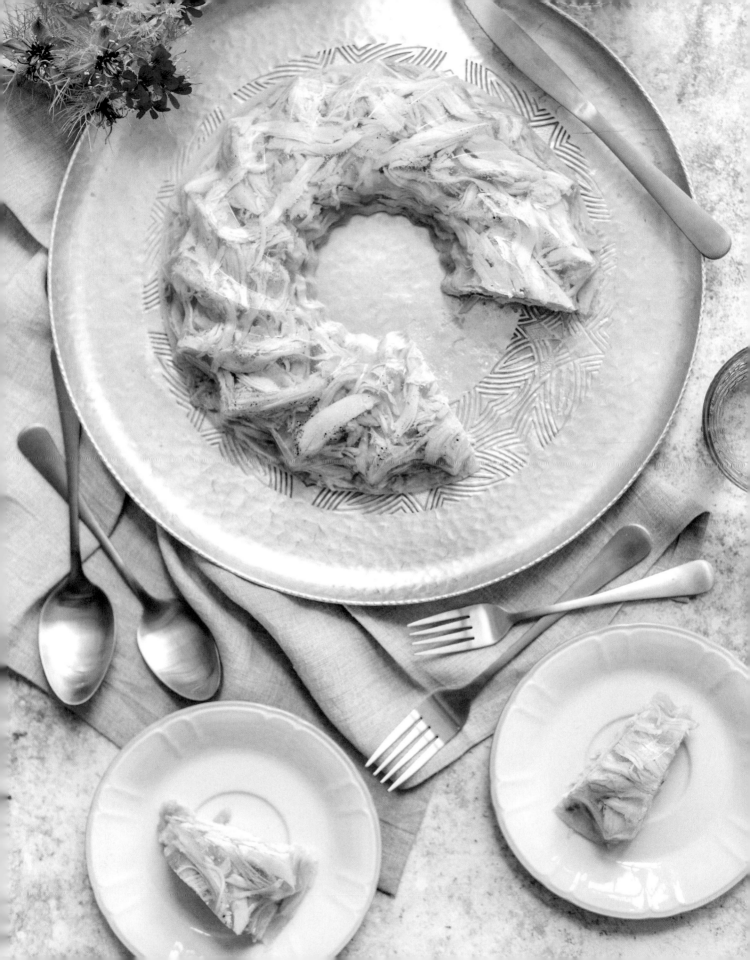

CHITTERLINGS

Yield: 12 servings
Prep Time: 15 minutes   **Cook Time:** 3 hours

Chitterlings, which are made from pig intestines, are a common Southern delicacy. The smell is intense and often turns people off, so it is important to make sure the chitterlings are really clean. You have to go through each piece to pick off anything that doesn't belong (if you know what I mean)—it doesn't matter that the bucket says they're already cleaned. Chitterlings can be hard to find in some areas, but your butcher can help.

5 pounds frozen cleaned chitterlings, thawed

6 cups cold water

2 teaspoons fine sea salt

1. Run the chitterlings under cold water to clean well, leaving the fat on. Soak in a very large pot filled with clean water for 5 minutes. If the water still has residue, soak the chitterlings a second time, replacing the water. Look through the chitterlings and pick off and discard any foreign materials.

2. Place the chitterlings in a large stockpot and add the cold water. Bring to a boil over medium-high heat; don't add the salt before the water boils or the chitterlings will get tough.

3. Reduce the heat to low, then season with the salt. Simmer for 3 hours, or longer if you prefer more tender chitterlings.

4. Use a slotted spoon to remove the chitterlings from the pot. Serve warm. Store in an airtight container in the refrigerator for up to 4 days. To reheat, place in a greased cast-iron skillet over medium-high heat for 1 minute, or until heated through.

Per Serving:

Calories: 430   Fat: 38 g   Protein: 23 g   Carbs: 0 g

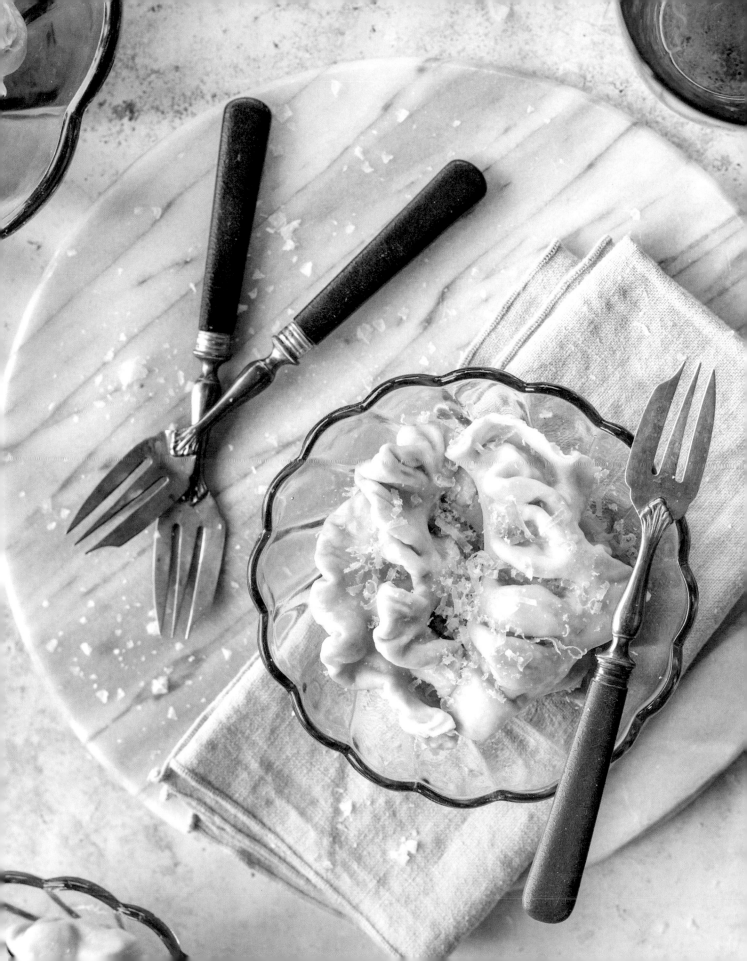

CHICKEN WINGS

Yield: 4 servings
Prep Time: 7 minutes   **Cook Time:** 32 minutes

1 pound chicken wings or drummies

1 teaspoon fine sea salt

1. Preheat the oven or an air fryer to 350°F. If using the oven, line a rimmed baking sheet with parchment paper.

2. Season the chicken wings on all sides with the salt. Place the wings on the lined baking sheet or in the air fryer basket in a single layer.

3. Cook for 25 minutes, flipping the wings over after 15 minutes.

4. After 25 minutes, increase the oven or air fryer temperature to 400°F and cook for 6 to 7 more minutes, or until the skin is browned and crisp.

5. Store in an airtight container in the refrigerator for up to 4 days. To reheat, place the wings in a preheated 350°F oven or air fryer for 5 minutes, then increase the temperature to 400°F and cook for 3 to 5 more minutes, or until warm to your liking and crispy.

Per Serving:

Calories: 325   Fat: 22 g   Protein: 30 g   Carbs: 0 g

1 2 3
CARNIVORE

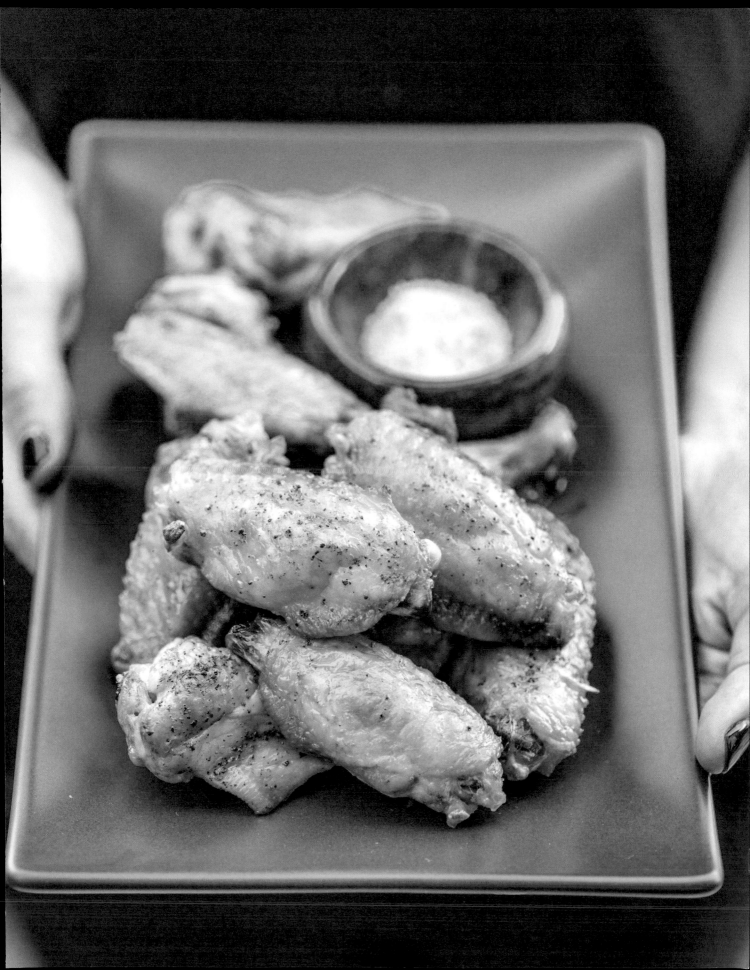

FRIED GOAT CHEESE RAVIOLI

Yield: 6 servings
Prep Time: 10 minutes   **Cook Time:** 10 minutes

Eat ravioli while carnivore? Yes, you can! These meaty raviolis are very tasty. The prosciutto adds a lot of saltiness, so there's no need to add extra salt.

12 thin slices prosciutto

10 ounces soft goat cheese

2 tablespoons lard or tallow (page 312)

1. To assemble the ravioli, lay a slice of prosciutto on a sheet of parchment paper so that a short end is facing you. Lay another slice across the center so you make a Greek cross with four "arms" to wrap around the filling.

2. Spoon about 1 heaping tablespoon of goat cheese into the center of the prosciutto cross. Fold one arm of the prosciutto over the filling. Continue folding the arms over the filling to form a square, making sure that the filling is covered well. Using your fingers, press down on the filling to evenly spread it into a square shape. Repeat with the remaining prosciutto and goat cheese to make 5 more ravioli.

3. Heat the lard in a cast-iron skillet over medium-high heat. Once hot, place the ravioli in the fat to cook for 3 minutes, or until the prosciutto is crispy, then turn them over and cook for another 2 minutes, or until crispy on the other side. Remove and place on a serving platter.

4. Store in an airtight container in the refrigerator for up to 4 days. To reheat, place the ravioli in a greased cast-iron skillet over medium-high heat for 1 minute per side, or until heated through.

Per Serving:

Calories: 236   Fat: 19 g   Protein: 18 g   Carbs: 2 g

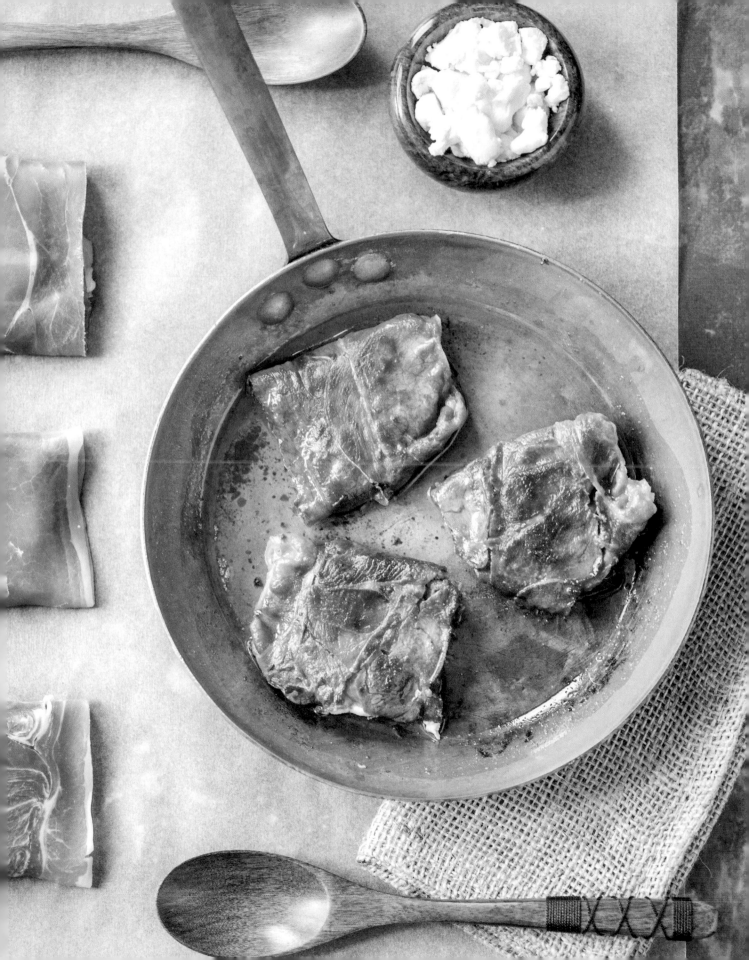

BACON-WRAPPED CHICKEN NUGGETS

Yield: 4 servings (6 nuggets per serving)
Prep Time: 8 minutes   **Cook Time:** 9 minutes

2 boneless, skinless chicken thighs, or 1 boneless, skinless chicken breast half (about 8 ounces), cut into 1-inch pieces

12 thin slices pork or beef bacon, cut in half crosswise

Ranch dressing, for dipping (optional)

1. Preheat the oven or an air fryer to 400°F. If using the oven, line a rimmed baking sheet with parchment paper. Set aside.

2. Cut the chicken into twenty-four 1-inch pieces. Wrap a piece of bacon around each piece of chicken and secure the ends of the bacon with a toothpick. Place on the lined baking sheet or in the air fryer basket in a single layer.

3. Cook for 7 to 9 minutes, flipping after 4 minutes, until the bacon is slightly crispy and the chicken is cooked through.

4. Serve with ranch dressing for dipping, if desired. Best served immediately.

Per Serving (without ranch dressing):

Calories: 270   Fat: 18 g   Protein: 25 g   Carbs: 0 g

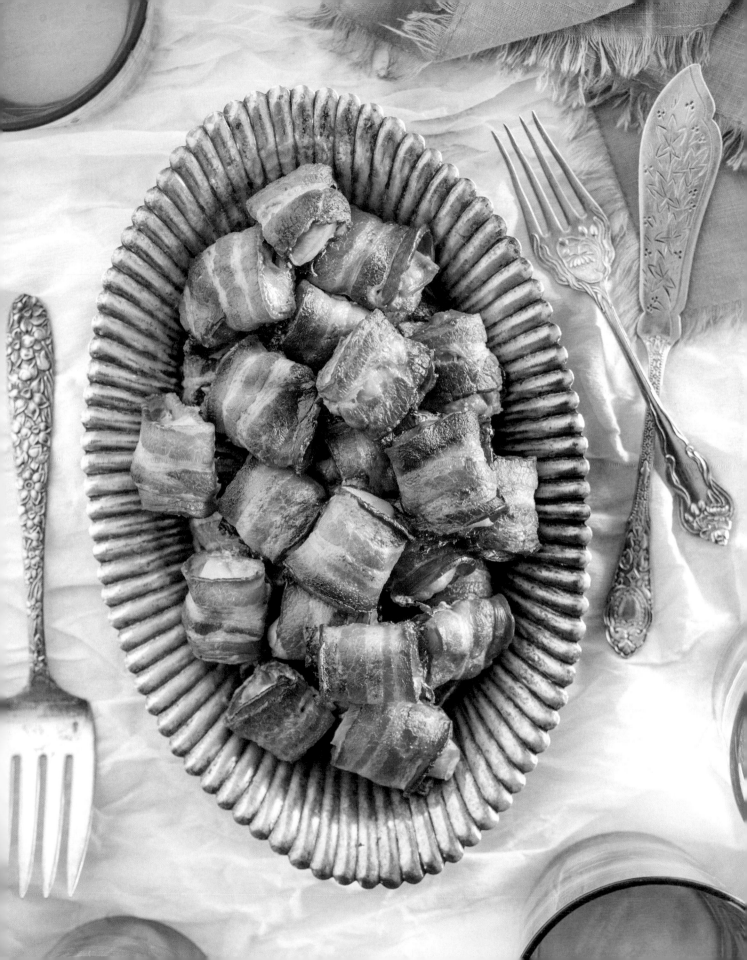

CARNIVORE MOZZARELLA STICKS

Yield: 8 sticks (1 per serving)
Prep Time: 8 minutes   **Cook Time:** 8 minutes

My boys love these meaty mozzarella sticks. They are a perfect finger food!

1 pound ground beef

1 teaspoon fine sea salt

8 mozzarella string cheese

8 thin slices pork or beef bacon

1. Preheat the oven or an air fryer to 400°F. If using the oven, line a rimmed baking sheet with parchment paper.

2. Place the ground beef in a large bowl and season with the salt. Use your hands to combine well. Divide the beef into 8 equal portions and form each portion into a ¼-inch-thick rectangle, about 3½ inches by 2 inches.

3. Place one string cheese in the center of a patty. Use your fingers to seal the patty around the cheese; be sure to seal the edges well or the cheese will melt out. Repeat with the remaining patties and cheese. Wrap a slice of bacon around the entire patty, then secure the ends of the bacon with toothpicks. Repeat with the remaining patties and pieces of bacon.

4. Place the wrapped patties on the lined baking sheet or in the air fryer basket in a single layer and cook for about 8 minutes, flipping after 4 minutes, until the bacon is cooked to your liking.

5. Remove the mozzarella sticks from the oven or air fryer and let cool for a few minutes before consuming, or the melted cheese will burn your mouth.

6. Store in an airtight container in the refrigerator for up to 4 days. To reheat, place in a preheated 400°F oven or air fryer for about 3 minutes, or until heated through.

Per Serving:

Calories: 274   Fat: 20 g   Protein: 24 g   Carbs: 0 g

1 2 3
CARNIVORE

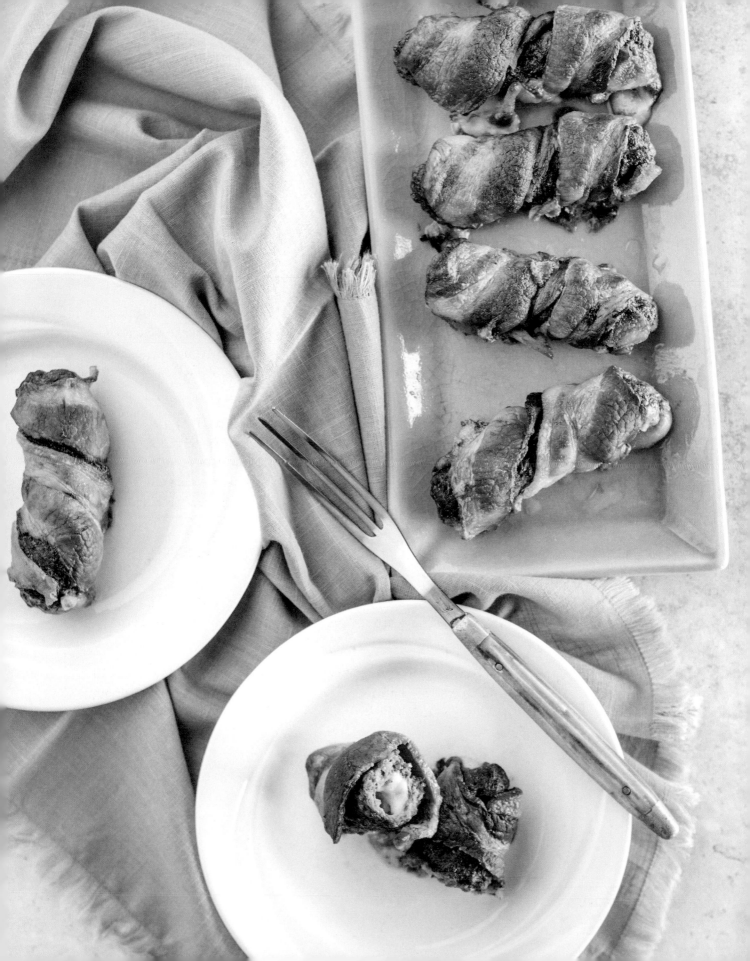

VENISON OR BEEF JERKY

Yield: 8 servings
Prep Time: 5 minutes, plus 1 hour to freeze   **Cook Time:** 6 to 8 hours

1 pound boneless venison or beef, preferably eye of round or rump roast

1 tablespoon smoked sea salt, store-bought or homemade (page 310)

1. Place the meat in the freezer for 1 hour to make it easier to slice cleanly. Slice the meat across the grain into long strips, 1 inch wide and ⅛ inch thick. Season the strips on all sides with the smoked salt.

2. Oven method: Preheat the oven to 160°F. Place a rimmed baking sheet on the bottom rack to catch drips. Arrange the strips of salted meat directly on the middle rack, not touching each other. Alternatively, place a wire rack on a rimmed baking sheet and arrange the strips of salted meat on the rack.

Dehydrator method: Place the strips of salted meat in a dehydrator, not touching each other, and set the dehydrator to low (170°F).

3. For both methods: Dehydrate the meat for 6 to 8 hours, or until the jerky dries to the desired chewiness. For a chewier jerky, dehydrate for less time.

4. Store in an airtight container in the refrigerator for up to 2 weeks or in the freezer for up to a month.

Per Serving:

Calories: 86   Fat: 1 g   Protein: 17 g   Carbs: 0 g

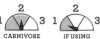

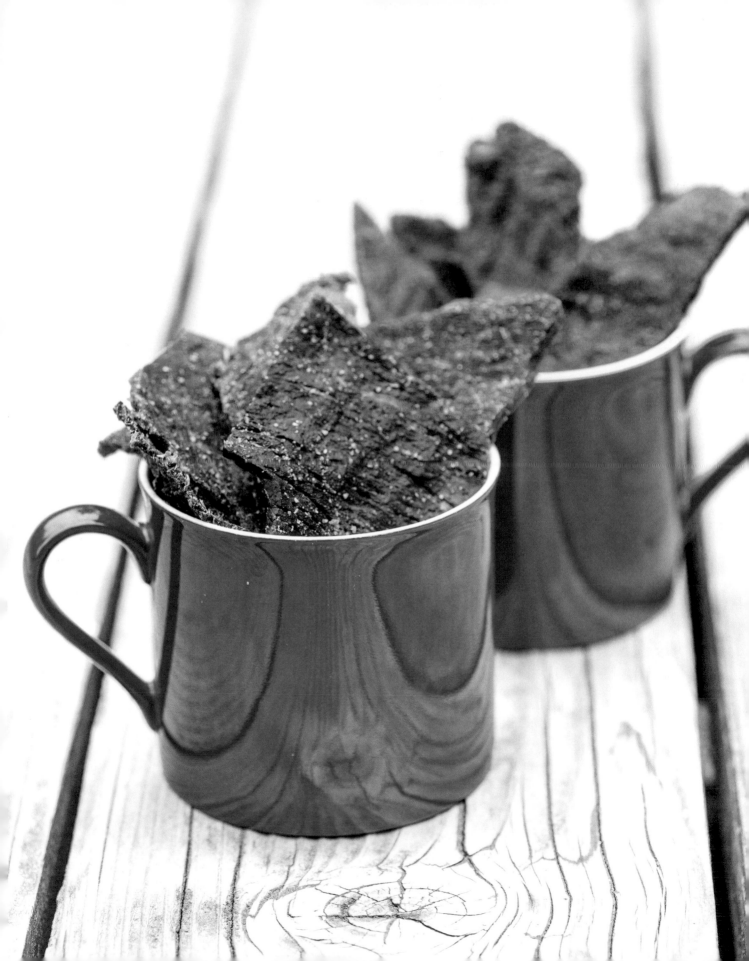

CARNIVORE GUMMIES

Yield: 12 servings
Prep Time: 5 minutes, plus 2 hours to chill   **Cook Time:** —

My boys love savory treats like these brothy gummies! They remind me of a savory Jell-O. You can easily scale this recipe up or down; just remember to use 1 tablespoon of gelatin for every 2 cups of broth.

1 tablespoon powdered grass-fed gelatin

2 cups Carnivore Bone Broth (page 308), beef or chicken version, warmed

Special Equipment:
4 silicone gummy molds (any shape)

1. Sprinkle the gelatin over the broth and whisk to combine.

2. Place the silicone mold on a rimmed baking sheet (for easy transport). Pour the broth into the mold. Place in the fridge until the gelatin is fully set, about 2 hours.

3. Release the gummies from the mold by gently pushing on the mold to pop them out. Store in an airtight container in the refrigerator for up to 5 days.

Per Serving:

Calories: 10   Fat: 0.2 g   Protein: 2 g   Carbs: 0 g

2
1 ⌇ 3   CARNIVORE
2
1 ⌇ 3   IF USING CHICKEN BROTH

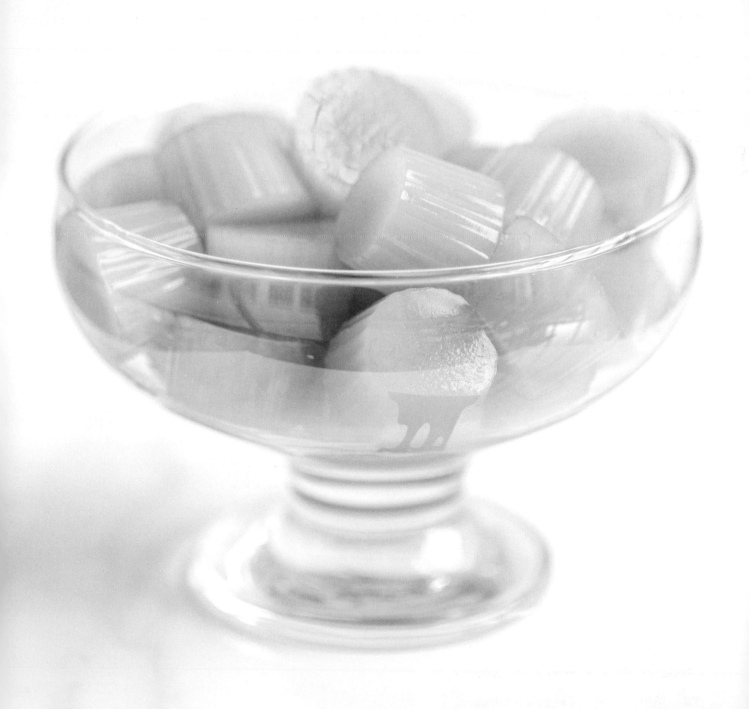

SAMOSAS

Yield: 6 servings
Prep Time: 10 minutes   **Cook Time:** 10 minutes

Samosas are typically a baked or fried pastry in a triangle shape with a savory filling. I think these carnivore samosas are even more delicious than traditional samosas. There's no need to salt the ground beef during cooking since the prosciutto adds enough salt.

2 tablespoons lard or tallow (page 312), divided

8 ounces ground beef

12 thin slices prosciutto

1. Heat 1 teaspoon of the lard in a cast-iron skillet over medium-high heat. Once hot, add the ground beef. Cook, crumbling the meat with a spatula to break up the clumps, for 5 minutes, or until no longer pink. Remove from the heat and set aside.

2. Assemble the samosas: Lay a slice of prosciutto on a sheet of parchment paper so that a short end is facing you. Lay another slice across the center of the prosciutto so you make a Greek cross with four "arms" to wrap around the filling.

3. Spoon about 1 heaping tablespoon of the ground beef into the center of the prosciutto cross. Fold one arm of the prosciutto over the filling. Continue folding the arms around the filling to form a square, making sure that the filling is covered well. Using your fingers, press down on the filling to evenly spread it into a square shape. Repeat with the remaining prosciutto and ground beef, making a total of 6 squares.

4. Heat the remaining lard in a cast-iron skillet over medium-high heat. Once hot, place the samosas in the fat to cook for 3 minutes, or until the prosciutto is crispy, then turn them over and cook for another 2 minutes, or until crispy on the other side. Remove and place on a serving platter. Cut in half diagonally to make triangles and serve.

5. Store in an airtight container in the refrigerator for up to 4 days. To reheat, place on a rimmed baking sheet in a 375°F oven for 1 minute per side, or until heated through.

Per Serving:

Calories: 237   Fat: 19 g   Protein: 16 g   Carbs: 0 g

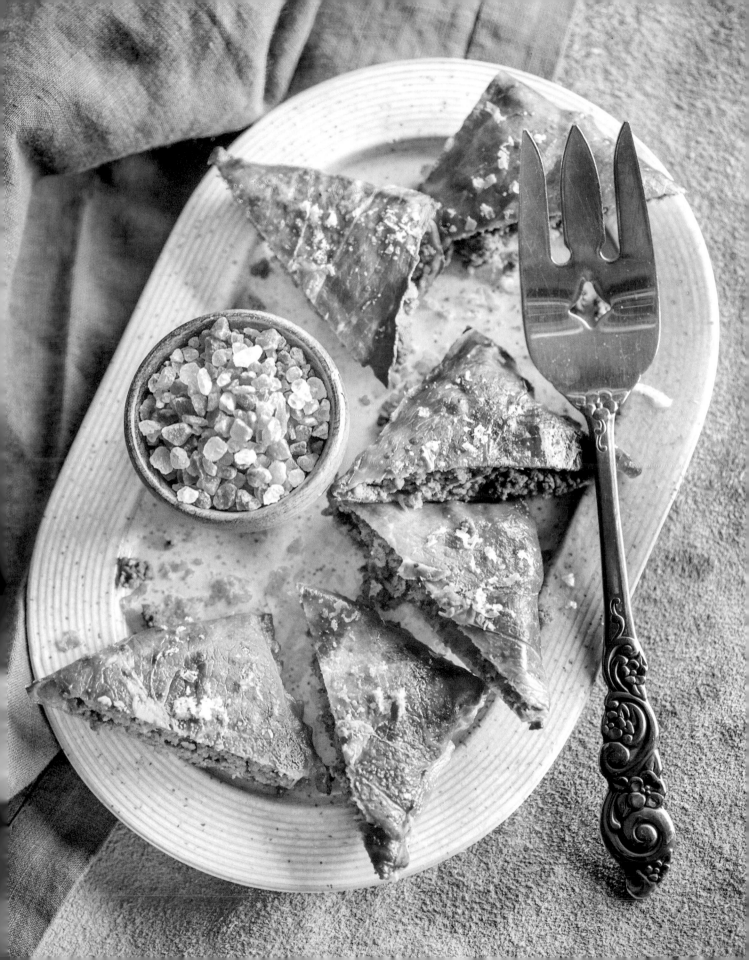

SMOKY CHICKEN PÂTÉ

Yield: 4 servings
Prep Time: 5 minutes, plus 2 hours to chill   **Cook Time:** 5 minutes

This creamy chicken pâté gets a delicious smoky flavor from the smoked salt.

½ cup plus 2 tablespoons bacon fat, duck fat, or tallow (page 312), divided

1 pound chicken livers, thinly sliced

1½ teaspoons smoked sea salt, store-bought or homemade (page 310), or fine sea salt

Pork rinds, for serving

1. Heat 2 tablespoons of the bacon fat in a large cast-iron skillet over medium-high heat. Once hot, add the sliced chicken livers and sauté for 5 minutes, or until the livers are cooked through.

2. Remove the livers from the skillet and place in a food processor with the remaining ½ cup of bacon fat and the smoked salt. Puree until smooth. Taste and adjust the seasoning to your liking. Place in the fridge to chill for at least 2 hours. Transfer to a serving dish and serve with pork rinds.

3. Store in an airtight container in the refrigerator for up to 4 days.

Per Serving:

Calories: 477   Fat: 39 g   Protein: 28 g   Carbs: 0 g

2
1 ◣ 3
CARNIVORE

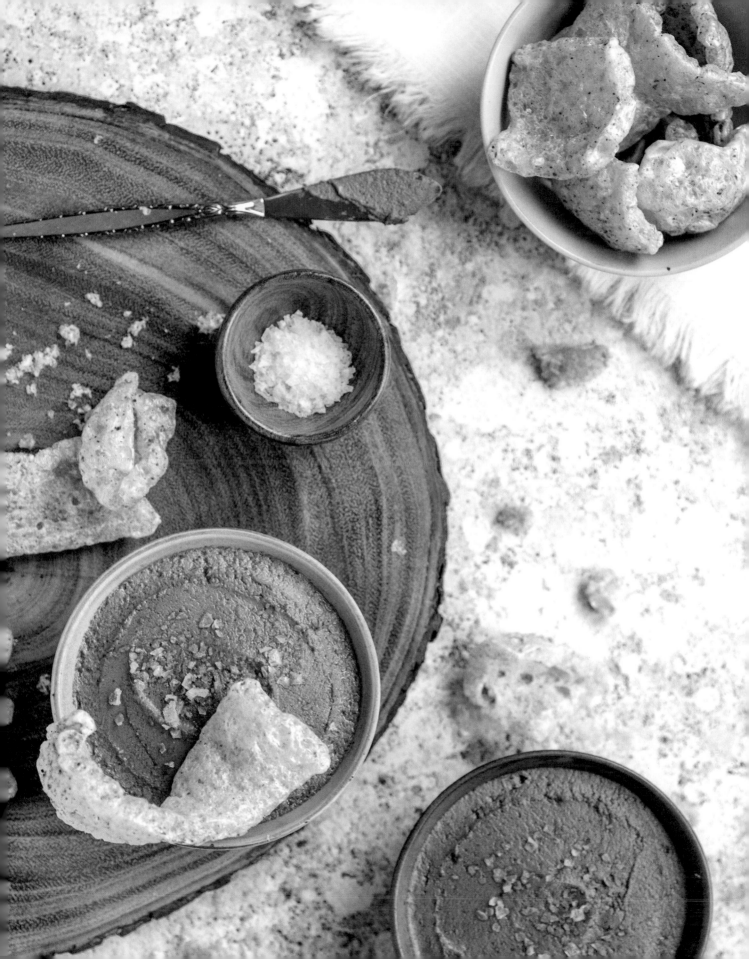

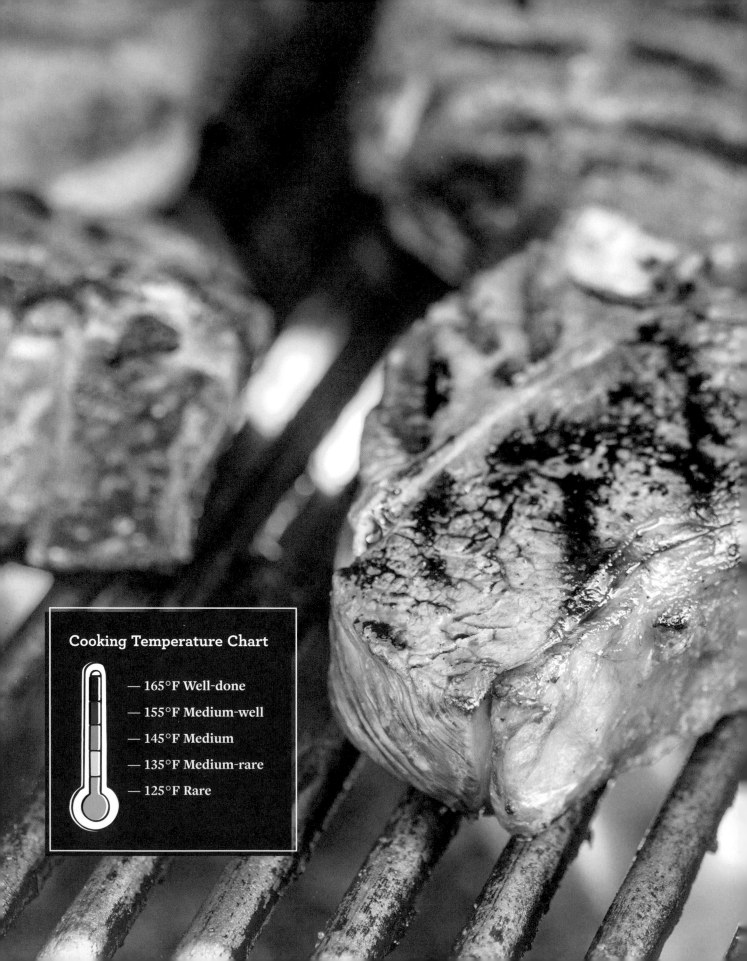

Cooking Temperature Chart

— 165°F Well-done

— 155°F Medium-well

— 145°F Medium

— 135°F Medium-rare

— 125°F Rare

BEEF & LAMB

REVERSE SEAR LONG-BONE

Yield: 2 servings   **Prep Time:** 7 minutes, plus 30 minutes to sit at room temperature   **Cook Time:** 47 minutes

The reverse sear method is particularly useful for extra thick cuts of steak. Baking at a lower temperature cooks the meat evenly so that you end up with a lovely pink color throughout the inside, and searing at the end gives you a nice crispy outside.

1 (1¼-pound) long-bone rib-eye steak, 2 inches thick

2 teaspoons fine sea salt

2 teaspoons lard or unsalted butter

1. Pat the steak dry with a paper towel and place on a rimmed baking sheet. Allow to sit at room temperature for 30 minutes to ensure even cooking.

2. Meanwhile, preheat the oven to 275°F.

3. Season the steak on all sides with the salt. Bake for 35 to 45 minutes, until the temperature in the thickest part of the steak reads 135°F to 140°F. Remove from the oven.

4. Heat the lard in a large cast-iron skillet over medium-high heat. Once hot, add the steak and sear for 1 minute, or until crispy and browned. Flip and cook for another minute to sear the other side. Remove from the skillet and serve.

Per Serving:

Calories: 911   Fat: 72 g   Protein: 70 g   Carbs: 0 g

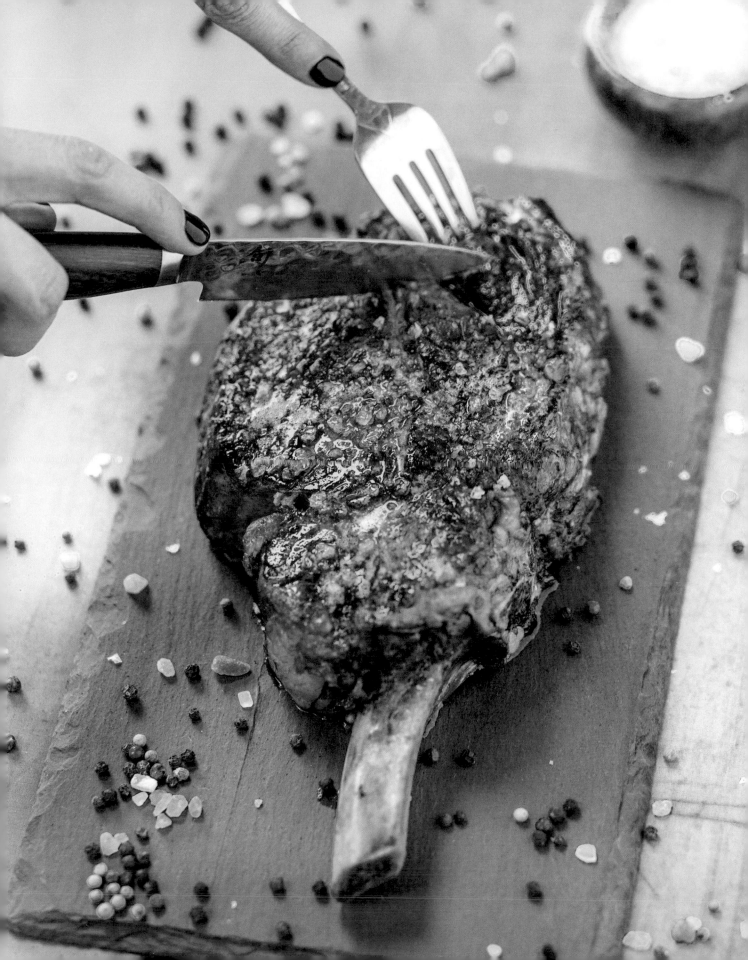

CARNIVORE SHABU SHABU

Yield: 4 servings
Prep Time: 5 minutes   **Cook Time:** less than 1 minute per slice

This is a fun dinner to eat with kids. To make this meal a communal activity, place the hot broth in the middle of the table. All you need is a way to keep the broth hot throughout the meal. There are specially designed Shabu Shabu pots for this purpose, but they are not required. I use a portable cast-iron pot that comes with its own flame burner/base, as shown in the photo. You could also set the saucepan of broth directly on a portable electric burner or use a fondue pot.

4 cups Carnivore Beef Bone Broth (page 308)

1 pound boneless beef chuck roast or rib-eye steak, very thinly sliced

2 teaspoons fine sea salt, divided

½ cup (1 stick) unsalted butter or ghee, melted, for dipping (optional)

Special Equipment:
Chopsticks

1. Bring the broth to a simmer in a medium saucepan over medium-low heat.

2. Meanwhile, lay the slices of beef on a platter. Season the slices with 1¾ teaspoons of the salt and set aside.

3. Place the melted butter in a serving dish. Season the butter with the remaining ¼ teaspoon of salt and set aside.

4. Use chopsticks to dip the slices of beef into the simmering broth, one slice at a time, for 10 seconds, or until cooked to your liking. Place the cooked beef on plates and serve with melted butter for dipping, if desired. Best served immediately.

Per Serving (with butter):

Calories: 587   Fat: 51 g   Protein: 30 g   Carbs: 0 g

CARNIVORE   WITHOUT BUTTER

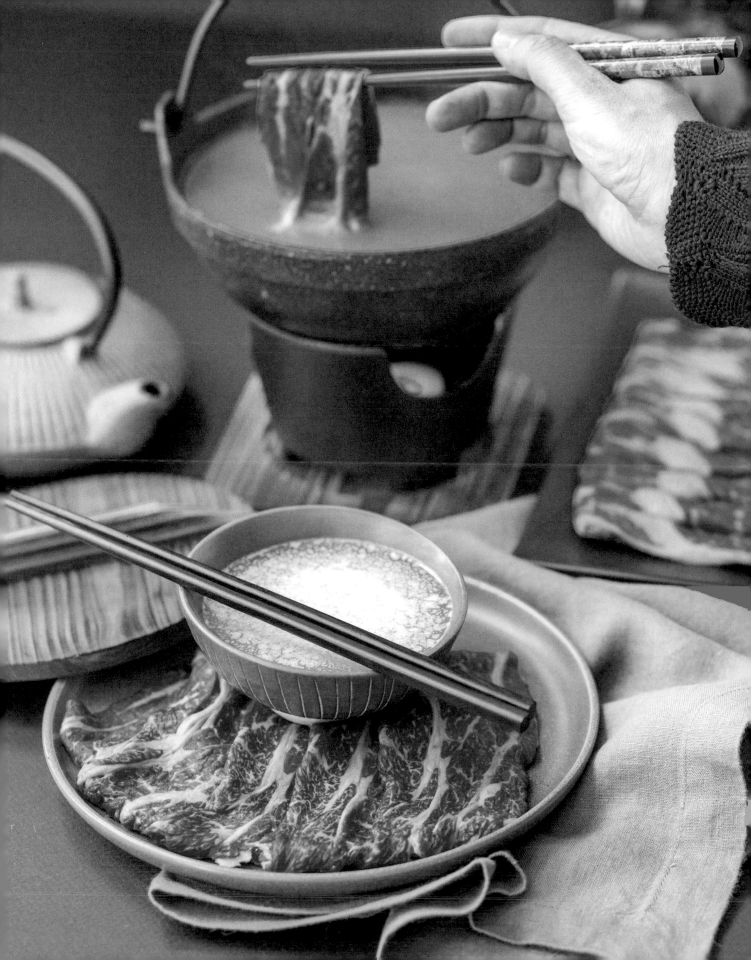

SALISBURY STEAK

Yield: 2 servings
Prep Time: 5 minutes   **Cook Time:** 6 minutes

I hadn't eaten Salisbury steak until I made this recipe. I never really knew what it was, and the name always made me think of a frozen TV dinner. Once I realized it was basically a large hamburger, I had to try it! You can easily double this recipe if you want to feed more people.

8 ounces ground beef

½ teaspoon fine sea salt

2 tablespoons lard

Blue cheese crumbles, ghee, unsalted butter, or Easy Carnivore Hollandaise (page 314), for serving (optional)

1. Place the ground beef and salt in a large bowl. Use your hands to mix until well combined. Form the meat mixture into 2 oval-shaped patties.

2. Heat the lard in a large cast-iron skillet over medium-high heat. Once hot, add the patties. Cook for 3 minutes, then gently flip and cook for another 3 minutes for medium doneness, or until cooked to your liking.

3. Remove the steaks from the skillet and serve with blue cheese crumbles, ghee, or hollandaise, if desired.

4. Store in an airtight container in the refrigerator for up to 4 days. To reheat, place on a lightly greased skillet over medium-high heat for 2 minutes per side, or until heated through.

Per Serving (without blue cheese):

Calories: 363   Fat: 30 g   Protein: 21 g   Carbs: 0 g

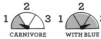

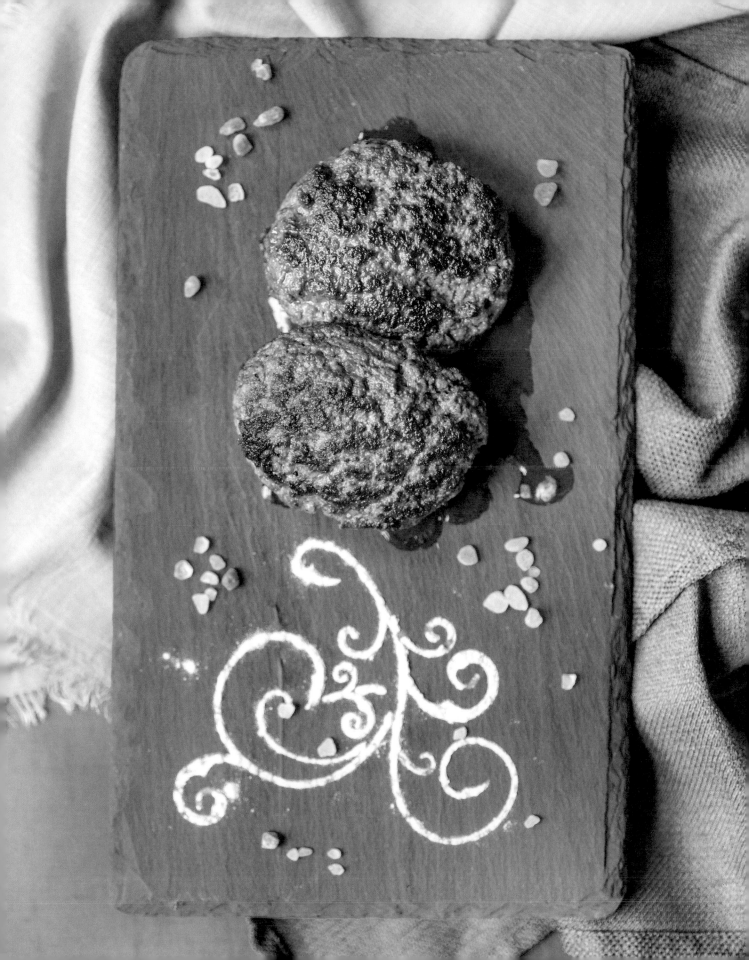

SLOW COOKER SHORT RIBS WITH BROWN BUTTER

Yield: 16 servings
Prep Time: 5 minutes   **Cook Time:** 7 to 8 hours

When served with brown butter, short ribs are extra delicious!

1 cup Carnivore Beef Bone Broth (page 308)

8 pounds bone-in beef short ribs

1 tablespoon fine sea salt

½ cup (1 stick) unsalted butter

1. Place the broth in a 6-quart slow cooker. Season the ribs on all sides with the salt and add to the slow cooker. Cover and cook on low for 7 to 8 hours, until the meat is tender and easily pulls away from the bone.

2. When the ribs are nearly done, make the brown butter: Melt the butter in a small saucepan over high heat. Whisk frequently until the butter froths up and then settles down with brown flecks. Keep whisking until the butter is dark brown (not black). Remove from the heat and set aside.

3. Remove the ribs from the slow cooker and place on a serving platter. Serve the ribs drizzled with the brown butter.

4. Store in an airtight container in the refrigerator for up to 4 days. To reheat, place on a rimmed baking sheet in a preheated 350°F oven for 7 minutes, or until heated through.

Per Serving:

Calories: 579   Fat: 53 g   Protein: 25 g   Carbs: 0 g

2
1 ➘ 3   CARNIVORE

2
1 ➘ 3   WITHOUT BUTTER

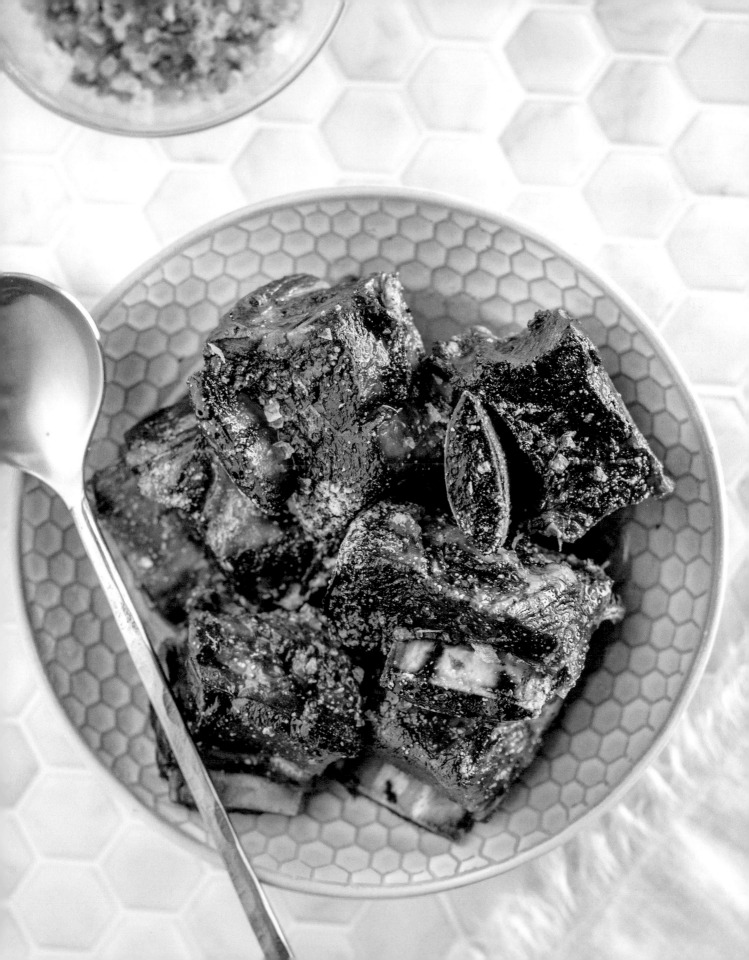

BRISKET

Yield: 8 servings   **Prep Time:** 4 minutes, plus 25 minutes to rest
Cook Time: 3½ to 4 hours

We usually smoke our brisket, but if you don't have a smoker, you don't need to feel left out. This recipe is not only simple but also gives the brisket an amazing smoky flavor.

1 (4-pound) brisket

2 tablespoons smoked sea salt, store-bought or homemade (page 310)

1½ cups Carnivore Beef Bone Broth (page 308)

1. Pat the brisket dry with a paper towel and place in a roasting pan that snugly fits the brisket. Allow the brisket to sit at room temperature for 10 to 15 minutes to ensure even cooking.

2. Meanwhile, preheat the oven to 350°F.

3. Season the brisket on all sides with the smoked salt. Use your hands to rub the salt into the meat. Cook, uncovered, for 1 hour.

4. Remove the brisket from the oven and pour the broth into the pan. Lower the oven temperature to 300°F, cover the pan, and cook for another 2½ hours to 3 hours, until the meat is fork-tender.

5. Remove the brisket from the pan and allow to rest for 10 minutes. Cut the brisket across the grain into ⅛-inch slices and serve.

6. Store in an airtight container in the refrigerator for up to 3 days. To reheat, place slices on a rimmed baking sheet in a preheated 350°F oven for 5 minutes, or until warmed through.

Per Serving:

Calories: 779   Fat: 59 g   Protein: 57 g   Carbs: 0 g

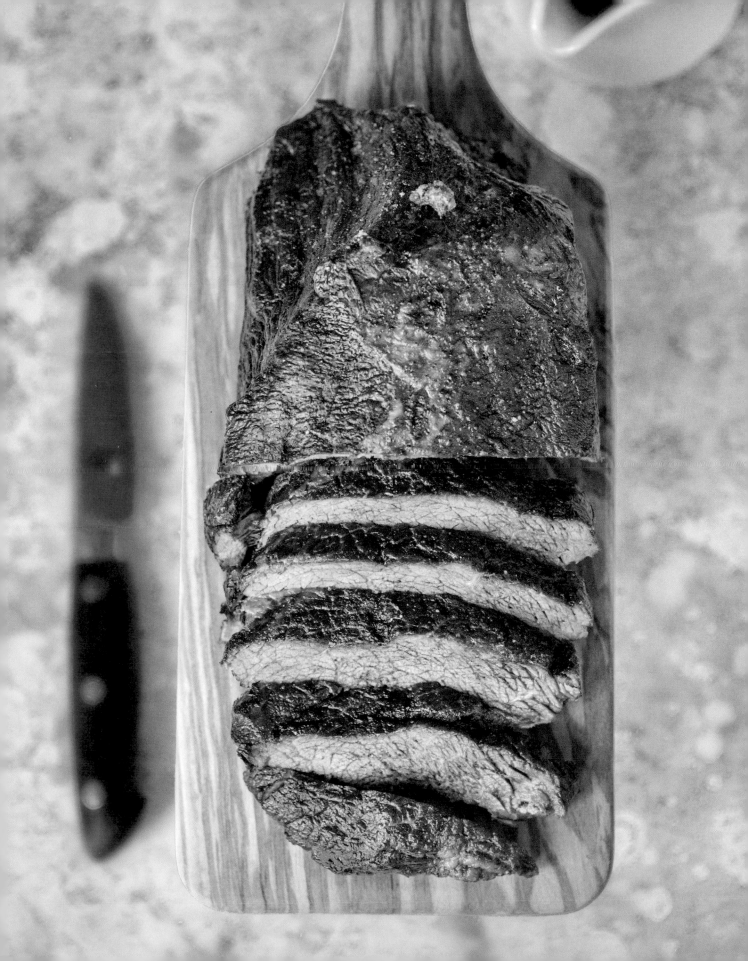

GRILLED LAMB CHOPS

Yield: 4 servings   **Prep Time:** 5 minutes, plus 15 minutes to sit at room temperature   **Cook Time:** 4 minutes

Lamb chops are a quick and tasty meal that can be cooked in just a few minutes.

8 lamb loin chops, about 1¼ inches thick

2 teaspoons fine sea salt

1. Pat the lamb chops dry with a paper towel and allow to sit at room temperature for 15 minutes to ensure even cooking.

2. Preheat a grill to high heat. Season the chops on both sides with the salt.

3. Once the grill is hot, place the chops on the grill and cook for 2 minutes per side for medium-rare, or until desired doneness. If your chops are thicker than 1¼ inches, cook them longer.

4. Remove the lamb chops from the grill and place on a serving platter.

5. Store in an airtight container in the refrigerator for 4 days. To reheat, place in a greased skillet over medium heat for 2 minutes per side, or until heated through.

Per Serving:

Calories: 510   Fat: 41 g   Protein: 30 g   Carbs: 0 g

1 — 2 — 3
CARNIVORE

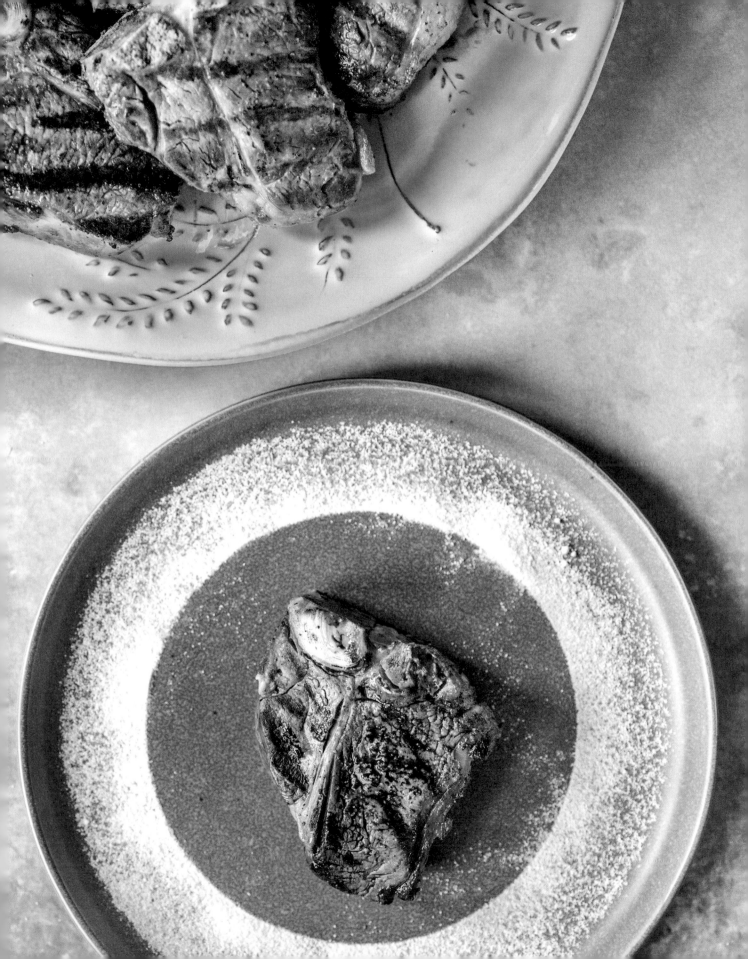

MEATBALLS

Yield: 12 meatballs (2 per serving)
Prep Time: 5 minutes   **Cook Time:** 12 minutes

I love meatballs, and so do my children. I often make a triple batch of these easy meatballs and freeze them unbaked for easy dinners later. They are delicious served with Carnivore Blue Cheese Dressing (page 316).

1½ pounds ground beef

4 ounces ground beef liver (or more ground beef)

1 large egg

2 teaspoons smoked sea salt, store-bought or homemade (page 310), or fine sea salt

1. Preheat the oven to 350°F.

2. Place the ground beef, ground liver, egg, and salt in a large bowl. Use your hands to thoroughly combine the meat mixture. Shape into twelve 1¼-inch balls, then set the meatballs on a rimmed baking sheet.

3. Bake for 10 to 12 minutes, until the meatballs are cooked through.

4. Store in an airtight container in the refrigerator for up to 4 days or in the freezer for up to a month. To reheat, place on a rimmed baking sheet in a preheated 350°F oven for 5 minutes, or until heated through.

Per Serving:

Calories: 281   Fat: 19 g   Protein: 26 g   Carbs: 1 g

1 — 2 — 3
CARNIVORE

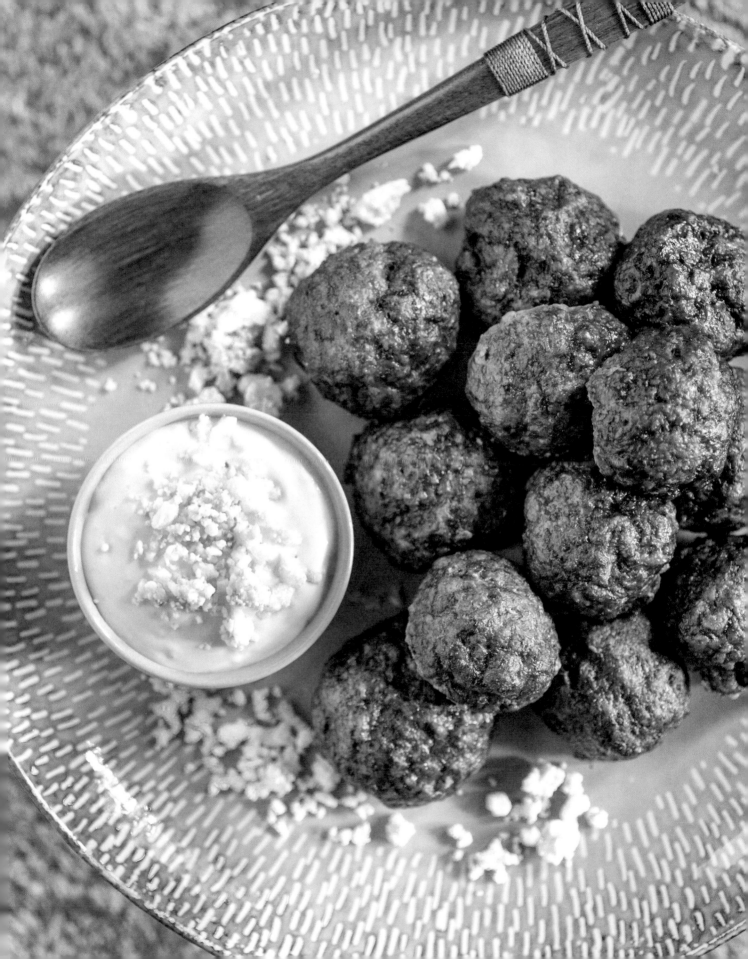

SMOKED MEATLOAF

Yield: 6 servings   **Prep Time:** 5 minutes, plus 30 minutes to soak wood chips (if using) and 10 minutes to rest   **Cook Time:** 3 hours

Smoked meatloaf is not like your mother's meatloaf! I dreaded meatloaf night when I was a kid, but smoking meatloaf takes it to a whole new level. I also like to sneak liver into my meatloaf for an extra nutrient-dense meal.

Be sure to read the manufacturer's directions for your smoker before you begin. There are wood, electric, propane, and charcoal smokers, and each type works differently. If you do not have a smoker, see page 79 for how to create a smoking technique using your oven or an outdoor grill.

1½ pounds ground beef

4 ounces ground beef liver (or more ground beef)

1 large egg

2 teaspoons fine sea salt

Special Equipment:
Smoker, wood chips
(optional)

1. If using wood chips, cover them with water and allow to soak for 30 minutes.

2. Place the ground beef, ground liver, egg, and salt in a large bowl. Mix until well combined and set aside.

3. Fold a long piece of heavy-duty aluminum foil in half to double the thickness, then use it to line a 9 by 5-inch loaf pan. Mold the foil sides to conform to the pan. Line the foil with parchment paper.

4. Place the meat mixture in the lined loaf pan and pat down evenly.

5. Smoke the meatloaf: Start the smoker, following the manufacturer's instructions. If your smoker has a water bowl, add water to it. When the temperature inside the smoker reaches 225°F to 250°F, you can start smoking the meatloaf.

6. Place the lined loaf pan on the smoker rack, not directly over the heat source, and secure the lid so that it is airtight and no smoke can escape. Smoke the meatloaf for 3 hours, or until the temperature in the thickest part of the meatloaf reaches 165°F.

7. Remove the meatloaf from the smoker and allow to rest for 10 minutes before slicing and serving.

Per Serving:

Calories: 281   Fat: 19 g   Protein: 26 g   Carbs: 1 g

1 — 2 — 3
CARNIVORE

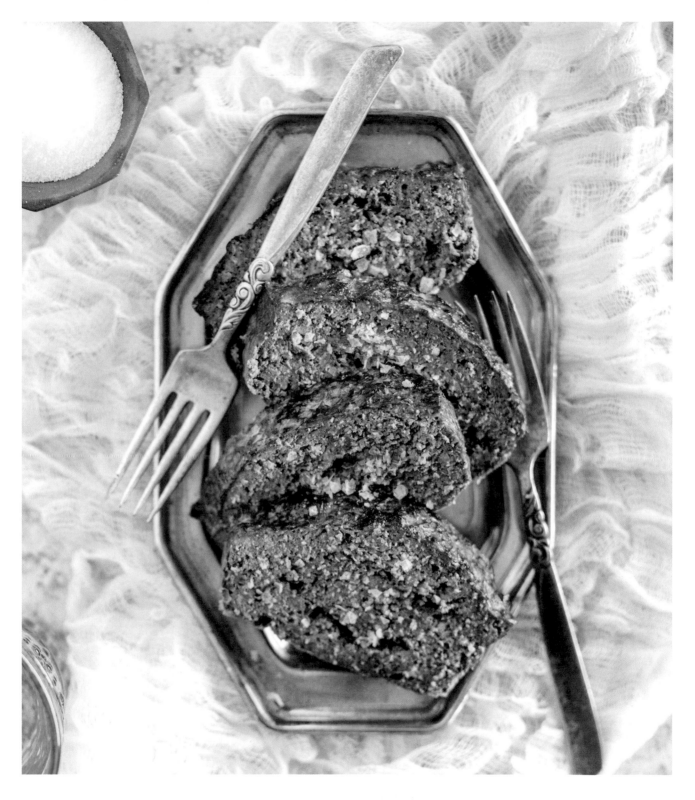

8. Store in an airtight container in the refrigerator for up to 4 days or in the freezer for up to a month. To reheat, place slices on a rimmed baking sheet in a preheated 350°F oven for 5 minutes, or until heated through.

BACON-WRAPPED JUICY LUCY

Yield: 4 servings
Prep Time: 8 minutes **Cook Time:** 20 minutes

If you've ever visited Minneapolis, you've probably heard about our classic Juicy Lucy, which is a mouthwatering burger with the cheese inside. Both the 5-8 Club and Matt's Bar claim to be the creator of the Juicy Lucy, and the two restaurants often have lighthearted battles over which of them makes the better version. They even had a televised battle on the Food Network!

1 pound ground beef

1 teaspoon fine sea salt

4 slices provolone or Munster cheese

8 thin slices pork or beef bacon

1. Preheat the oven or an air fryer to 400°F. If using the oven, line a rimmed baking sheet with parchment paper.

2. Place the ground beef in a large bowl and season with the salt. Use your hands to combine well. Divide the beef into 8 equal portions and form each portion into a ¼-inch-thick patty, about 3½ inches in diameter.

3. Fold the cheese slices in half and then in half again so that each slice is about 1½ inches square. Place a stack of cheese squares in the center of a patty and top with another patty. Use your fingers to seal the patty around the cheese; be sure to seal the edges well or the cheese will melt out. Repeat with the remaining patties and cheese.

4. Take a slice of bacon and wrap it around the top and sides of a patty. Wrap another slice of bacon around the patty, making an X on top with the first bacon slice. Secure the bacon with a toothpick and place the patty on the lined baking sheet or in the air fryer basket. Repeat with the remaining patties and bacon.

5. Cook for 15 to 20 minutes, flipping after 10 minutes, until the bacon is cooked to your liking.

6. After removing the burgers from the oven or air fryer, let cool for a few minutes before consuming or the melted cheese will burn your mouth.

7. Store in an airtight container in the refrigerator for up to 4 days. To reheat, place on a rimmed baking sheet in a preheated 400°F oven for 3 minutes, or until heated through.

Per Serving:

Calories: 498   Fat: 35 g   Protein: 42 g   Carbs: 0 g

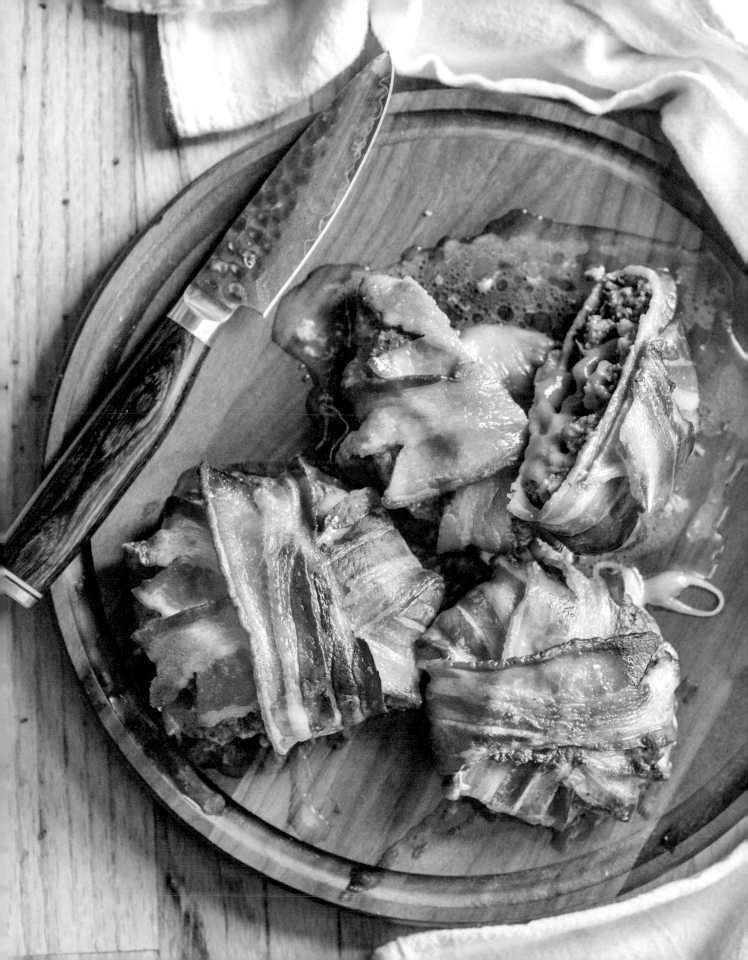

BAKED LAMB AND FETA PATTIES

Yield: 6 servings
Prep Time: 5 minutes   **Cook Time:** 12 minutes

This delicious twist on a cheeseburger patty combines lamb and feta cheese for a classic Greek flavor.

1½ pounds ground lamb

4 ounces feta cheese, crumbled

2 teaspoons smoked sea salt, store-bought or homemade (page 310), or fine sea salt

1. Preheat the oven to 350°F.

2. Place the ingredients in a large bowl and use your hands to thoroughly combine. Shape the mixture into eight 2½-inch-diameter patties, then place them on a rimmed baking sheet.

3. Bake for 10 to 12 minutes, until the patties are cooked through.

4. Store in an airtight container in the refrigerator for up to 4 days or in the freezer for up to a month. To reheat, place on a rimmed baking sheet in a preheated 350°F oven for 5 minutes, or until heated through.

Per Serving:

Calories: 327   Fat: 25 g   Protein: 22 g   Carbs: 1 g

1 2 3
CARNIVORE

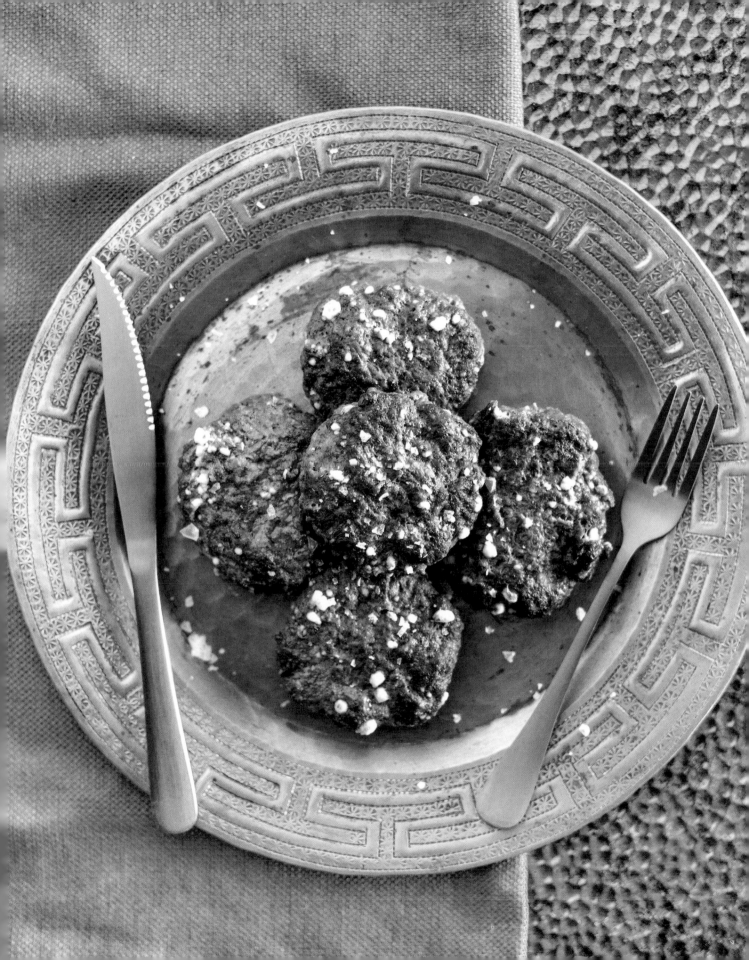

BACON-WRAPPED FILET MIGNONS

Yield: 2 servings **Prep Time:** 5 minutes, plus 20 minutes to rest
Cook Time: 15 minutes

What is more delicious than a filet mignon? A filet wrapped in bacon! If you use beef bacon and omit the butter, this recipe is Carnivore Level 1.

2 (4-ounce) filet mignons, about 1¼ inches thick

1½ teaspoons fine sea salt

2 thin slices pork or beef bacon

2 pats of unsalted butter, for topping (optional)

1. Allow the filets to sit at room temperature for 15 minutes to ensure even cooking.

2. Preheat the oven or an air fryer to 400°F.

3. Pat the filets dry with a paper towel and season the top and bottom of the filets with the salt. Wrap a piece of bacon around the sides of each filet and secure with a toothpick.

4. Place the bacon-wrapped filets on a rimmed baking sheet in the oven or in the air fryer basket. Cook for 15 minutes for medium-rare, or continue to cook until done to your liking (see the chart on page 180). Thicker filets will take longer.

5. Remove the filets from the baking sheet or air fryer and allow to rest for 5 minutes before serving. Top each with a pat of butter, if desired.

Per Serving (with butter):

Calories: 237   Fat: 13 g   Protein: 27 g   Carbs: 0 g

CARNIVORE   WITHOUT BUTTER

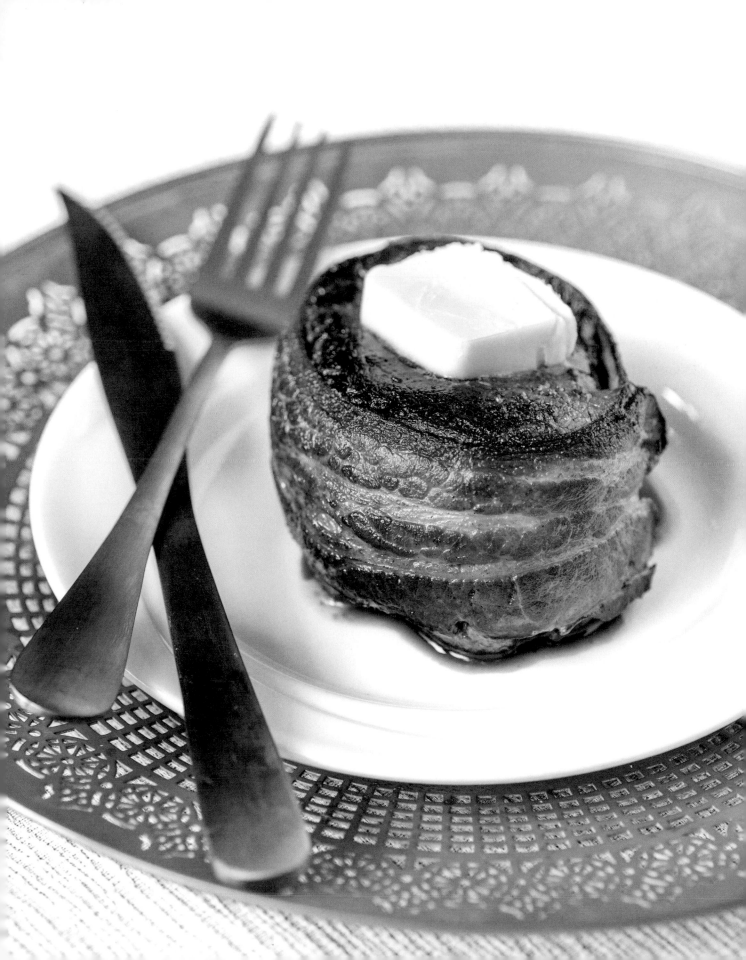

EGG-CELLENT MEATLOAF CUPCAKES

Yield: 4 servings
Prep Time: 10 minutes   **Cook Time:** 20 minutes

My boys love my meatloaf cupcakes! They are not only cute, but also delicious.

1 pound ground beef

1 teaspoon smoked sea salt, store-bought or homemade (page 310)

4 large hard-boiled eggs, peeled

8 thin slices pork or beef bacon

1. Preheat the oven or an air fryer to 400°F. If using the oven, line a rimmed baking sheet with parchment paper.

2. Place the ground beef and salt in a large bowl. Use your hands to mix until well combined. Divide the mixture into 4 balls, then flatten each ball into a ¼-inch-thick patty. Place an egg in the center of each patty and wrap the meat completely around the egg.

3. Take a slice of bacon and wrap it around the top and sides of a patty. Wrap another slice of bacon around the patty, making an X on top with the first bacon slice. Secure the bacon with a toothpick and place the patty on the lined baking sheet or in the air fryer basket. Repeat with the remaining patties, eggs, and bacon.

4. Cook for 15 to 20 minutes, or until the meatloaves are cooked through and the bacon is crisp. Remove the meatloaves from the oven or air fryer and serve.

5. Store in an airtight container in the refrigerator for up to 3 days or in the freezer for up to a month. To reheat, place in a preheated 350°F oven or air fryer for 4 minutes, or until heated through.

Per Serving:

Calories: 488   Fat: 35 g   Protein: 43 g   Carbs: 0 g

1 2 3
CARNIVORE

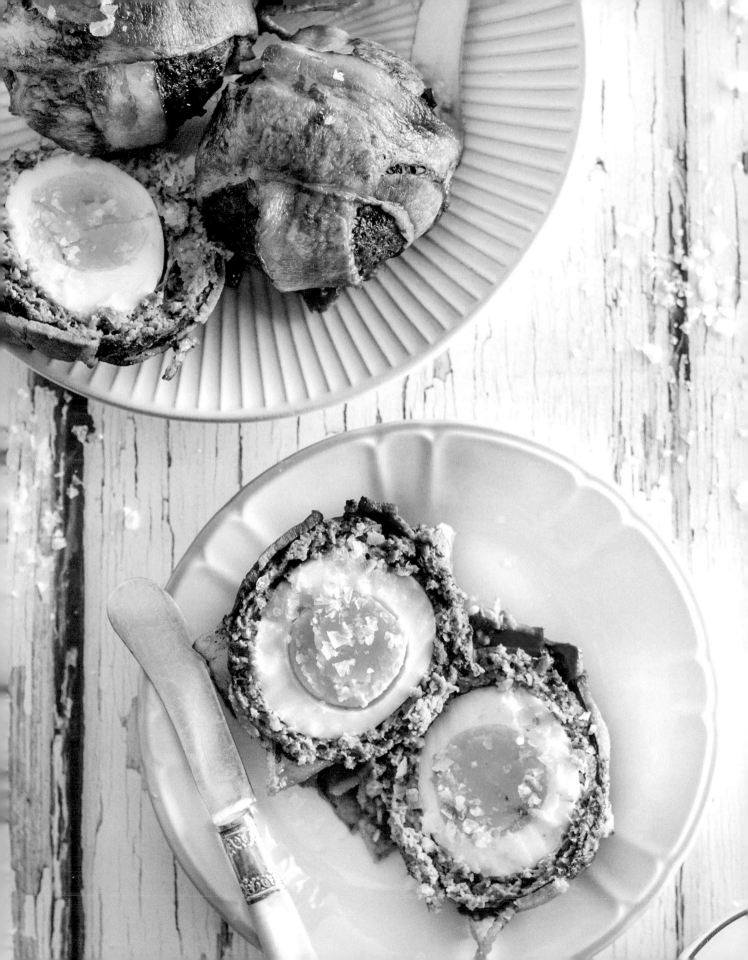

ROAST BEEF

Yield: 8 servings   **Prep Time:** 5 minutes, plus 40 minutes to sit at room temperature   **Cook Time:** 45 minutes

Roast beef is a classic Sunday supper that I ate often growing up. This recipe yields a lot of meat, but it makes great leftovers!

1 (2-pound) boneless beef roast

1 tablespoon tallow (page 312), melted

1 tablespoon fine sea salt

1. Remove the roast from the fridge and allow it to come to room temperature for 30 minutes.

2. Preheat the oven or an air fryer to 375°F. If using the oven, line a rimmed baking sheet with parchment paper.

3. Rub the roast all over with the melted tallow. Sprinkle all sides of the roast with the salt. Place the roast on the lined baking sheet or in the air fryer basket.

4. Cook for 45 minutes, or until the internal temperature reads 165°F for medium-rare beef, or continue cooking until cooked to your liking (see the chart on page 180).

5. Remove the roast from the oven or air fryer and allow to rest on a cutting board for 10 minutes before slicing and serving.

6. Store in an airtight container in the refrigerator for up to 4 days. Serve chilled, or reheat slices in a preheated 350°F oven or air fryer for 3 minutes, or until heated through.

Per Serving:

Calories: 321   Fat: 21 g   Protein: 29 g   Carbs: 0 g

1 2 3 CARNIVORE

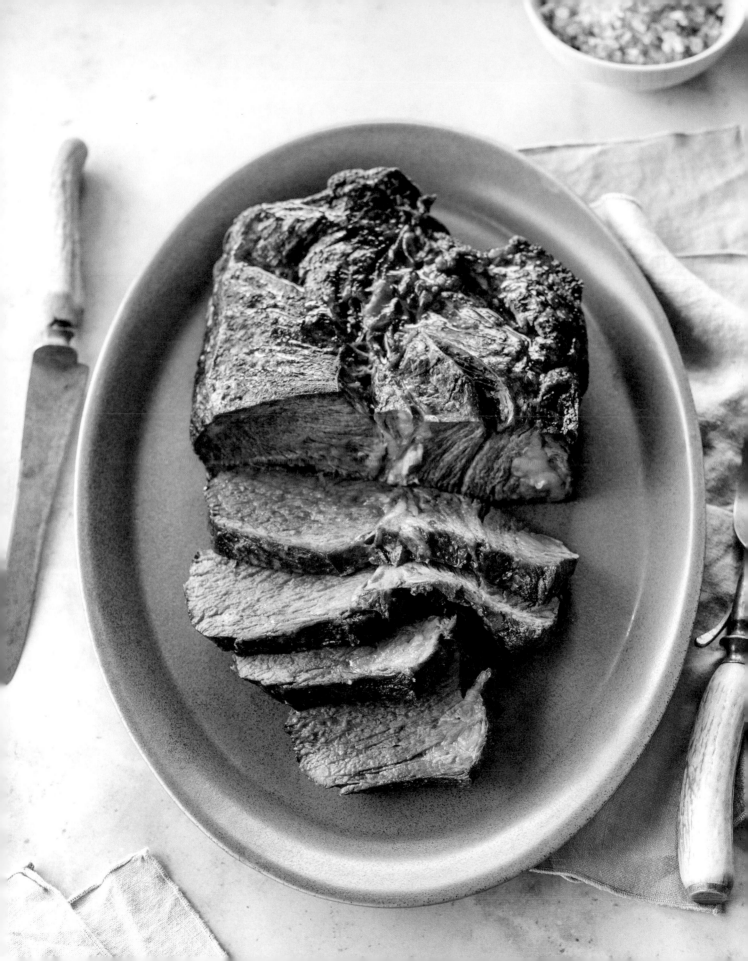

BACON-WRAPPED TENDERLOIN

Yield: 4 servings **Prep Time:** 8 minutes, plus 25 minutes to rest
Cook Time: 15 minutes

If you've never had tenderloin, you are in for a very juicy and soft steak! But it must not be overcooked, or you will end up with a chewy loin. I highly suggest cooking tenderloin rare to medium-rare. My kids were a little afraid of the pink color at first, but after they took their first bites, they smiled and gobbled it up.

1 pound venison or beef tenderloin

1½ teaspoons fine sea salt

4 slices pork or beef bacon

1. Remove the tenderloin from the fridge and allow to come to room temperature for 15 minutes.

2. Preheat the oven or an air fryer to 400°F. If using the oven, line a rimmed baking sheet with parchment paper.

3. Season the tenderloin on all sides with the salt. Wrap the bacon slices snugly around the tenderloin and place with the ends of the bacon under the tenderloin so the bacon is secured around the loin. Place on the lined baking sheet or in the air fryer basket.

4. Cook for 15 minutes, flipping after 10 minutes, for medium-rare meat.

5. Remove the tenderloin from the baking sheet or air fryer basket and allow to rest on a cutting board for 10 minutes before slicing. To serve, cut the tenderloin into ½-inch slices and place on a platter.

6. Store in an airtight container in the refrigerator for up to 3 days. To reheat, place in a preheated 350°F oven or air fryer for 4 minutes, or until heated through.

Per Serving:

Calories: 242   Fat: 9 g   Protein: 38 g   Carbs: 0 g

1 2 3 CARNIVORE   1 2 3 IF USING BEEF

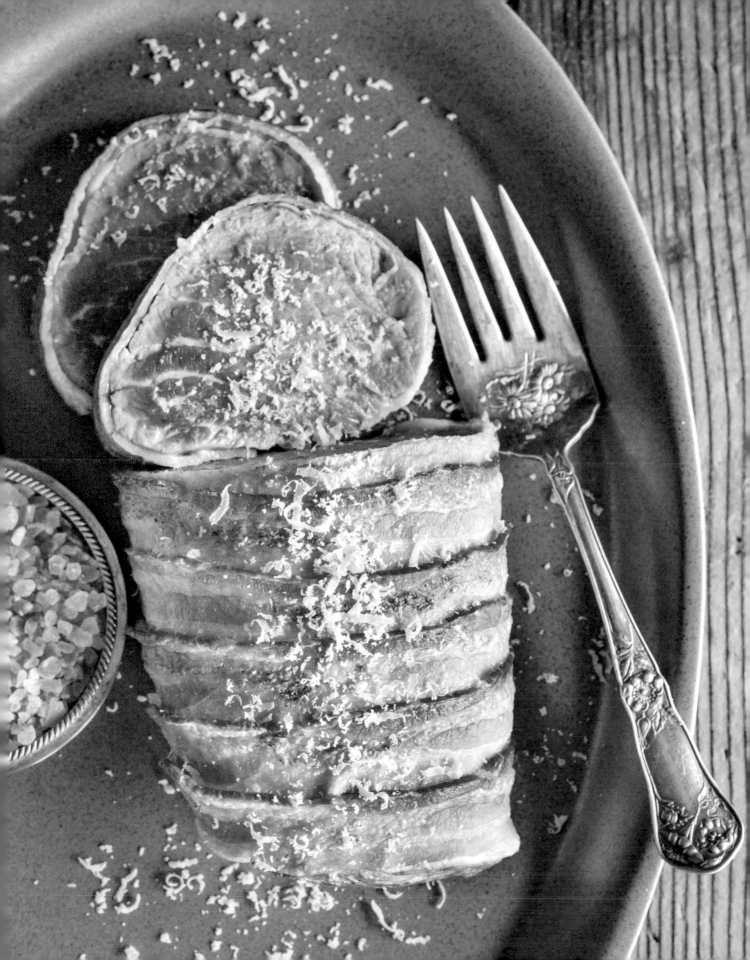

BASTED TOP SIRLOIN

Yield: 1 serving **Prep Time:** 6 minutes, plus 20 minutes to rest
Cook Time: 12 minutes

Basting steak is a great way to infuse it with flavor and get a crispy outside.

1 (8-ounce) top sirloin steak, about 1¼ inches thick

1 teaspoon fine sea salt

1 tablespoon tallow (page 312) or duck fat

3 tablespoons unsalted butter (or more tallow for dairy-free), for dipping

1. Allow the steak to sit at room temperature for 15 minutes to ensure even cooking. Then pat the steak dry with a paper towel and season with the salt.

2. Heat the tallow in a large cast-iron skillet over medium-high heat. Once hot, sear the steak for 2 minutes, without moving it, then flip it over and sear it for another 2 minutes.

3. Lower the heat to medium-low and add the butter. Use a spoon to constantly pour the butter over the steak. Continue to baste and cook the steak for about 4 more minutes per side for medium-rare. The exact timing will depend on the thickness of the steak or your desired doneness.

4. Remove the steak from the pan and allow to rest for 5 minutes before slicing. Pour the butter into a small serving dish for dipping the steak and serve.

Per Serving (with butter):

Calories: 570 Fat: 47 g Protein: 34 g Carbs: 0 g

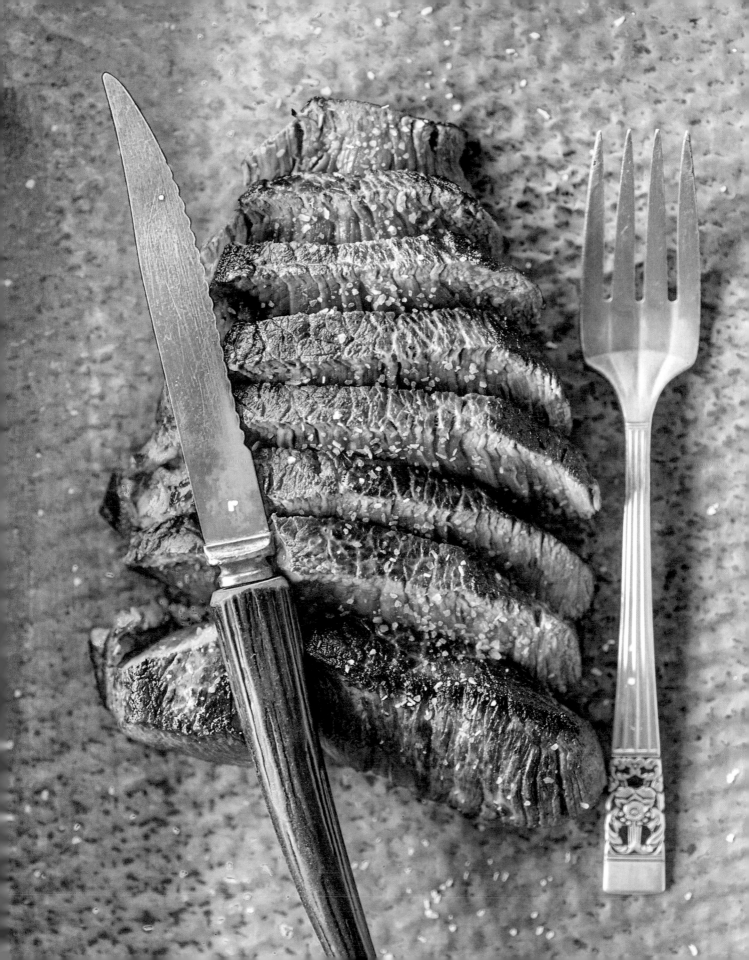

AIR-FRIED T-BONE STEAKS WITH SMOKED BUTTER

Yield: 2 servings   **Prep Time:** 7 minutes, plus 10 minutes to rest
Cook Time: 12 minutes

If you don't have an air fryer, you can still make this delicious dish in your oven.

2 (8-ounce) T-bone steaks, about ¾ inch thick

2 teaspoons fine sea salt

¼ cup (½ stick) unsalted butter, softened, for serving (optional)

⅛ teaspoon smoked sea salt, store-bought or homemade (page 310)

1. Preheat an air fryer or the oven to 400°F.

2. Remove the steaks from the refrigerator and allow to sit at room temperature for 10 minutes to ensure even cooking. Season the steaks on both sides with the salt.

3. Place the steaks in the air fryer basket, or on a rimmed baking sheet if using the oven, and cook for 12 minutes, flipping after 6 minutes, for medium-rare steaks; if you prefer a different level of doneness, see the chart on page 180.

4. Meanwhile, make the smoked butter, if using: Place the butter and smoked salt in a small dish and stir well to combine.

5. Remove the steaks from the air fryer or oven and allow to rest for 10 minutes before serving. Top with the smoked butter.

Per Serving (with butter):

Calories: 680   Fat: 54 g   Protein: 44 g   Carbs: 0 g

CARNIVORE   WITHOUT BUTTER

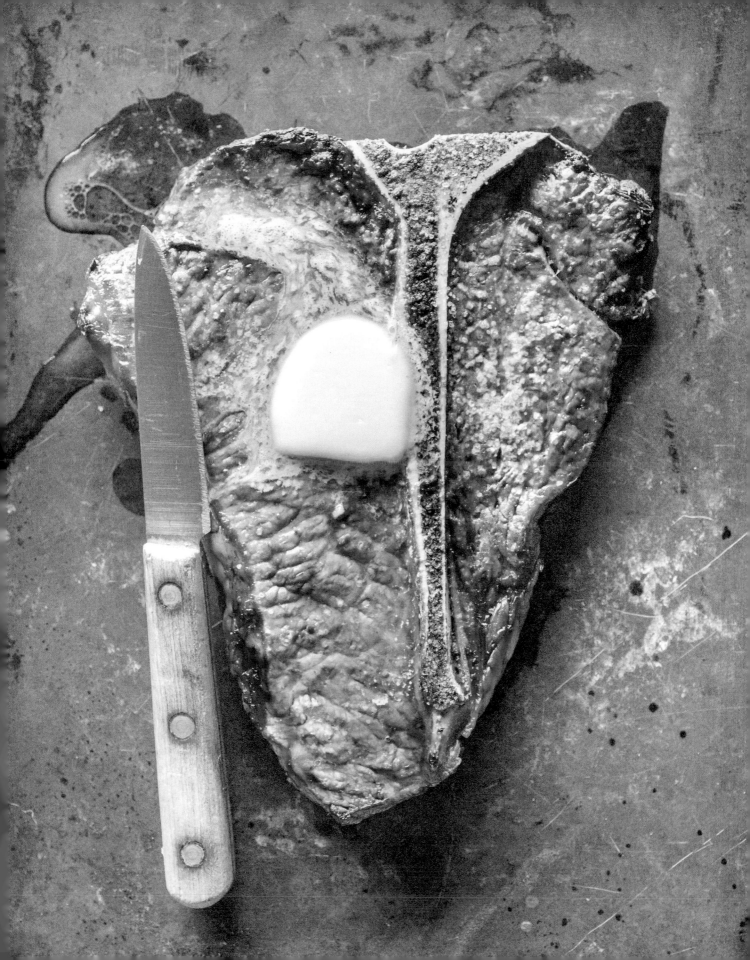

SMOKY BEEF TARTARE

Yield: 4 servings
Prep Time: 10 minutes, plus 1 hour to chill   **Cook Time:** —

Using smoked salt gives beef tartare a nice flavor. If you prefer a more traditional tartare, however, feel free to use regular sea salt instead. Please note that eating tartare is not recommended for infants, pregnant women, or people with weakened immune systems.

1 (1-pound) top round steak

1 teaspoon smoked sea salt, store-bought or homemade (page 310)

1 large egg yolk, plus 4 yolks for garnish if desired

Special Equipment:
3-inch round cookie cutter

1. Put the steak in the freezer for about 1 hour to make it easier to cut.

2. Place the chilled steak on a cutting board and slice it against the grain into very thin strips. Then cut the strips into a fine dice. Continue to chop until you have finely chopped steak.

3. Place the chopped steak in a large bowl. Add the salt and egg yolk and mix thoroughly with your hands. Taste and adjust the salt to your liking.

4. Divide the meat mixture into 4 equal portions. Place 1 portion in the center of a 3-inch cookie cutter. Press with your hands to form a tight mound. Remove the cookie cutter and repeat with the remaining meat mixture.

5. Top each mound with an egg yolk, if desired. Serve immediately.

Per Serving:

Calories: 297   Fat: 15 g   Protein: 38 g   Carbs: 1 g

2
1 3
CARNIVORE

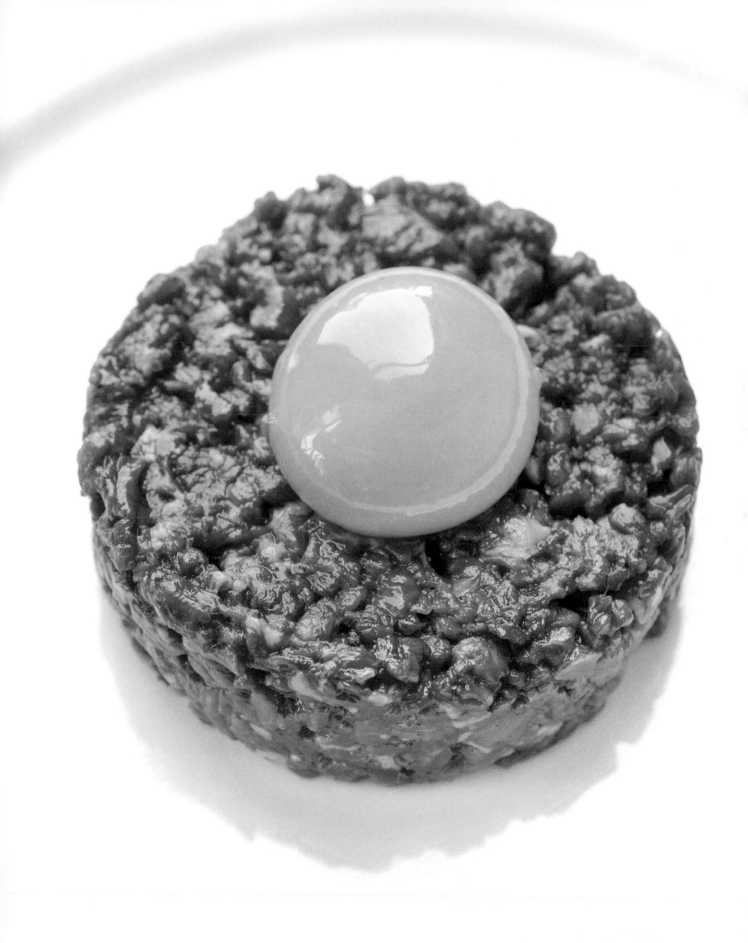

BEEF TONGUE

Yield: 4 servings
Prep Time: 5 minutes   **Cook Time:** 1 hour

I had the great pleasure to teach people about keto while traveling through Italy last spring. One of the participants who came on my tour was a carnivore from South Africa who loves beef tongue. This recipe is in honor of my lovely friend Amy.

1 (2-pound) beef tongue

1 tablespoon fine sea salt

Easy Carnivore Hollandaise (page 314), for serving (optional)

1. Place the beef tongue in a large pot. Fill the pot with water so that the tongue is completely covered. Add the salt.

2. Turn the heat to high and bring the water to a boil. Cover, reduce the heat to medium-low, and simmer for 1 hour, or until the skin slides off easily.

3. Remove the tongue from the pot and let cool slightly. Once cool enough to handle, remove the skin and cut the tongue into ¼-inch slices. Serve warm, topped with hollandaise, if desired.

4. Store in an airtight container in the refrigerator for up to 4 days. To reheat, place in a pot of boiling water for 5 minutes, or until heated through.

Per Serving (without hollandaise):

Calories: 512   Fat: 50 g   Protein: 44 g   Carbs: 0 g

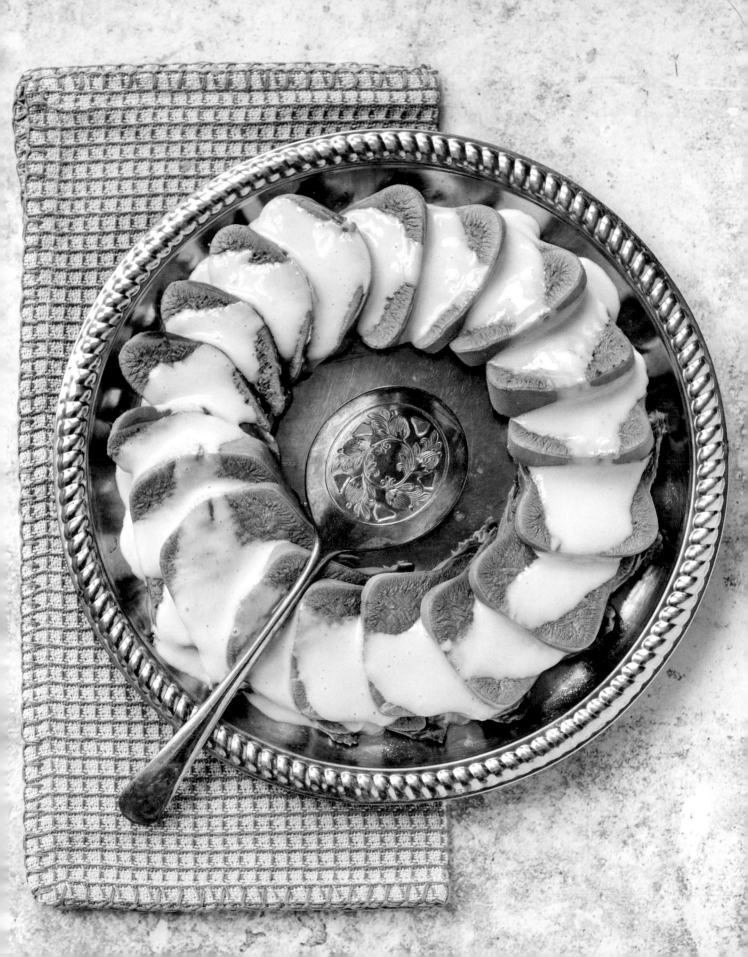

BUTTER BURGERS

Yield: 4 servings
Prep Time: 8 minutes   **Cook Time:** 6 minutes

I am from Wisconsin, and we are known for our love of beef and our love of butter. If you've ever visited the Badger State, you've probably heard about our butter burgers—mouthwatering burgers with the butter enclosed inside! It is the most juicy and delicious carnivore meal I have ever had.

1 pound ground beef

½ cup (1 stick) unsalted butter, cut into 4 chunks

1 teaspoon fine sea salt

1 tablespoon bacon fat

1. Using your hands, divide the ground beef into 8 equal portions. Form each portion into a ¼-inch-thick patty, about 3½ inches in diameter. Then make a circular indentation in the middle of each patty using your thumb.

2. Place a pat of butter in the center of a patty and top with another patty. Use your fingers to seal the patty around the butter; be sure to seal the edges well. Repeat with the remaining patties and butter. Season the patties on both sides with the salt.

3. Heat the bacon fat in a large cast-iron skillet over medium-high heat. Once the skillet is hot, fry the patties for 3 minutes per side for medium-done burgers, or cook longer if you prefer well-done burgers.

4. Remove the burgers from the skillet and let cool for at least 3 minutes before consuming or the melted butter will burn your mouth.

5. Store in an airtight container in the refrigerator for up to 4 days. To reheat, place in a lightly greased skillet over medium heat for 3 minutes, or until heated through.

Per Serving:

Calories: 446   Fat: 40 g   Protein: 21 g   Carbs: 0 g

1 2 3
CARNIVORE

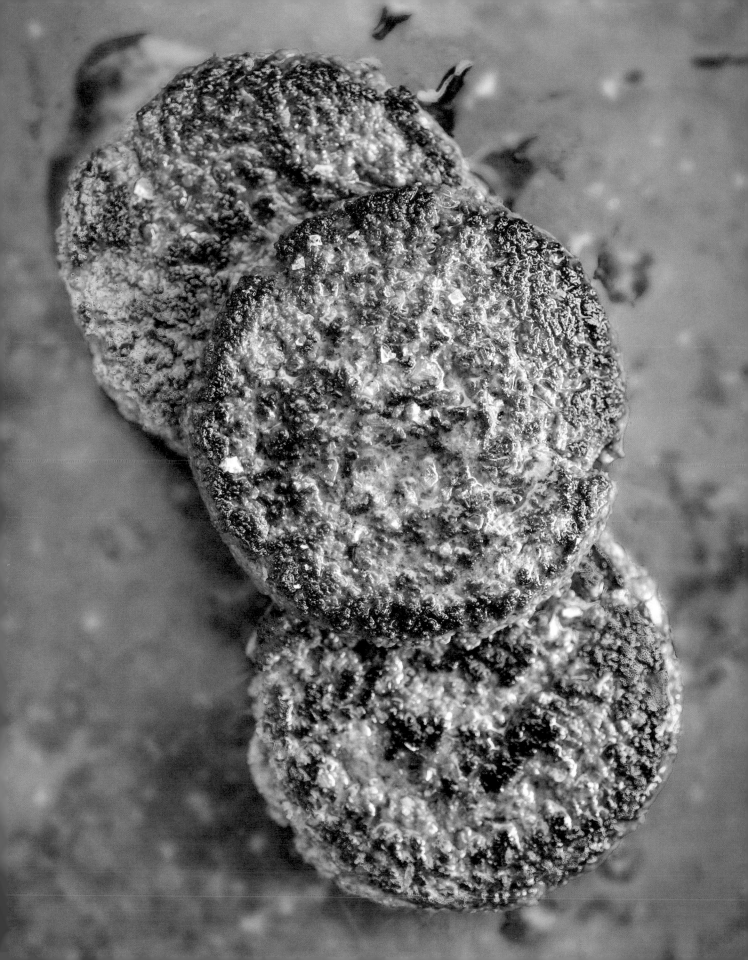

GRILLED LAMB KOFTA

Yield: 4 servings (3 koftas per person)
Prep Time: 5 minutes   **Cook Time:** 8 minutes

This delicious grilled lamb kofta recipe is a twist on a traditional kofta. These koftas taste great with melted soft goat cheese. If you make this recipe with ground beef and beef tallow and omit the cheese, it is Carnivore Level 1.

1 pound ground lamb or ground beef

1¾ teaspoons fine sea salt

Melted tallow (page 312) or lard, for greasing

Soft goat cheese, melted, for serving (optional)

Special Equipment:
12 (8-inch) metal or wooden skewers

1. If using wooden skewers, soak them in water for 10 minutes. Preheat a grill to medium heat.

2. Make the kofta: Place the ground beef and salt in a large bowl and mix until well combined. Use your hands to form the mixture into 12 balls. Place each ball around a skewer and use your hands to flatten it, making it about 6 inches long and 1¼ inches thick.

3. Grease the hot grill grates with melted tallow. Place the skewers on the grill and cook for about 4 minutes per side for medium-done kofta, or until cooked to your liking.

4. Serve with goat cheese on the side, if desired.

5. Store in an airtight container in the refrigerator for up to 4 days. To reheat, place in a lightly greased skillet over medium heat for 4 minutes or until heated through.

Per Serving:

Calories: 283   Fat: 22 g   Protein: 19 g   Carbs: 0 g

CARNIVORE   WITH CHEESE

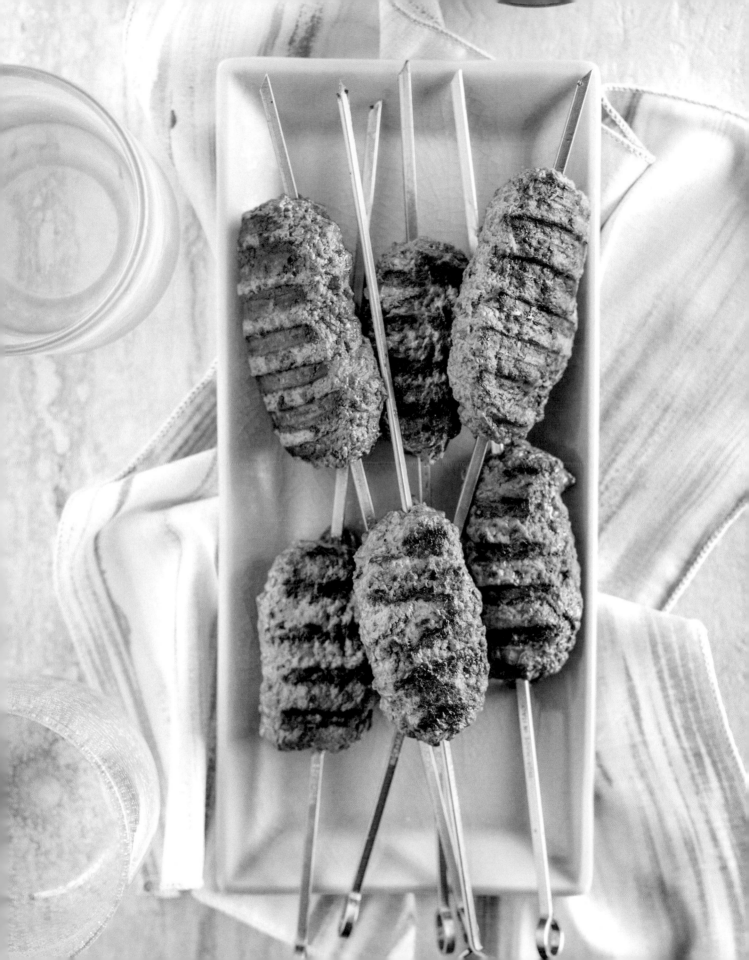

GRILLED PORTERHOUSE

Yield: 2 servings   **Prep Time:** 5 minutes, plus 25 minutes to come to room temperature and rest   **Cook Time:** 8 minutes

I love a big porterhouse steak! This cut of beef is so easy to make and so flavorful.

1 (1¼-pound) porterhouse steak, about ¾ inch thick

2 teaspoons fine sea salt

1. Allow the steak to sit at room temperature for 15 minutes to ensure even cooking.

2. Preheat a grill to high heat. Pat the steak dry with a paper towel and season on both sides with the salt.

3. Once the grill is hot, place the steak on the grill and cook for 6 to 8 minutes, flipping after 3 minutes, until the steak reaches your desired doneness (see the chart on page 180).

4. Remove from the grill and allow to rest for 10 minutes before serving.

Per Serving:

Calories: 600   Fat: 41 g   Protein: 55 g   Carbs: 0 g

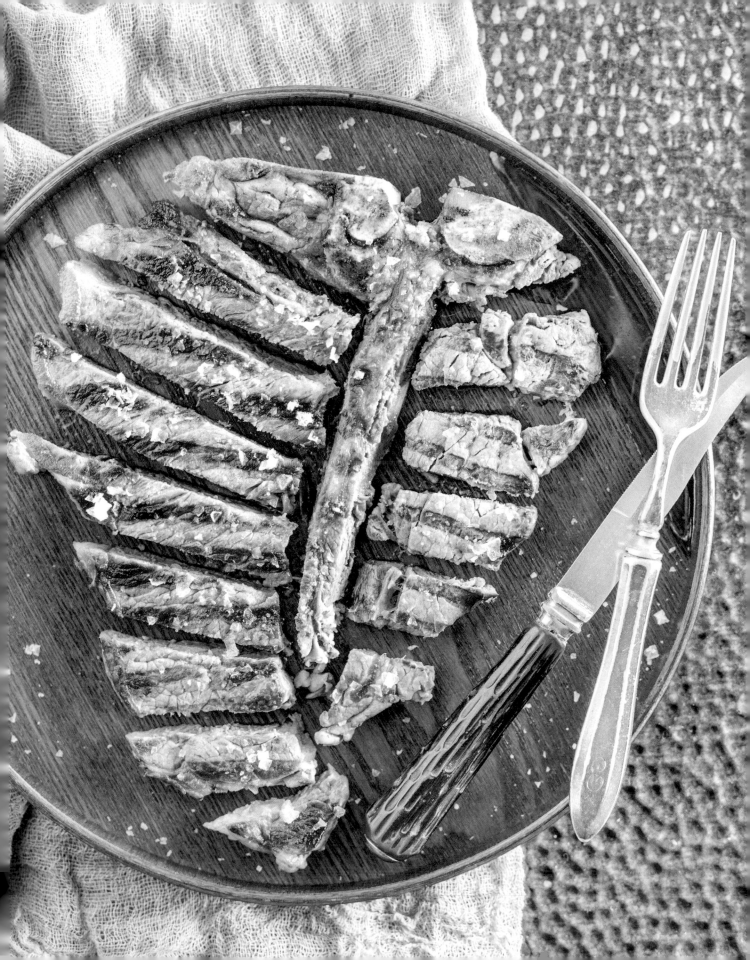

BLACK 'N' BLUE STRIP STEAK

Yield: 2 servings   **Prep Time:** 5 minutes, plus 25 minutes to come to room temperature and rest   **Cook Time:** 7 minutes

The combination of steak, bacon fat, and blue cheese makes this meal a family dinner classic.

2 (10-ounce) New York strip steaks, about ¾ inch thick

2 tablespoons bacon fat

2 teaspoons fine sea salt

2 ounces blue cheese crumbles, divided

1. Remove the steaks from the fridge 15 minutes before cooking to allow to come to room temperature.

2. Heat the bacon fat in a large cast-iron skillet over medium-high heat.

3. Pat the steaks dry and season on all sides with the salt. Once the skillet is hot, add the steaks and cook for 3 minutes, then flip and cook for 3 minutes on the other side, or until cooked to your liking.

4. Top each steak with 1 ounce of the blue cheese. Cover and cook for another minute to melt the cheese. Remove from the skillet and allow to rest for 10 minutes before serving.

Per Serving:

Calories: 781   Fat: 64 g   Protein: 50 g   Carbs: 0 g

1 — 2 — 3
CARNIVORE

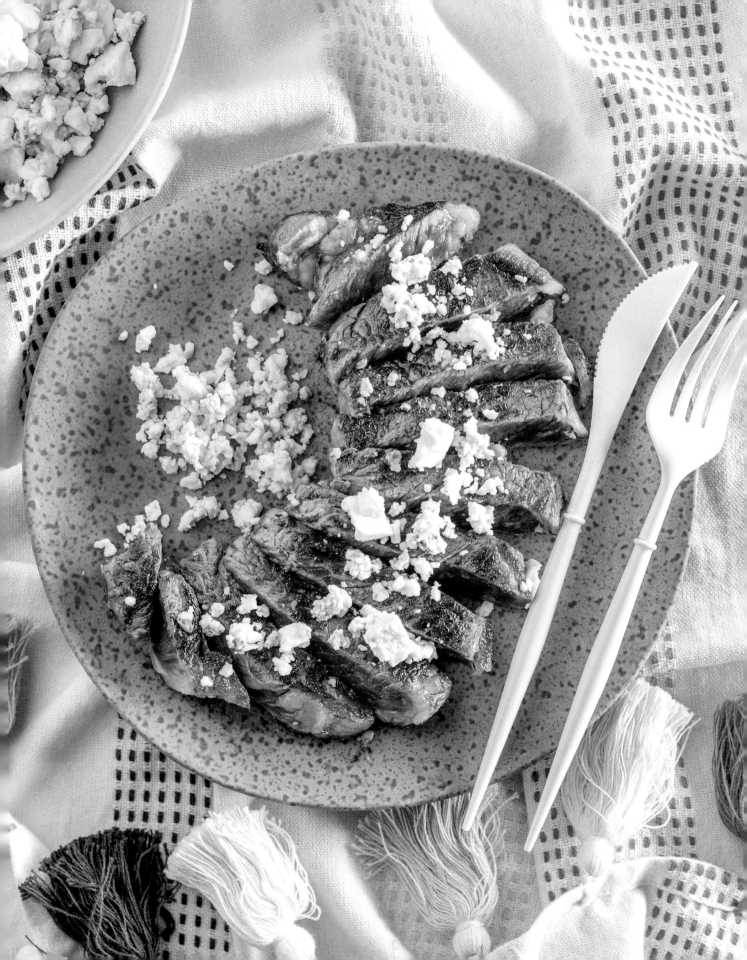

CREAMY PARMESAN BEEF TIPS

Yield: 10 servings
Prep Time: 5 minutes   **Cook Time:** 6 hours

OPTION

At our wedding, we served beef tips. It is a common wedding meal in Wisconsin. I wish that our beef tips had been prepared in this mouthwatering way!

1 cup heavy cream

1 cup Carnivore Beef Bone Broth (page 308)

4 ounces Parmesan cheese, grated (about 1 cup)

1½ teaspoons fine sea salt

1 (5-pound) boneless top sirloin or rump roast, cut into 1-inch cubes

2 Salt-Cured Egg Yolks (page 320), grated, for garnish (optional)

1. Place the cream, broth, Parmesan, and salt in a 4-quart or larger slow cooker and stir to combine. Place the cubed roast on top of the broth mixture. Cover and cook on low for 6 hours, or until the meat is very tender and falls apart easily. Serve the meat with the sauce from the slow cooker and garnish with cured egg yolks, if desired.

2. Store in an airtight container in the refrigerator for up to 3 days. To reheat, place in a large cast-iron skillet over medium heat, stirring occasionally, for 5 minutes, or until warmed through.

Per Serving (with egg yolks):

Calories: 543   Fat: 36 g   Protein: 52 g   Carbs: 1 g

1 2 3
CARNIVORE

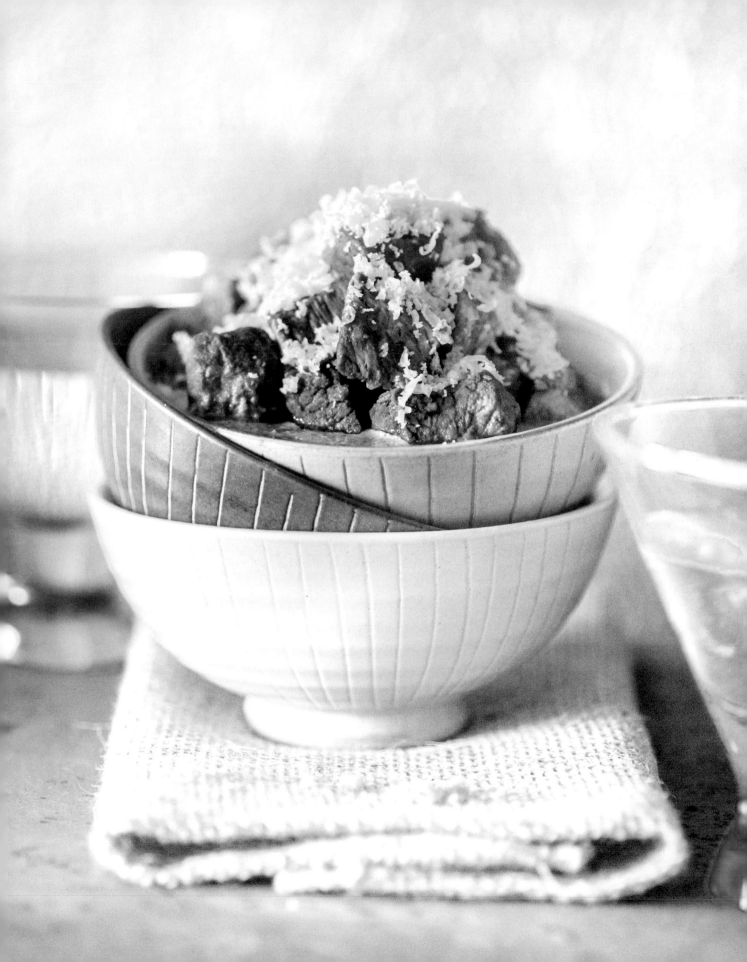

SHREDDED BEEF WITH BROWN BUTTER JUS

Yield: 10 servings
Prep Time: 5 minutes   **Cook Time:** 4 to 8 hours

I like using my slow cooker to make delicious family dinners. If you're pressed for time, cook the roast on high; however, "low and slow" will give you more tender and juicier meat.

3 cups Carnivore Beef Bone Broth (page 308)

2¼ teaspoons fine sea salt

1 (5-pound) boneless rump roast

½ cup (1 stick) unsalted butter

1. Pour the broth into a 4-quart or larger slow cooker. Add the salt and stir to combine.

2. Place the roast in the slow cooker. Cover and cook on low for 8 hours or on high for 4 hours, until the meat is very tender and falls apart easily.

3. Meanwhile, make the brown butter: Melt the butter in a saucepan over high heat. Whisk frequently until it froths up, then settles down with brown flecks visible. Keep whisking until the butter is a dark brown. Remove the pan from the heat and set aside.

4. Remove the beef from the slow cooker and place on a serving platter. Shred with two forks.

5. Pour 1 cup of the cooking liquid from the slow cooker into the saucepan with the brown butter and whisk to combine. Serve the brown butter jus with the shredded beef.

6. Store in an airtight container in the refrigerator for up to 4 days or in the freezer for up to a month. To reheat, place slices in a casserole dish with the brown butter jus in a preheated 350°F oven for 5 minutes, or until heated through.

Per Serving:

Calories: 519   Fat: 34 g   Protein: 51 g   Carbs: 0 g

2 1 2
1 3 1 3
CARNIVORE WITHOUT BROWN
BUTTER JUS

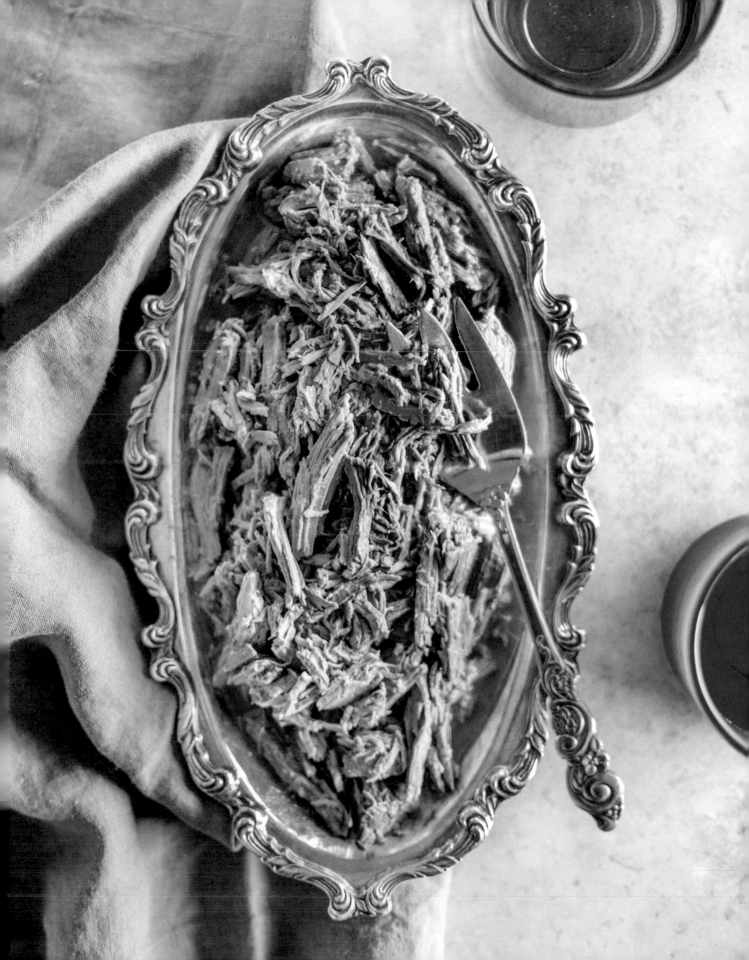

OXTAIL

Yield: 8 servings
Prep Time: 5 minutes   **Cook Time:** 2 hours 6 minutes

Oxtail is the tail of a cow, and it has a rich gelatin-filled meat. It works great when prepared in a slow cooker or slowly braised.

¼ cup tallow (page 312) or unsalted butter

2 pounds oxtails, cut into 1-inch segments

2 teaspoons fine sea salt

2 cups Carnivore Beef Bone Broth (page 308)

1. Heat the tallow in a large cast-iron skillet over medium-high heat.

2. Pat the pieces of oxtail dry with a paper towel and season on all sides with the salt. Once the skillet is hot, add the oxtail and sauté for 6 minutes, or until browned.

3. Pour in the broth, cover, and simmer over medium-low heat for 2 hours, or until the oxtail is tender. Serve the meat with the pan sauce.

4. Store in an airtight container in the refrigerator for up to 4 days. To reheat, place in a cast-iron skillet over medium-high heat for 5 minutes, or until heated through.

Per Serving:

Calories: 360   Fat: 25 g   Protein: 31 g   Carbs: 0 g

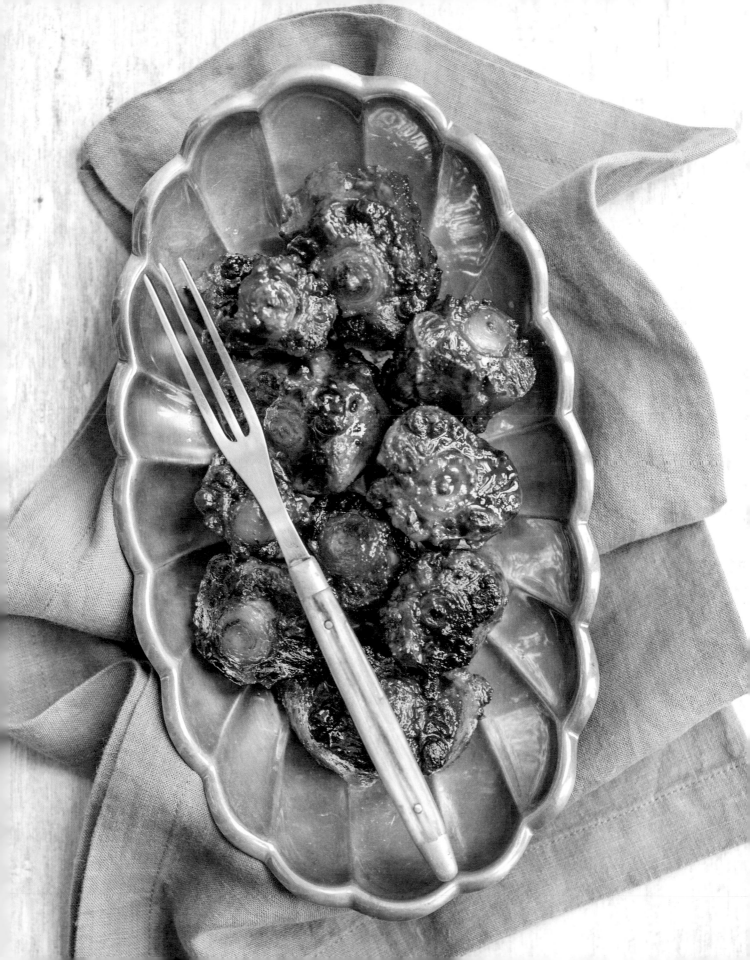

ROULADEN

Yield: 12 servings   **Prep Time:** 10 minutes
Cook Time: 2 hours 8 minutes, plus 10 minutes for creamy broth

I am a typical German girl who loves traditional German food. Rouladen is a German dish made with thin slices of beef that are rolled with bacon and braised until tender. The original recipe is often served with onions, pickles, and mustard, but in this carnivore version, the meat remains the star of the show. If you prefer a more complex flavor profile, you can add cream to the sauce.

2 pounds rump steak, sliced ¼ inch thick

2 teaspoons fine sea salt

12 slices pork or beef bacon

2 tablespoons tallow (page 312) or ghee

½ cup Carnivore Beef Bone Broth (page 308), plus more if needed

1 cup heavy cream (optional)

1. Lay the steak slices on a work surface and sprinkle on all sides with the salt.

2. Lay a slice of bacon in the center of each steak slice. If the bacon is longer than the steak, cut the bacon at the end of the steak and place it on another open area of the steak. Roll up like a jelly roll, starting at one end. Tie with kitchen twine to hold it shut. Repeat with the remaining steak and bacon slices.

3. Heat the tallow in a large Dutch oven over medium-high heat. Add the roll-ups and brown on all sides for 2 minutes per side.

4. Add the broth, making sure to add enough liquid to be ½ inch deep in the pot. Cover and cook over low heat for 2 hours, or until the beef is very tender. If desired, remove the lid, add the cream, if using, and cook for 10 more minutes to heat the cream. Serve the rouladen with the sauce from the pot.

5. Store in an airtight container in the refrigerator for up to 4 days or in the freezer for up to a month. To reheat, place in a casserole dish with the sauce in a preheated 350°F oven for 5 minutes, or until heated through.

Per Serving (with cream):

Calories: 260   Fat: 20 g   Protein: 21 g   Carbs: 0 g

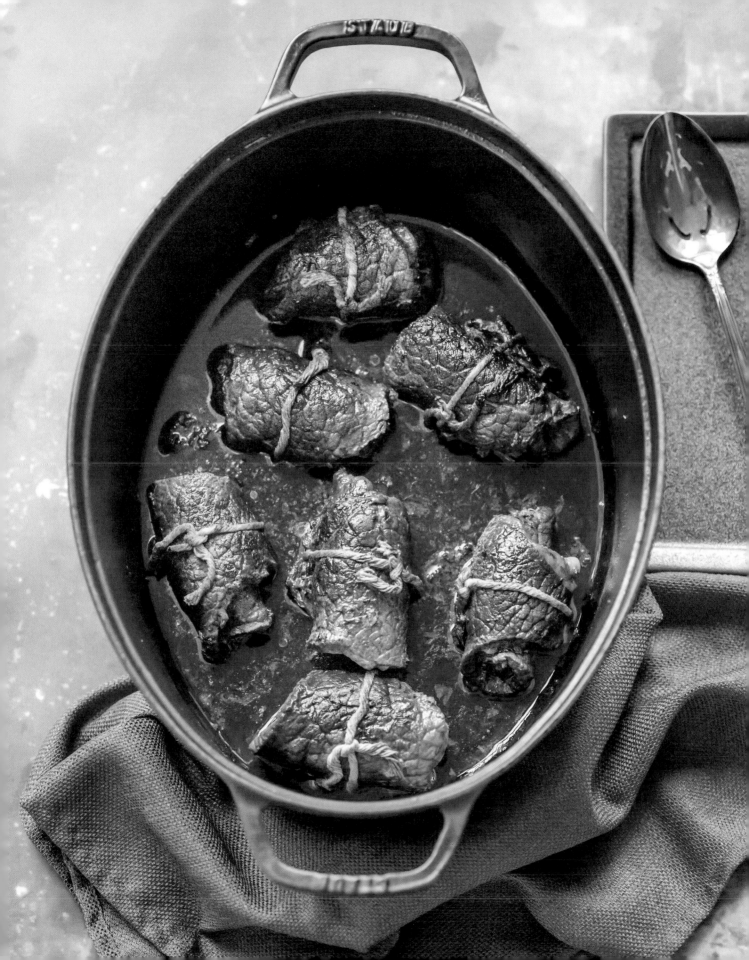

GRILLED SWEETBREADS

Yield: 4 servings
Prep Time: 10 minutes, plus 5 minutes to rest   **Cook Time:** 16 minutes

Sweetbreads sound like a carb-heavy nightmare, don't they? But don't be fooled; this recipe is not filled with either sugar or bread. Sweetbreads are the thymus or pancreas of an animal, usually calf or lamb, but sometimes cow or pig. Honestly, they are a delicious and super nutritious treat, and I suggest not even telling your dinner guests what they are until they try them.

1 pound sweetbreads

3 tablespoons plus
2 teaspoons fine sea salt,
divided

2 tablespoons tallow (page
312) or ghee, melted, plus
more for serving

Special Equipment:
4 (8-inch) metal or wooden
skewers

1. If using wooden skewers, soak them in water for 10 minutes.

2. Bring a pot of water with 3 tablespoons of the salt to a boil over medium-high heat. Add the sweetbreads, reduce the heat to medium-low, and simmer for 10 minutes. Using a slotted spoon, transfer the sweetbreads from the pot to a bowl of ice-cold water to stop the cooking.

3. When the sweetbreads are completely cool, drain and pat dry with paper towels. Using your fingers, peel away as much of the membrane as possible from the sweetbreads and discard. Separate the sweetbreads into nuggets.

4. Preheat a grill to medium-high heat. Place the sweetbreads in a bowl. Add the melted tallow and toss well to coat. Season on all sides with the remaining 2 teaspoons of salt. Thread onto the skewers.

5. Place the skewers on the hot grill and cook, turning occasionally, until golden brown on all sides, about 6 minutes.

6. Remove the sweetbreads from the grill and place on a serving platter to rest for 5 minutes before serving. Serve with additional melted tallow, if desired.

7. Store in an airtight container in the refrigerator for up to 4 days. To reheat, place on a rimmed baking sheet in a preheated 350°F oven for 5 minutes, or until heated through.

Per Serving:

Calories: 429   Fat: 35 g   Protein: 36 g   Carbs: 0 g

1 2 3 CARNIVORE   1 2 3 IF USING GHEE

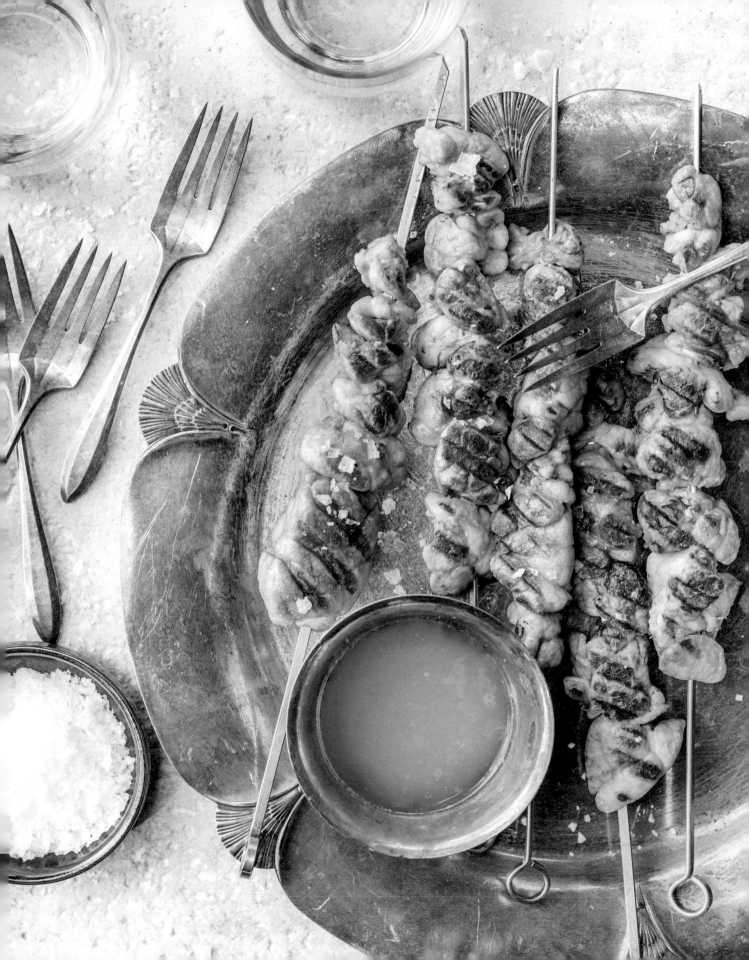

TRADITIONAL TERRINE

Yield: 8 servings   **Prep Time:** 15 minutes, plus 2 hours to rest and chill
Cook Time: 1 hour 35 minutes

A terrine is a French pâté dish that can be served warm or chilled. I prefer it chilled.

2 pounds beef or venison tenderloin, cut into ½-inch pieces

3 teaspoons fine sea salt, divided

2 tablespoons tallow (page 312) or lard

1 pound ground beef or ground pork

1 large egg

¼ cup Carnivore Beef Bone Broth (page 308)

12 slices pork or beef bacon

1. Preheat the oven to 325°F. Grease a 5-cup terrine mold or a 4 by 8-inch loaf pan.

2. Season the pieces of tenderloin on all sides with 1 teaspoon of the salt.

3. Heat a large cast-iron skillet over medium-high heat with the tallow. Once hot, sear the tenderloin pieces on all sides until browned, about 5 minutes. Remove from the skillet and set aside.

4. Place the ground meat, egg, broth, and remaining 2 teaspoons of salt in a large bowl. Use your hands to combine well.

5. Line the bottom and sides of the terrine mold with the bacon slices, allowing the ends to hang over the sides. Place one-third of the ground meat mixture on top of the bacon. Layer half of the tenderloin on top of the ground meat. Repeat the layers, finishing with a layer of ground meat. Wrap the overhanging bacon over the top of the meat mixture. Cover with the lid to the terrine (or cover the loaf pan tightly with aluminum foil) and place the mold in a large roasting pan. Fill the roasting pan with water so the water comes about halfway up the sides of the terrine mold. Bake for 1½ hours, or until the internal temperature in the center of the loaf reaches 185°F.

6. Remove from the oven. Place the terrine mold on a rimmed baking sheet. Remove the lid and place a brick wrapped in foil or something heavy and clean on top of the meat to weight down and compress it for the proper texture. Allow to sit at room temperature for 1 hour. Place in the refrigerator with the brick still compressing the terrine and chill for at least 1 hour before serving.

Per Serving:

Calories: 442   Fat: 25 g   Protein: 51 g   Carbs: 0 g

2
1 ◣ 3
CARNIVORE

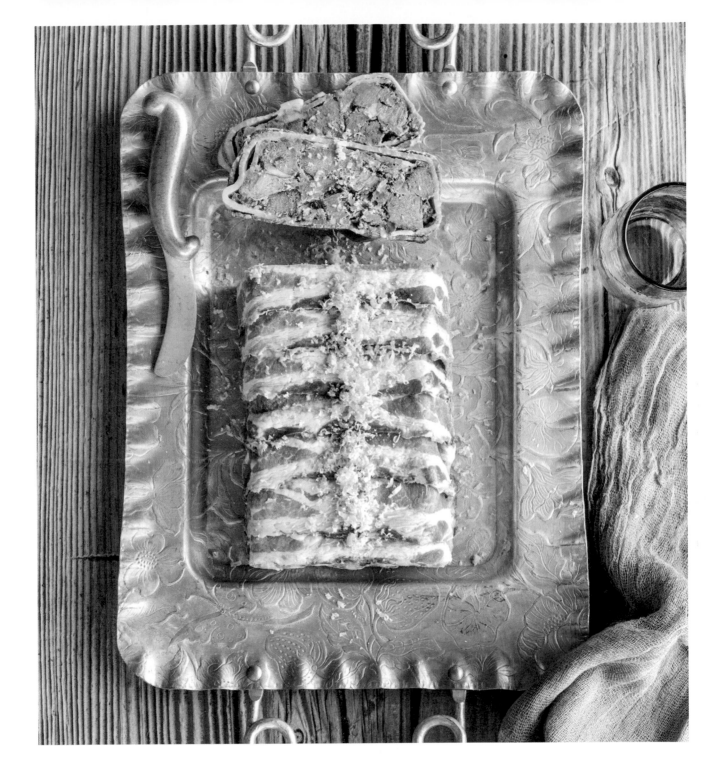

7. To serve, remove the terrine from the mold and cut into ¾-inch slices. Serve chilled or at room temperature.

8. Store in an airtight container in the refrigerator for up to 4 days.

SHORT RIB TERRINE

Yield: 8 servings   **Prep Time:** 10 minutes, plus 1 hour to sit at room temperature
(not including time to make ribs)   **Cook Time:** —

*I use my leftover short ribs to make this delicious terrine. I top it with grated salt-cured egg
yolk for a delicious addition and a pop of color.*

4 cups leftover Smoked
Short Ribs (page 242)

½ cup duck fat or ghee,
softened

½ teaspoon fine sea salt

2 Salt-Cured Egg Yolks
(page 320), grated, for
garnish (optional)

1. Shred the short ribs into very small pieces, then cut into small dice.
Place the chopped short ribs, duck fat, and salt in a large bowl and stir to
combine.

2. Scoop the short rib mixture into a 5-cup terrine mold or crock dish.
Pack it down well using your hands. Refrigerate until ready to serve;
the terrine can be made up to 2 days ahead. Before serving, remove the
terrine from the refrigerator and allow to sit at room temperature for 1
hour. Serve slices garnished with cured egg yolks, if desired.

3. Store in an airtight container in the refrigerator for up to 4 days.

Per Serving (with salt-cured egg yolks):

Calories: 687   Fat: 64 g   Protein: 26 g   Carbs: 0 g

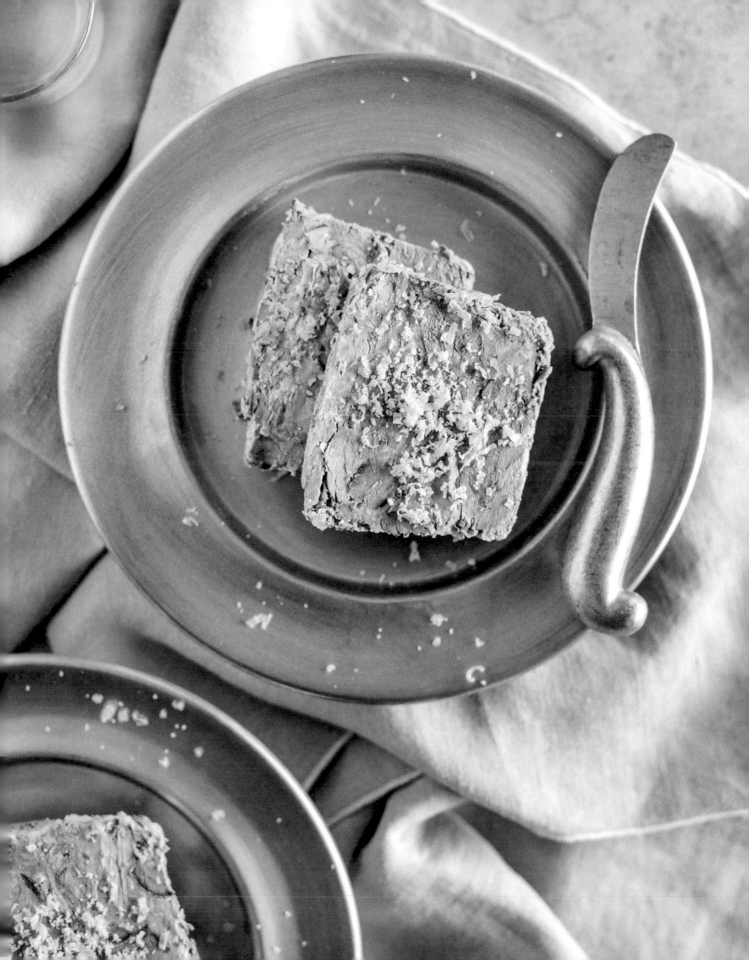

SMOKED BEEF ROAST

Yield: 12 servings   **Prep Time:** 5 minutes, plus 30 minutes to soak wood chips (if using) and 10 minutes to rest   **Cook Time:** 3 hours

Be sure to read the manufacturer's directions for your smoker before you begin. There are wood, electric, propane, and charcoal smokers, and each type works differently. If you do not have a smoker, see page 79 for how to create a smoking technique using your oven or an outdoor grill.

1 (5-pound) boneless beef roast

2½ tablespoons fine sea salt

Special Equipment:
Smoker, wood chips (optional)

1. If using wood chips, cover them with water and allow to soak for 30 minutes. Season the roast on all sides with the salt.

2. Smoke the roast: Start the smoker, following the manufacturer's instructions. If your smoker has a water bowl, add water to it. When the temperature inside the smoker reaches 225°F to 250°F, you can start smoking the roast.

3. Place the roast directly on the smoker rack and secure the lid so that it is airtight and no smoke can escape. Smoke the meat for 3 hours, or until the temperature in the thickest part reaches 135°F for medium-rare meat, or cook longer until it reaches the desired doneness (see the chart on page 180).

4. Remove the roast from the smoker and allow to rest for 10 minutes before slicing.

5. Store in an airtight container in the refrigerator for up to 4 days or in the freezer for up to a month. To reheat, place slices on a rimmed baking sheet in a preheated 350°F oven for 5 minutes, or until heated through.

Per Serving:

Calories: 507   Fat: 33 g   Protein: 49 g   Carbs: 0 g

1 — 2 3 CARNIVORE

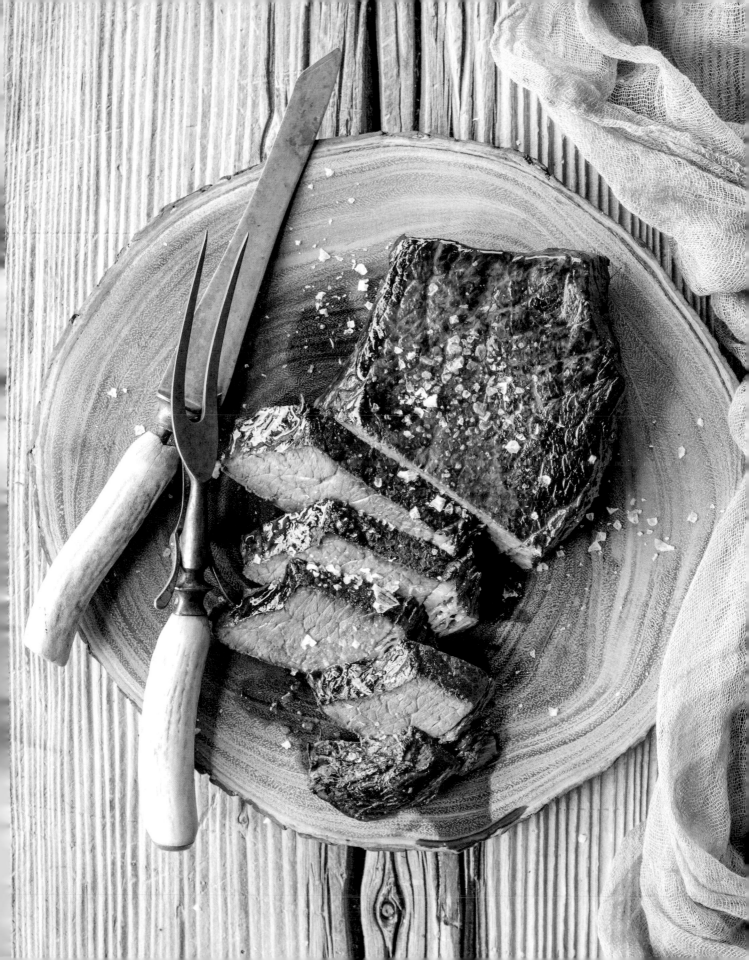

SMOKED SHORT RIBS

Yield: 8 servings   **Prep Time:** 10 minutes, plus 30 minutes to soak wood chips (if using)   **Cook Time:** 4 to 5½ hours

When smoking ribs, I often make extra. After smoking the ribs, I freeze them for easy meals later. I finish the ribs in the oven, which makes them fall apart tender and delicious!

Be sure to read the manufacturer's directions for your smoker before you begin. There are wood, electric, propane, and charcoal smokers, and each type works differently. If you do not have a smoker, see page 79 for how to create a smoking technique using your oven or an outdoor grill.

8 pounds short ribs

Fine sea salt

½ cup Carnivore Beef Bone Broth (page 308), for drizzling

Grated Salt-Cured Egg Yolks (page 320), for garnish (optional)

Special Equipment: Smoker, wood chips (optional)

1. If using wood chips, cover them with water and allow to soak for 30 minutes. Season the ribs on both sides with salt.

2. Smoke the ribs: Start the smoker, following the manufacturer's instructions. If the smoker has a water bowl, add water to it. When the temperature inside the smoker reaches 225°F to 250°F, you can start smoking the ribs.

3. Place the ribs in the smoker and secure the lid so that it is airtight and no smoke can escape. Every so often, check the temperature and adjust the air vents to maintain a temperature of 225°F to 250°F.

4. Smoke the ribs for 2 to 3 hours, depending on how smoky you like them; the longer you smoke them, the more intense the smoke flavor will be. Add more fuel to the smoker if needed to maintain the temperature, or add more soaked wood chips, if using, if the smoke starts to dissipate.

5. Remove the ribs from the smoker. At this point, the meat still needs to be fully cooked at a higher temperature, which is best done on a grill or in the oven. You can either cook the entire amount now or divide the ribs into portions for quick-and-easy meals later. Make packets of ribs and broth as described in Step 6 and store the extra packet(s) in the fridge for up to 3 days or in the freezer for up to a month. (I always have wrapped ribs in my freezer for easy meals I can just toss in the oven.)

Per Serving (without salt-cured egg yolks):

Calories: 560   Fat: 50 g   Protein: 26 g   Carbs: 0 g

CARNIVORE   WITH EGG YOLKS

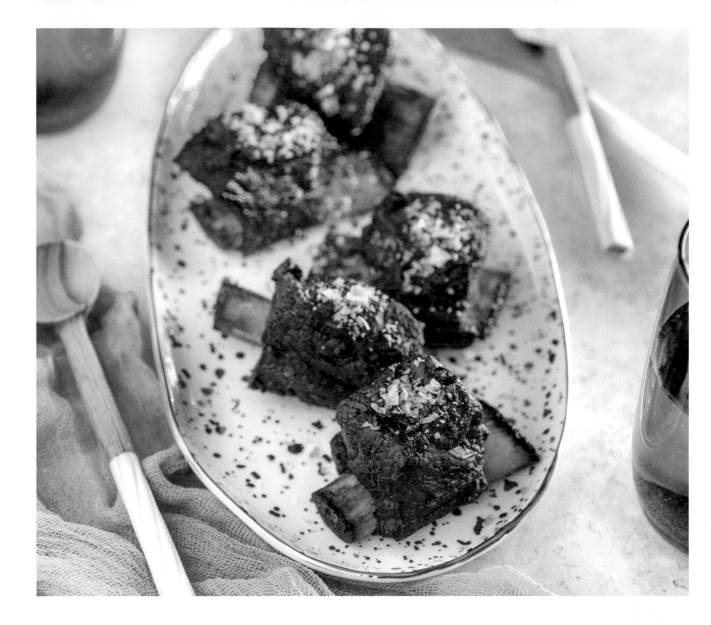

6. Prepare the ribs for cooking: Place a long sheet of aluminum foil on the counter, then cover the foil with a sheet of parchment paper. Transfer the ribs to the parchment-lined foil. Generously sprinkle the ribs with the broth, then tightly seal the foil around the ribs to make a packet. Make sure that there are no holes in the foil or the ribs will dry out.

7. Cook the ribs: Preheat the oven or a grill to 275°F (or medium-low). Place the tightly wrapped ribs in the oven or on the grill and cook for 2 to 2½ hours, until the meat is tender.

8. Remove the foil packets from the oven or grill and turn up the oven or grill to broil/high. Remove the ribs from the foil packets, then place back in the oven with the meaty side up or on the grill with the meaty side down. Broil or grill for 5 minutes to crisp the edges on one side. Serve the ribs garnished with cured egg yolks, if desired.

9. Store extras wrapped tightly in foil in the refrigerator for up to 4 days or in the freezer for up to a month. To reheat, place in a preheated 350°F oven for 8 minutes, or until heated through.

BEEF HEART STEAKS

Yield: 2 servings   **Prep Time:** 5 minutes, plus 2 hours to soak if desired and 15 minutes to come to room temperature and rest   **Cook Time:** 10 minutes

This recipe makes super juicy steaks! Including organ meat in your diet is essential when eating carnivore. If you have a hard time finding beef heart, you can ask your butcher to order it for you. Always request grass-fed meats. I highly suggest soaking the heart slices in Carnivore Bone Broth before cooking to reduce the blood flavor.

2 (8-ounce) slices beef heart, 1 inch thick

1 cup Carnivore Beef Bone Broth (page 308) (optional)

2 teaspoons fine sea salt

2 tablespoons tallow (page 312) or ghee, plus more for serving if desired

1. If you want to soak the heart steaks, put the slices in a casserole dish and pour in the broth. Cover and place in the refrigerator to soak for at least 2 hours. Remove the steaks from the broth and pat dry with a paper towel. Allow to come to room temperature for 10 minutes.

2. If desired, cut the heart steaks into strips. Season them on both sides with the salt.

3. Heat the tallow in a large cast-iron skillet over medium-high heat. Once hot, place the heart steaks in the skillet and cook for 5 minutes. Flip and cook for 5 minutes on the other side, or until cooked to your liking (see the chart on page 180).

4. Remove the steaks from the skillet and allow to rest for 5 minutes before serving. Serve with melted tallow, if desired.

Per Serving (with broth):

Calories: 509   Fat: 25 g   Protein: 63 g   Carbs: 0 g

2
1 ╱╲ 3   1 ╱╲ 3
CARNIVORE   IF USING GHEE

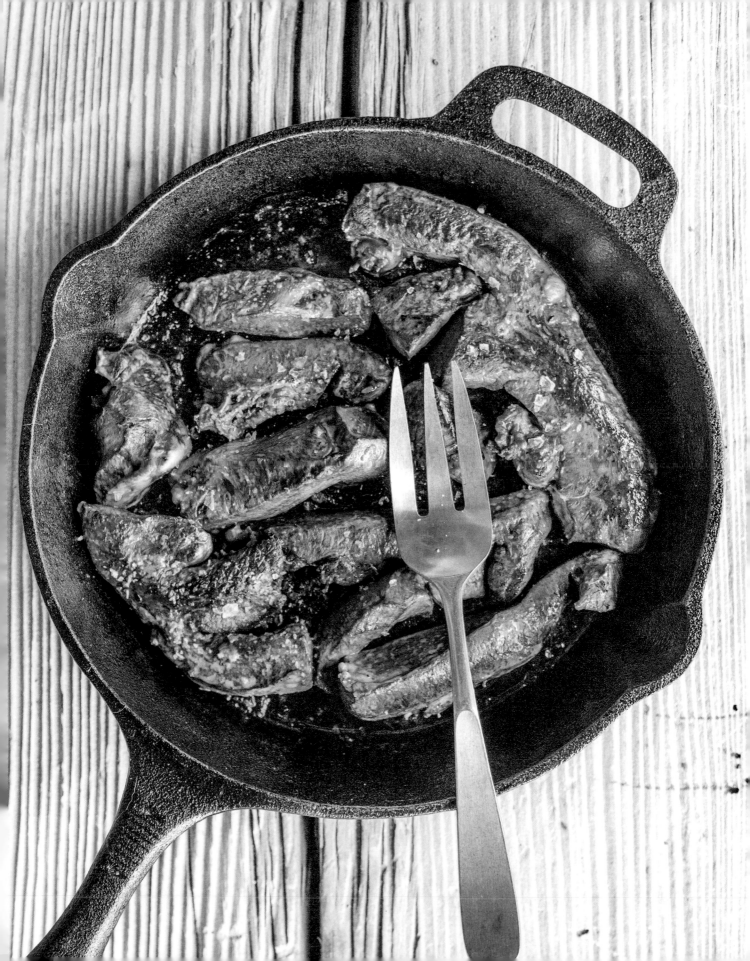

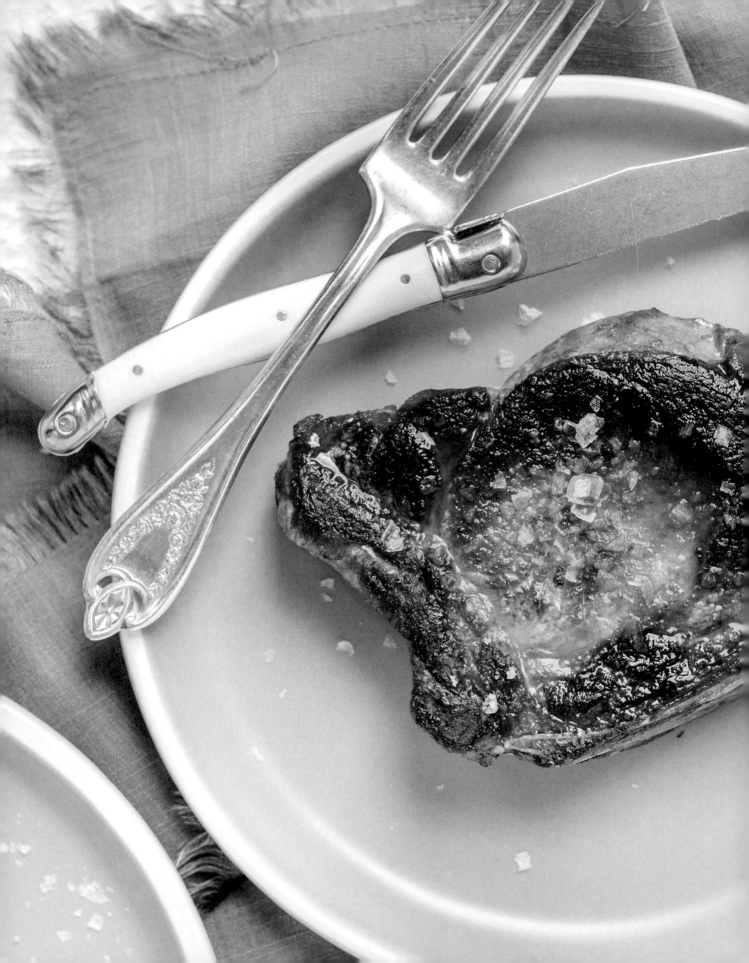

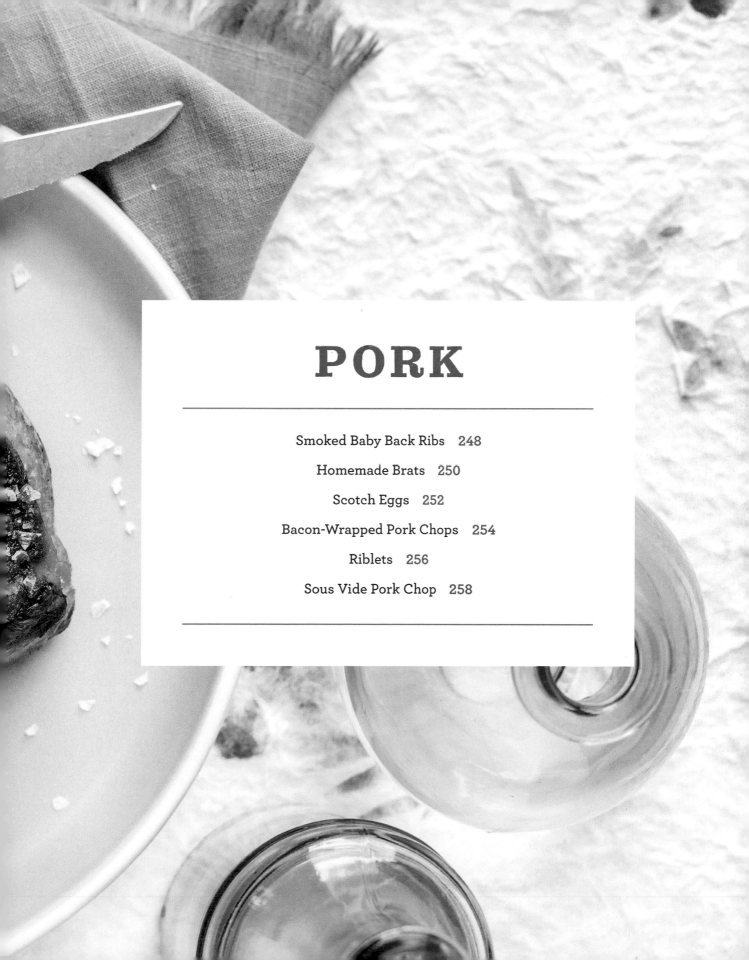

PORK

SMOKED BABY BACK RIBS

Yield: 8 servings **Prep Time:** 10 minutes, plus 30 minutes to soak wood chips (if using) **Cook Time:** 4 to 5½ hours

Be sure to read the manufacturer's directions for your smoker before you begin. There are wood, electric, propane, and charcoal smokers, and each type works differently. When slow-cooking meat, it is essential that you have a thermometer to monitor the temperature inside the smoker. If you do not have a smoker, see page 79 for how to create a smoking technique using your oven or an outdoor grill.

4 full racks baby back ribs

Fine sea salt

½ cup Carnivore Beef Bone Broth (page 308), for drizzling

Special Equipment:
Smoker, wood chips (optional)

1. If using wood chips, cover them with water and allow to soak for 30 minutes. Liberally season the ribs on both sides with salt.

2. Smoke the ribs: Start the smoker, following the manufacturer's instructions. If your smoker has a water bowl, add water to it. When the temperature inside the smoker reaches 225°F to 250°F, you can start smoking the ribs.

3. Place the ribs in the smoker and secure the lid so that it is airtight and no smoke can escape. Every so often, check the temperature and adjust the air vents to maintain a temperature of 225°F to 250°F.

4. Smoke the ribs for 2 to 3 hours, depending on how smoky you like them; the longer you smoke them, the more intense the smoke flavor will be. Add more fuel to the smoker if needed to maintain the temperature, or add more soaked wood chips, if using, if the smoke starts to dissipate.

5. Remove the ribs from the smoker. At this point, the meat still needs to be fully cooked at a higher temperature, which is best done on a grill or in the oven. You can either cook the entire amount now or divide the ribs into portions and store what you're not going to eat right away for quick-and-easy meals later. Make packets of ribs and broth as described in Step 6 and store the extra packet(s) in the fridge for up to 3 days or in the freezer for up to a month. (I always have wrapped ribs in my freezer for easy meals I can just toss in the oven.)

Per Serving:

Calories: 702 Fat: 54 g Protein: 54 g Carbs: 0 g

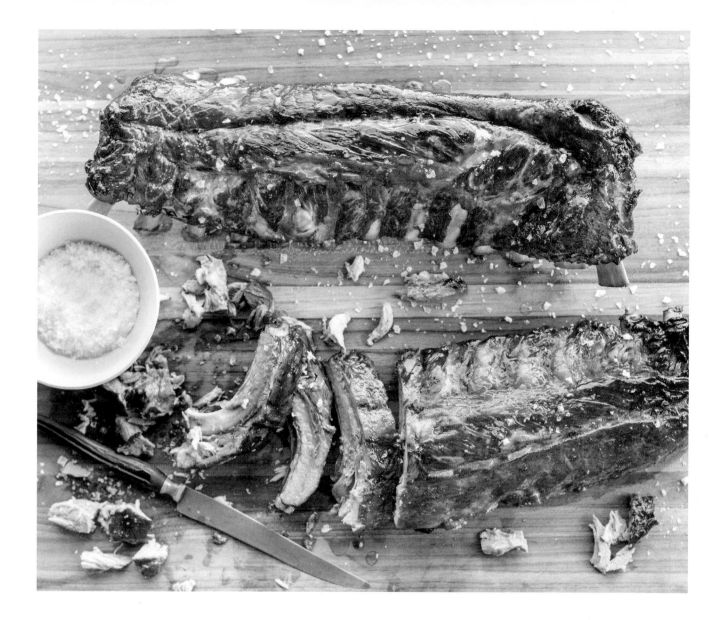

6. Prepare the ribs for cooking: Place a long sheet of aluminum foil on the counter, then cover the foil with a sheet of parchment paper. Transfer the ribs to the parchment-lined foil. Evenly sprinkle the ribs with the broth, then tightly seal the foil around the ribs to make a packet. Make sure that there are no holes in the foil or the ribs will dry out.

7. Cook the ribs: Preheat the oven or a grill to 275°F (or medium-low). Place the tightly wrapped ribs in the oven or on the grill and cook for 2 to 2½ hours, until the meat is tender.

8. Remove the foil packets from the oven or grill and turn up the oven or grill to broil/high. Remove the ribs from the foil packets, then place back in the oven with the meaty side up or on the grill with the meaty side down. Broil or grill for 5 minutes to crisp the edges on one side.

9. Store extras wrapped tightly in foil in the refrigerator for up to 4 days or in the freezer for up to a month. To reheat, place in a preheated 350°F oven for 8 minutes, or until heated through.

HOMEMADE BRATS

Yield: twelve 4½-ounce brats (1 per serving)
Prep Time: 20 minutes, plus 4 hours to chill   **Cook Time:** 10 minutes

If you use cold meat and fat when making bratwurst and other types of sausage, the sausage won't turn mushy. In fact, commercial sausage makers often add dry ice to the meat to keep it cold. After cubing the meat, place it either in the freezer for 1 hour or in the refrigerator for 4 hours or up to overnight before grinding. After grinding, place the bowl in the freezer for 30 minutes to keep the meat cold while stuffing the casings.

Liquid is needed to bind protein to fat. The more liquid you add to your sausage, the more fat you can add. For great flavor and added nutrients, homemade Carnivore Bone Broth is best for the liquid. But good-quality store-bought broth will work, too. If the brats pop out of the casings when you bite into them, you cooked them too fast and at too high a heat.

2 pounds pork butt

8 ounces pork fatback

6 feet medium hog casings (optional)

8 ounces ground beef

⅓ cup ice-cold Carnivore Beef Bone Broth (page 308)

1 tablespoon fine sea salt

1 tablespoon lard or tallow (page 312), for the pan

Special Equipment:
Meat grinder (or grinder attachment on stand mixer); sausage stuffer (optional)

1. Line a rimmed baking sheet with parchment paper. Cut the pork butt and fatback into 1-inch cubes and spread out on the lined baking sheet. Freeze for 1 hour.

2. Meanwhile, fill a large bowl with 2 quarts of water. Soak the casings in the liquid for 30 minutes.

3. Remove the pork butt and fatback from the freezer and grind it using the coarse disk of a meat grinder (or grinder attachment on a stand mixer). Transfer the ground pork butt and fatback to a large bowl.

4. Add the ground beef, broth, and salt to the bowl with the ground pork mixture and mix everything together until evenly combined. Put a small dab of the meat mixture in a skillet over medium heat and cook until no longer pink inside, then taste the sausage. Add more salt to the sausage mixture, if desired.

5. Load a sausage stuffer, or a sausage stuffer attachment on a stand mixer, with the presoaked casings and stuff the sausages by pushing the meat mixture through the stuffer. Twist the brats into links about 5 inches in length. (*Note:* If you do not have a sausage stuffer, you can form the meat into 12 large patties.)

Per Serving:

Calories: 310   Fat: 25 g   Protein: 20 g   Carbs: 0 g

1 2 3
CARNIVORE

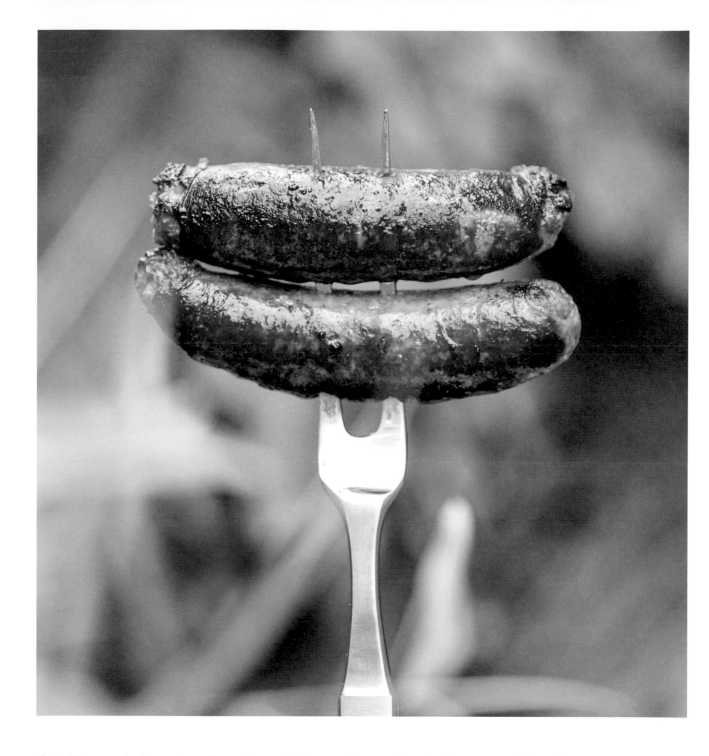

6. Refrigerate the brats for at least 3 hours before cooking to allow the flavors to meld; cook them within 3 days.

7. To cook the brats, melt the lard in a large skillet over medium heat. Poke a few small holes in each brat. Cook for 10 minutes, until the outsides of the brats are browned and the internal temperature reaches 160°F.

8. Store the cooked brats in an airtight container in the refrigerator for up to 5 days or in the freezer for up to a month.

SCOTCH EGGS

Yield: 4 servings
Prep Time: 12 minutes   **Cook Time:** 15 minutes

2 pounds ground pork or ground beef

2 teaspoons fine sea salt

8 large soft-boiled eggs, peeled (see page 266)

8 thin slices prosciutto

1. Preheat the oven or an air fryer to 400°F. If using the oven, line a rimmed baking sheet with parchment paper.

2. Place the ground pork in a large bowl and add the salt. Use your hands to work the salt into the meat. Divide the seasoned pork into 8 equal portions.

3. Flatten each portion of the seasoned pork into a patty and place a peeled egg in the center. Mold the pork around the egg. Wrap a slice of prosciutto around each pork-wrapped egg. Repeat with the remaining pork, eggs, and prosciutto.

4. Place the wrapped eggs on the lined baking sheet or in the air fryer basket. Cook for 15 minutes, or until the pork is cooked through and the prosciutto is crispy.

5. Store in an airtight container in the refrigerator for up to 1 week or in the freezer for up to a month. To reheat, place in a preheated 400°F oven or air fryer for 3 minutes, or until heated through.

Per Serving:

Calories: 793   Fat: 60 g   Protein: 78 g   Carbs: 1 g

1 2 3
CARNIVORE

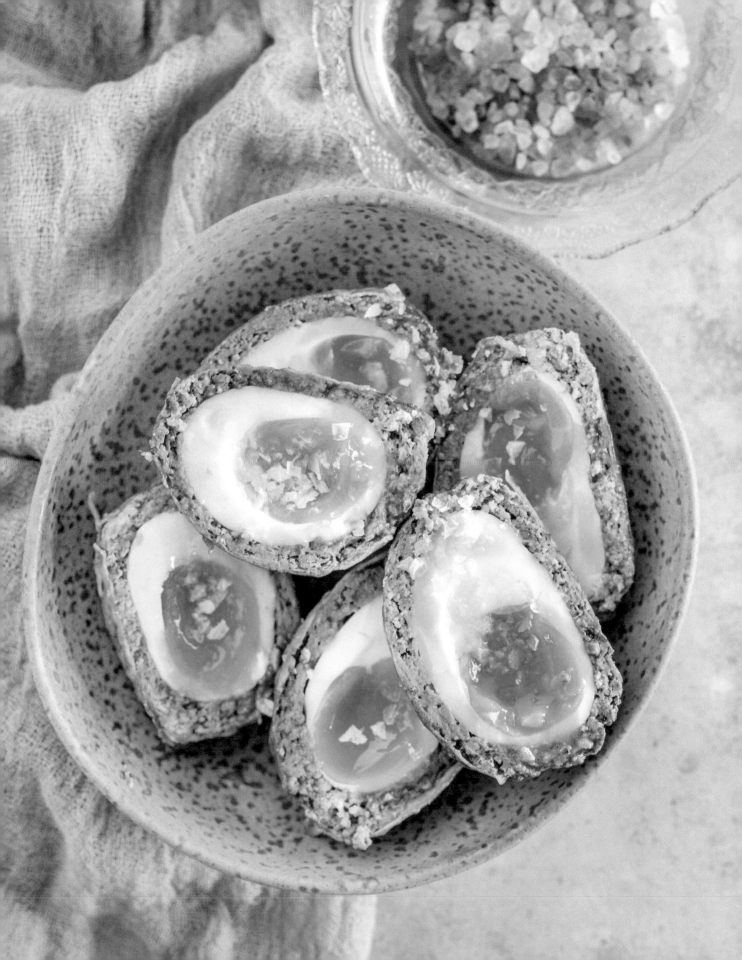

BACON-WRAPPED PORK CHOPS

Yield: 4 servings
Prep Time: 10 minutes   **Cook Time:** 20 minutes

8 thin slices pork or beef bacon

4 boneless pork chops, about ¾ inch thick

1. Preheat the oven or an air fryer to 400°F.

2. Wrap 2 strips of bacon around each pork chop and secure the ends with toothpicks. Place the bacon-wrapped chops on a rimmed baking sheet or in the air fryer basket. Cook for 18 to 20 minutes, flipping the chops over after 10 minutes, until the bacon is crisp and the pork is cooked through.

3. Store in an airtight container in the refrigerator for up to 3 days. To reheat, place on a rimmed baking sheet in a preheated 400°F oven or air fryer for 5 minutes, or until warmed through.

Per Serving:

Calories: 380   Fat: 28 g   Protein: 30 g   Carbs: 0 g

1 2 3
CARNIVORE

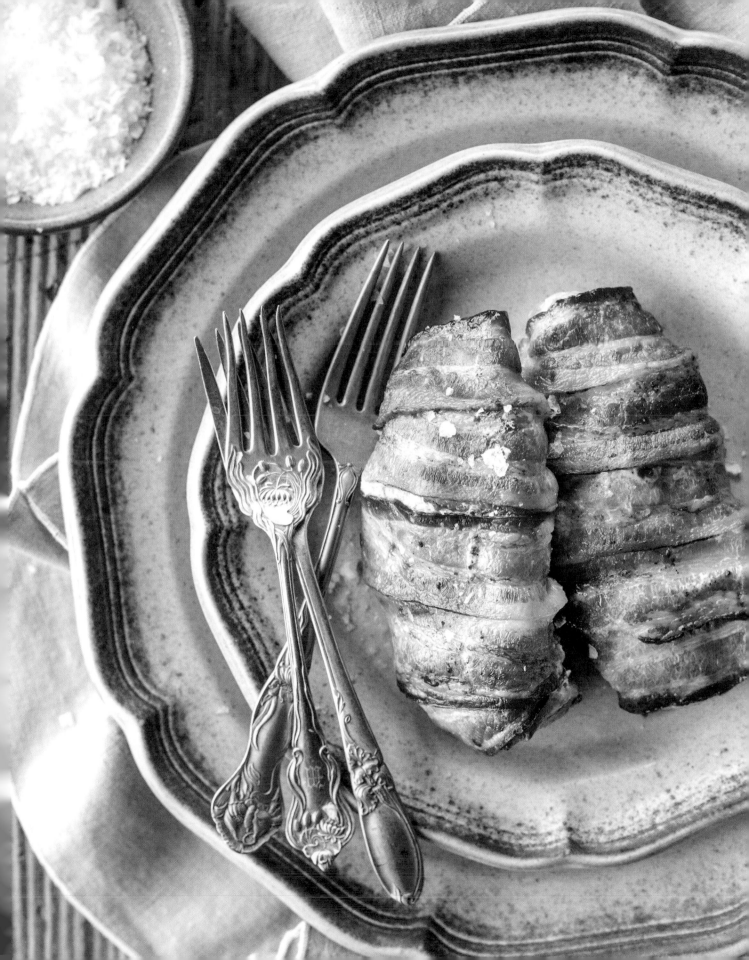

RIBLETS

Yield: 4 servings
Prep Time: 10 minutes **Cook Time:** 25 minutes

1 rack pork spare ribs

3 teaspoons smoked sea salt, store-bought or homemade (page 310), divided

½ cup Carnivore Beef Bone Broth (page 308)

1. Preheat the oven to 350°F. Cut the rack of ribs into individual riblets with one bone each.

2. Season the riblets on all sides with 2 teaspoons of the salt and place in a casserole dish. Bake for 10 minutes.

3. Add the broth and the remaining 1 teaspoon of smoked salt to the casserole dish, place the dish back in the oven, and bake for another 15 minutes, or until the pork is cooked through and the internal temperature reaches 145°F.

4. Store in an airtight container in the refrigerator for up to 4 days. To reheat, place in a casserole dish in a preheated 350°F oven or air fryer for 5 minutes, or until heated through.

Per Serving:

Calories: 297 Fat: 25 g Protein: 17 g Carbs: 0 g

1 — 2 — 3
CARNIVORE

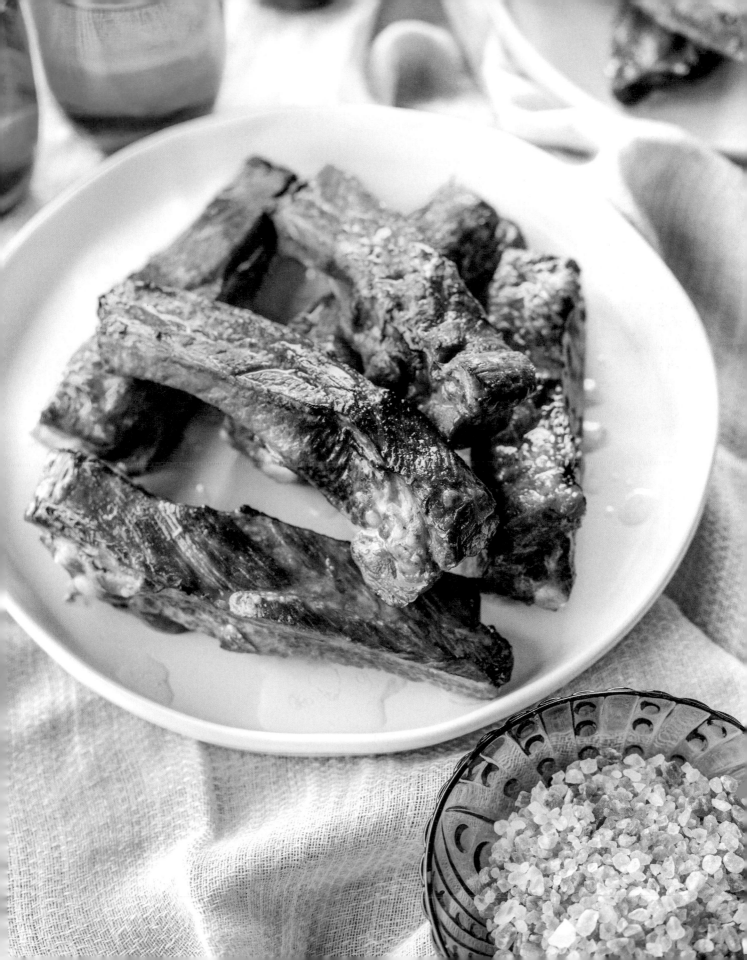

SOUS VIDE PORK CHOP

Yield: 1 serving
Prep Time: 5 minutes **Cook Time:** 47 minutes

If you grew up eating chewy pork chops like I did, you simply must try this way of cooking them! You will have the juiciest chops you've ever tasted. If you don't have a sous vide machine, however, I've also provided oven directions below.

Using a sous vide machine is one way to make meats moist and tender. I am not a gadget girl, but I do love cooking in my sous vide. If you do invest in a sous vide machine, I highly suggest downloading the free app called Joule. It helps guide you in whatever you are cooking. You just select the meat (pork chop, chicken breast, tenderloin) and how you want it cooked (rare, medium-rare, medium, medium-well, or well-done), and the app will tell you when the meat has finished cooking.

With this app on my phone, I can leave the house without worrying that the meat is overcooking while I'm gone. The first time I used my sous vide machine, I made a venison tenderloin. I placed it in the machine, set my Joule app, and then went out to bow hunt. My phone alerted me when the tenderloin was finished and told me that the machine would hold it at that temperature without overcooking the tenderloin for 90 minutes. If you have ever cooked a tenderloin, you know that it's very easy to overcook. When I finished hunting, I came back home to enjoy a delicious juicy tenderloin.

1 bone-in pork chop, about ¾ inch thick

¾ teaspoon fine sea salt

1½ teaspoons tallow (page 312) or bacon fat

1. Fill a large pot with water. Set the sous vide machine to 140°F and place it into the pot of water. Season the pork chop on both sides with the salt. Place the chop in the sous vide bag. Seal the bag, making sure no air pockets remain in the bag.

2. Select Pork Chop on the Joule app on your phone, if using, then select your desired doneness. Place the bag in the water bath. Cook until done, about 45 minutes. (*Note:* The machine will hold the chop at the perfect temperature for 90 minutes, so don't worry if you are not home when it is finished.)

3. Heat the tallow in a cast-iron skillet over medium-high heat. Once the skillet is hot, remove the pork chop from the bag and place in the hot oil. Sear on both sides, about 1 minute per side, until golden brown and a crust forms. Remove from the heat, allow to rest for 5 minutes, and serve.

Per Serving:

Calories: 305 Fat: 23 g Protein: 22 g Carbs: 0 g

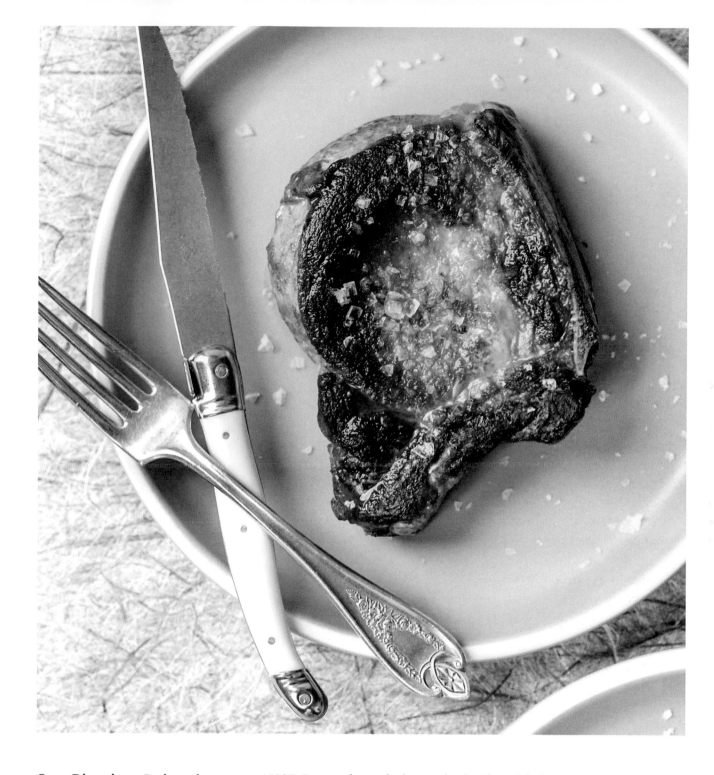

Oven Directions: Preheat the oven to 450°F. Season the pork chop on both sides with the salt. Heat the tallow in a cast-iron skillet over medium-high heat. Once the skillet is hot, add the seasoned chop and cook for 1½ minutes, or until golden brown, then flip and cook for another 1½ minutes. Use a potholder to transfer the skillet to the oven to cook for 5 minutes. Remove from the oven and allow the chop to rest for 5 minutes before serving.

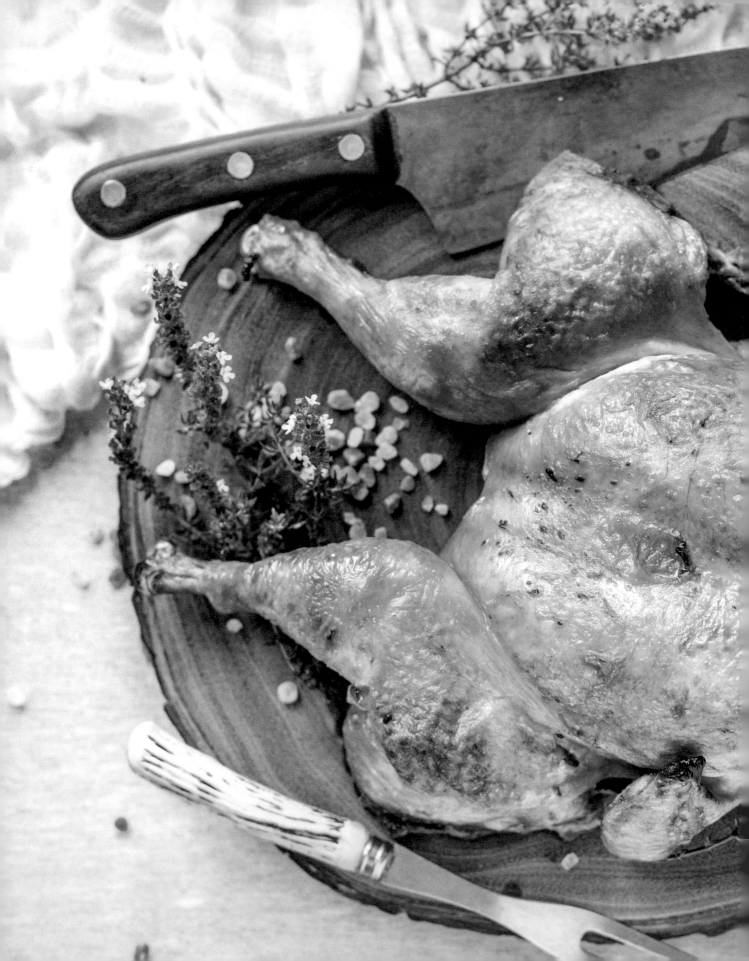

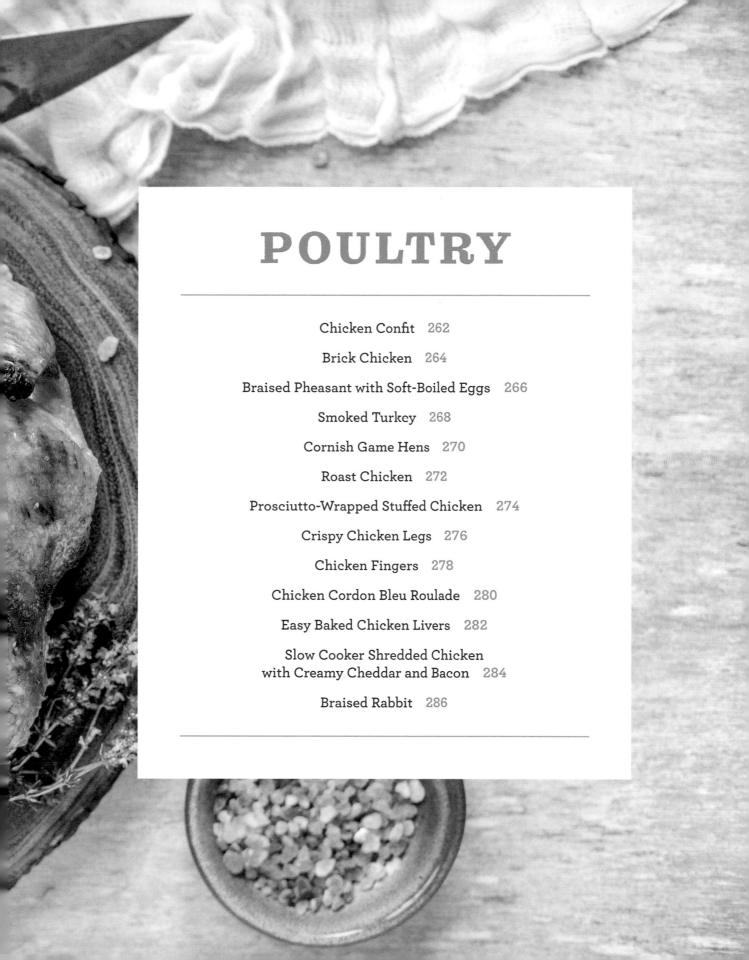

POULTRY

CHICKEN CONFIT

Yield: 4 servings   **Prep Time:** 8 minutes, plus up to 2 days to cure
Cook Time: 3 hours 5 minutes

I love duck confit, but sometimes duck is hard to find, so I make chicken confit instead. It is a delicious way to prepare chicken. The duck fat makes it so tender and delicious! I like to make a double batch and freeze the extras in two containers for easy dinners later.

3 tablespoons fine sea salt, divided

4 chicken legs with thighs, patted dry

4¼ cups duck fat or lard, divided

1. Sprinkle 1 tablespoon of the salt in a dish large enough to lay the chicken legs in a single layer. Place the chicken in the dish skin side up, then sprinkle the remaining 2 tablespoons of salt over the legs. Cover and refrigerate for 1 to 2 days to help draw moisture into the chicken.

2. When ready to cook the chicken, preheat the oven to 225°F.

3. Melt 4 cups of the duck fat in a medium saucepan over medium heat. Remove the dish containing the chicken from the refrigerator and wipe the salt off the chicken. Place the chicken legs close together, in a single layer, in a 10-inch square baking dish with high sides. Pour the melted fat over the chicken so that all the pieces are covered.

4. Bake the chicken for 2½ to 3 hours, until fork-tender. Remove the chicken from the baking dish. Let the duck fat cool and store for later use; it will keep in the pantry for up to 5 days or in the refrigerator for up to 4 weeks.

5. Heat the remaining ¼ cup of duck fat in a large cast-iron skillet over high heat. Once hot, place the chicken skin side down in the skillet and fry until golden brown, about 5 minutes, flipping halfway through. Remove from the skillet and serve.

6. Store in an airtight container in the refrigerator for up to 4 days or in the freezer for up to 3 months. To reheat, place in a greased skillet over medium-high heat for 5 minutes, flipping halfway through, or until heated through.

Per Serving:

Calories: 373   Fat: 28 g   Protein: 19 g   Carbs: 0 g

CARNIVORE

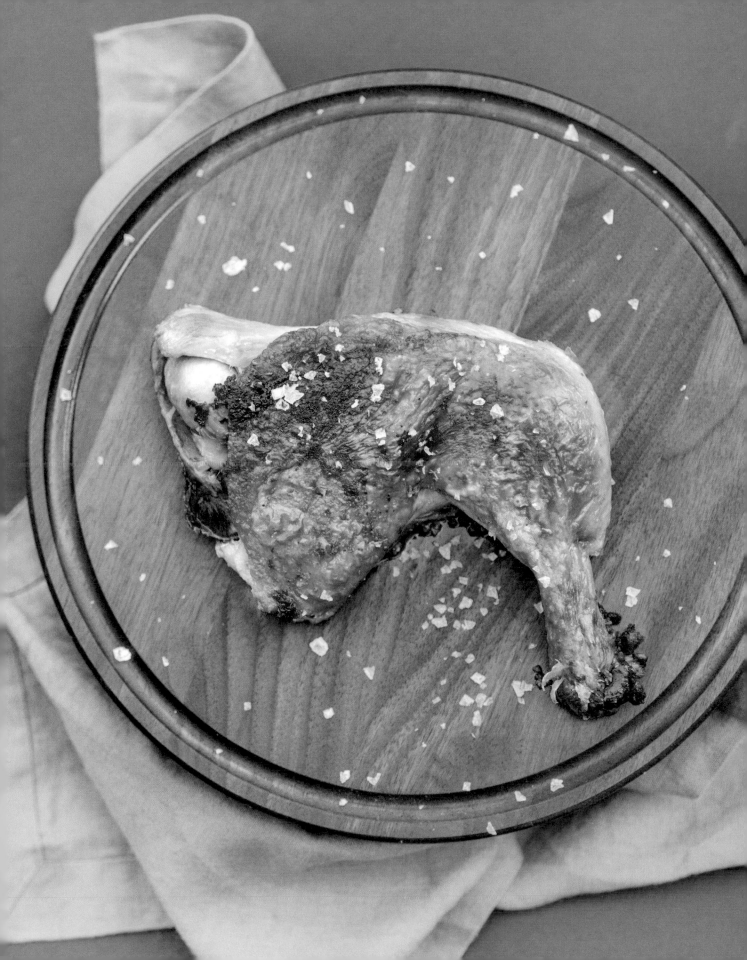

BRICK CHICKEN

Yield: 6 servings
Prep Time: 10 minutes, plus 10 minutes to rest   **Cook Time:** 30 minutes

Brick chicken is a great way to get a crispy skin by weighting it down with a heavy object. I use bricks that are wrapped in aluminum foil, but you could use a heavy salt block or other heavy object instead.

1 (3-pound) chicken

3 tablespoons ghee, softened, divided

3½ teaspoons fine sea salt

1. Preheat the oven to 500°F. Wrap two large bricks in aluminum foil.

2. Clean the chicken and pat it dry with a paper towel. Use kitchen shears to cut down both sides of the backbone of the chicken. Remove the backbone and discard. From the inside, cut through the breastbone until the chicken opens easily.

3. Place the chicken skin side down on a cutting board and, using your hands, press down hard to open the chicken like a book, making it as flat as possible. Rub the chicken all over with 2 tablespoons of the ghee. Season all over with the salt.

4. Heat the remaining tablespoon of ghee in a large cast-iron skillet over medium-high heat. Once hot, put the chicken skin side down in the skillet. Place the wrapped bricks on top of the chicken and press into the skillet. Cook for 5 minutes.

5. Leaving the bricks on the chicken, carefully transfer the skillet to the oven. Bake for 15 minutes.

6. Remove the skillet from the oven, then remove the bricks. Flip the chicken over, return the skillet to the oven, and cook for another 8 to 10 minutes, until the chicken is cooked through and no longer pink inside and the internal temperature in the breast reaches 170°F.

7. Remove the chicken from the skillet and allow to rest for 10 minutes before slicing and serving.

8. Store in an airtight container in the refrigerator for up to 4 days. To reheat, place in a lightly greased skillet over medium-high heat for 3 minutes per side, or until heated through.

Per Serving:

Calories: 615   Fat: 40 g   Protein: 63 g   Carbs: 0 g

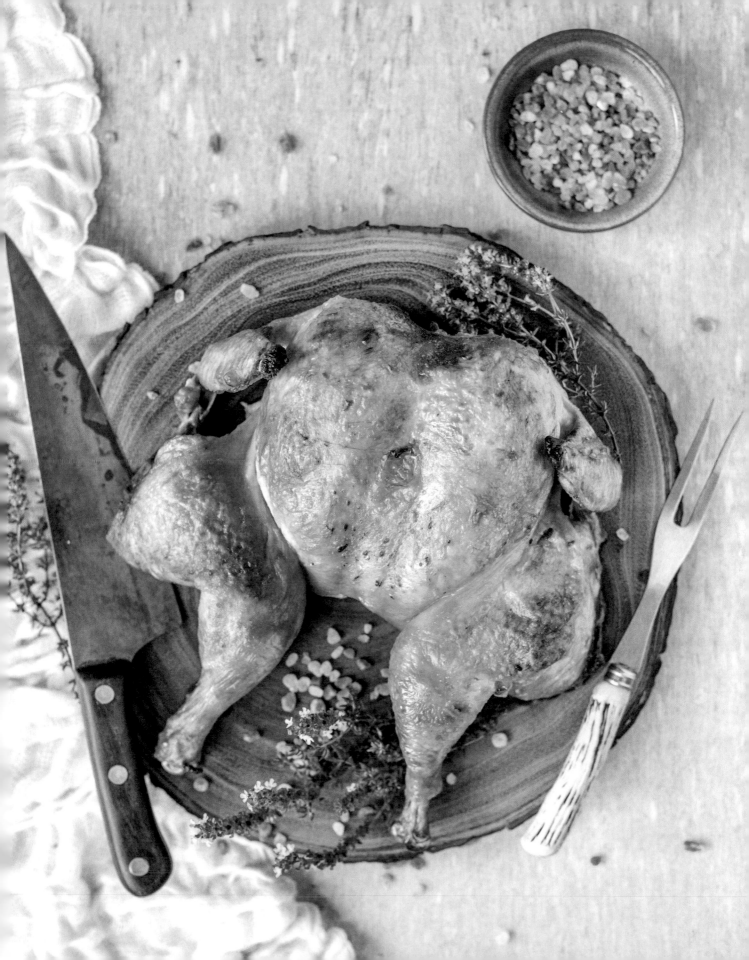

BRAISED PHEASANT WITH SOFT-BOILED EGGS

Yield: 4 servings
Prep Time: 10 minutes   **Cook Time:** 36 minutes

I grew up hunting pheasant, and this is one of my favorite recipes that uses it. If you can't find pheasant, you can substitute chicken thighs.

2 ounces pancetta or bacon, diced

8 skin-on pheasant thighs or chicken thighs

1½ teaspoons smoked sea salt, store-bought or homemade (page 310)

1 cup Carnivore Chicken Bone Broth (page 308)

4 large eggs

1. Heat a large cast-iron skillet over medium heat. When the skillet is hot, add the pancetta and cook for 3 minutes, or until crispy. Remove the pancetta, leaving the drippings in the skillet.

2. Pat the pheasant dry with a paper towel. Season the pheasant thighs with the salt. Place the thighs skin side down in the skillet and cook for 4 minutes, or until the skin is browned and crispy. Flip the thighs over and cook for 4 minutes on the other side.

3. Pour in the broth and reduce the heat to low. Simmer, uncovered, for 20 to 25 minutes, until the thighs are cooked through and tender and the internal temperature reaches 170°F.

4. Meanwhile, soft-boil the eggs: Fill a medium saucepan about halfway with water. Bring to a boil, then add the eggs. Cover, turn off the heat, and allow the eggs to cook in the hot water for 6 minutes. After 6 minutes, remove the eggs and rinse under cold water. Gently peel the eggs.

5. Place the cooked pheasant thighs with the pan drippings on a serving platter and garnish with the pancetta. Cut the soft-boiled eggs in half to serve with the pheasant.

6. Store in an airtight container in the refrigerator for up to 4 days. To reheat, place in a lightly greased skillet over medium-high heat for 3 minutes per side, or until heated through.

Per Serving:

Calories: 461   Fat: 26 g   Protein: 53 g   Carbs: 0.4 g

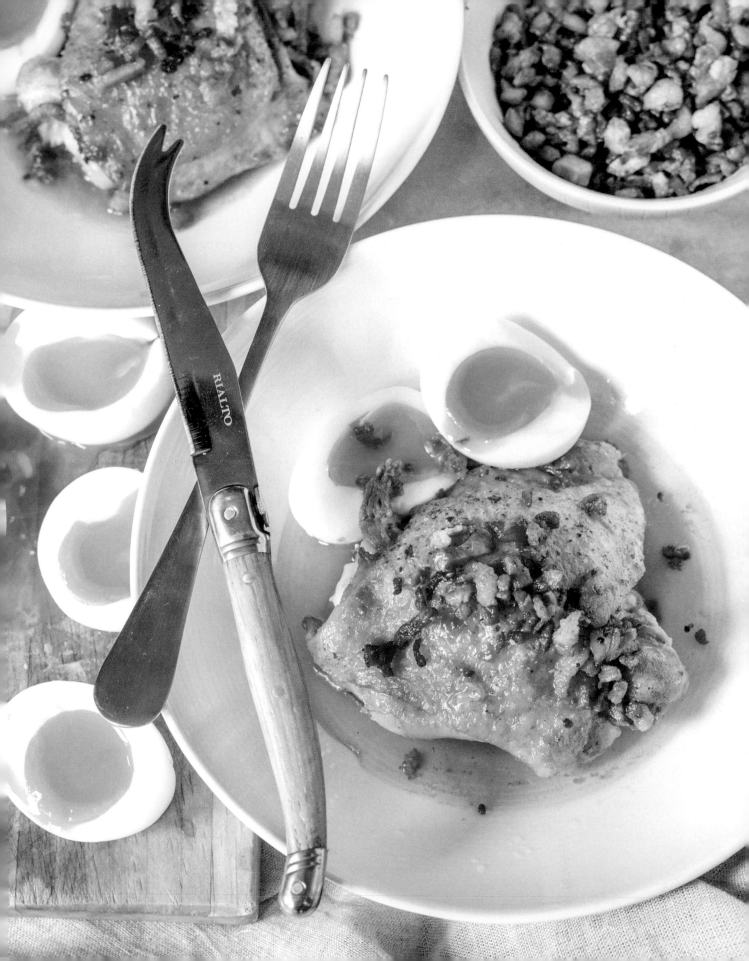

SMOKED TURKEY

Yield: 12 servings   **Prep Time:** 10 minutes, plus 30 minutes to soak wood chips (if using)   **Cook Time:** 10 hours

I'm not a fan of plain turkey, but smoked turkey is amazing! I like to make smoked turkey for Thanksgiving. Be sure to read the manufacturer's directions for your smoker before you begin. There are wood, electric, propane, and charcoal smokers, and each type works differently. If you do not have a smoker, see page 79 for how to create a smoking technique using your oven or an outdoor grill.

1 (10-pound) turkey

2 tablespoons fine sea salt

Special Equipment:
Smoker, wood chips
(optional)

1. If using wood chips, cover them with water and allow to soak for 30 minutes.

2. Clean the turkey and pat it dry with paper towels. Sprinkle the salt all over the turkey.

3. Smoke the turkey: Start the smoker, following the manufacturer's instructions. If your smoker has a water bowl, add water to it. When the temperature inside the smoker reaches 225°F to 250°F, you can start smoking the turkey.

4. Place the turkey in the smoker and secure the lid so that it is airtight and no smoke can escape. Smoke the turkey for 10 hours, or until the internal temperature in the thickest part of the breast reaches 180°F. Every so often, check the temperature and adjust the air vents to maintain a temperature of 225°F to 250°F. Add more fuel to the smoker if needed to maintain the temperature, or add more soaked wood chips if the smoke starts to dissipate.

5. Remove the turkey from the smoker. Slice and serve.

6. Store in an airtight container in the refrigerator for up to 4 days or in the freezer for up to a month. Serve warm or chilled. To reheat, place in a preheated 300°F oven for 8 minutes, or until heated through.

Per Serving:

Calories: 453   Fat: 11 g   Protein: 82 g   Carbs: 0 g

1 2 3
CARNIVORE

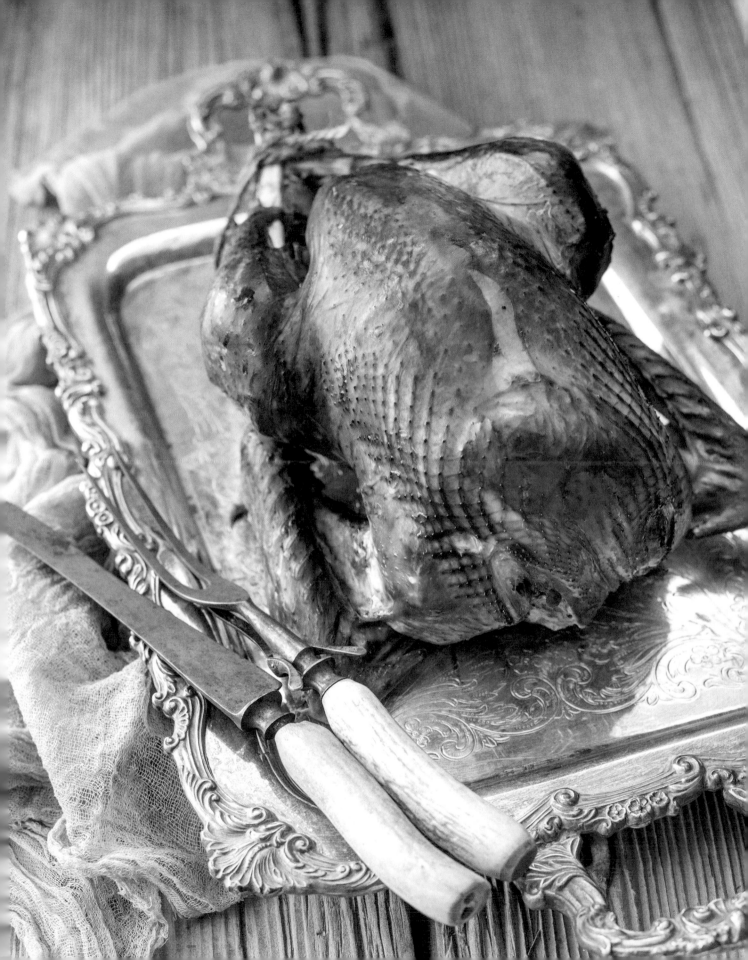

CORNISH GAME HENS

Yield: 4 servings
Prep Time: 12 minutes, plus 10 minutes to rest   **Cook Time:** 25 minutes

This is a lovely dish that would be great to serve at a dinner party. I like Cornish game hens because they are much more tender than most other poultry.

2 (1-pound) Cornish game hens

2 tablespoons lard or tallow (page 312), melted

3 teaspoons smoked sea salt, store-bought or homemade (page 310), or fine sea salt

1. Preheat the oven or an air fryer to 400°F.

2. Clean the hens and pat them dry with a paper towel. Brush them with the melted lard, then season them with the salt.

3. Place the hens on a rimmed baking sheet or in the air fryer basket with the breasts facing up. Cook for 25 minutes, flipping after 15 minutes, or until the skin is golden brown and the internal temperature in the breast reaches 170°F.

4. Remove the hens from the oven or air fryer and allow to rest for 10 minutes before slicing and serving.

5. Store in an airtight container in the refrigerator for up to 5 days or in the freezer for up to a month. To reheat, place in a baking dish in a preheated 350°F oven or air fryer for 5 minutes, or until heated through.

Per Serving:

Calories: 454   Fat: 34 g   Protein: 34 g   Carbs: 0 g

1 — 2 — 3
CARNIVORE

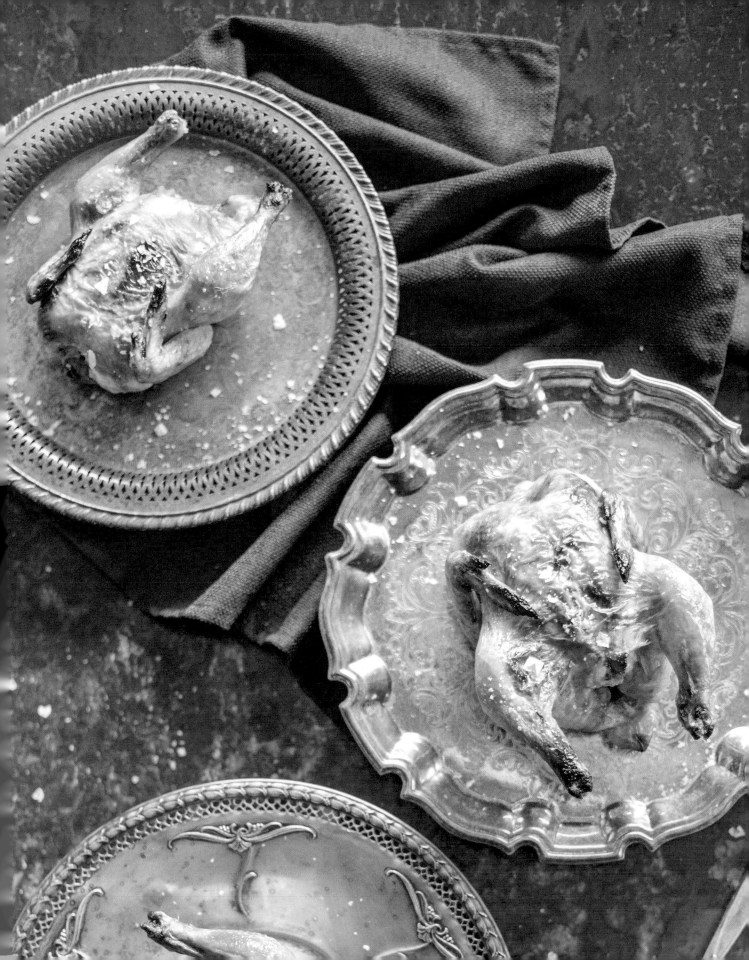

ROAST CHICKEN

Yield: 12 servings
Prep Time: 5 minutes   **Cook Time:** 55 minutes

This roasting recipe gives you a rotisserie-style chicken without using a rotisserie!

1 (4½-pound) chicken

2 tablespoons lard or tallow (page 312), melted, plus more if needed

1½ tablespoons smoked sea salt, store-bought or homemade (page 310), or fine sea salt

1. Preheat the oven or an air fryer to 325°F. If using the oven, line a rimmed baking sheet with parchment paper. If using an air fryer, grease the air fryer basket with lard.

2. Clean the chicken and pat it dry with a paper towel. Brush the bird with the melted lard and season it with the salt.

3. Place the chicken on the lined baking sheet or in the greased air fryer basket with the breast facing up. Cook for 30 minutes, then use heat-safe kitchen gloves to flip the chicken so that the legs are facing up. Cook for another 25 minutes, or until the internal temperature in the breast reaches 165°F.

4. Store in an airtight container in the refrigerator for up to 4 days or freeze for up to a month. To reheat, place in a preheated 350°F oven or air fryer for 5 minutes, or until warmed through.

Per Serving:

Calories: 384   Fat: 28 g   Protein: 32 g   Carbs: 0 g

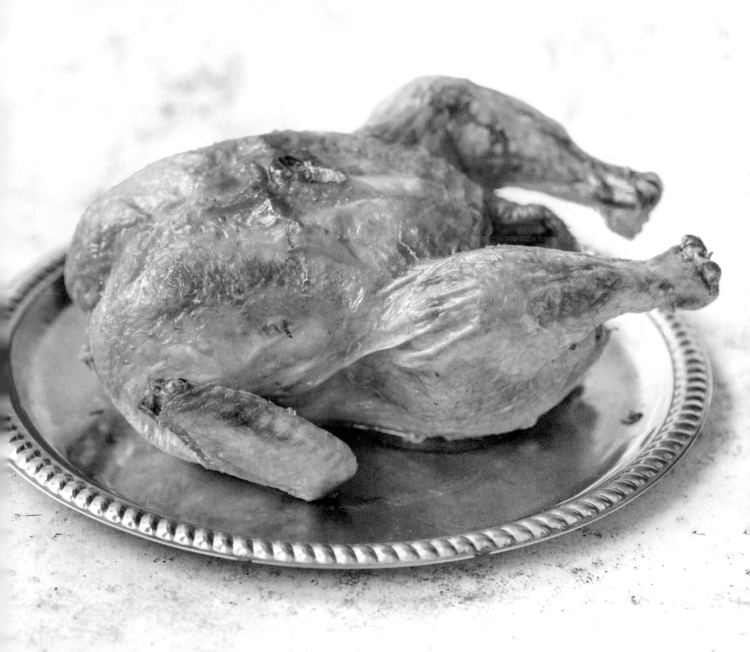

PROSCIUTTO-WRAPPED STUFFED CHICKEN

Yield: 4 servings
Prep Time: 10 minutes   **Cook Time:** 20 minutes

4 (8-ounce) boneless, skinless chicken breast halves

8 ounces Brie, rind removed

8 thin slices prosciutto

1. Preheat the oven or an air fryer to 400°F.

2. Place a chicken breast on a cutting board. Take a sharp knife and, holding it parallel to the chicken, make a 1-inch-wide incision at the top of the breast. Carefully cut into the breast to form a large pocket, leaving a ½-inch border along the sides and bottom. Repeat with the remaining breasts.

3. Use a large spoon to stuff the cheese into the pockets in the chicken, dividing the cheese evenly among them. Wrap 2 strips of prosciutto around each breast and secure the ends with toothpicks.

4. Place the wrapped chicken on a rimmed baking sheet or in the air fryer basket. Cook for 18 to 20 minutes, flipping after 10 minutes, until the prosciutto is crisp, the chicken is cooked through, and the internal temperature in the breast reaches 170°F.

5. Store in an airtight container in the refrigerator for up to 4 days. To reheat, place in a preheated 400°F oven or air fryer for 5 minutes, or until warmed through.

Per Serving:

Calories: 684   Fat: 39 g   Protein: 78 g   Carbs: 0 g

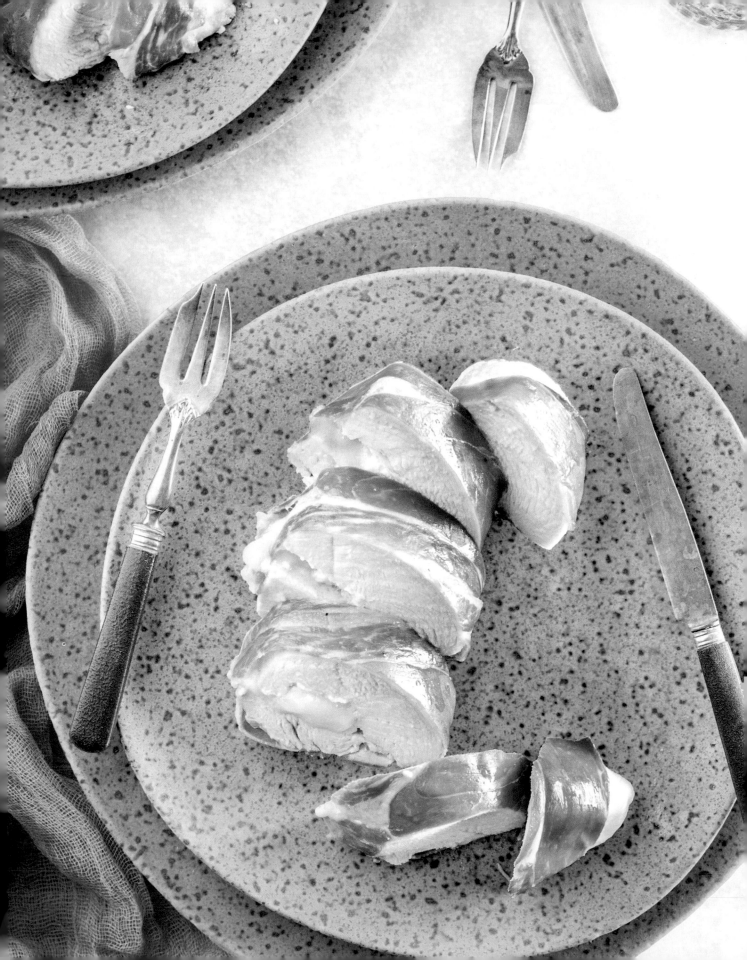

CRISPY CHICKEN LEGS

Yield: 2 servings (2 legs per serving)
Prep Time: 8 minutes   **Cook Time:** 25 minutes

This recipe uses a carnivore-friendly Parmesan cheese coating to make a "fried" chicken without all the carbs! (Use pork dust instead if you need to be dairy-free.)

Duck fat or lard, for greasing the air fryer

1 large egg

½ cup powdered Parmesan cheese or pork dust (for dairy-free)

4 chicken legs

1. Preheat the oven or an air fryer to 400°F. If using the oven, line a rimmed baking sheet with parchment paper. If using an air fryer, grease the air fryer basket with duck fat.

2. Place the egg in a shallow bowl and lightly beat with a fork. Place the powdered Parmesan cheese in a separate shallow bowl. Dip the chicken legs into the beaten egg, then into the Parmesan. Use your hands to press the cheese onto the chicken to form a nice crust.

3. Place the chicken legs on the lined baking sheet or in the air fryer basket. Cook for 25 minutes, flipping after 15 minutes, or until the chicken is cooked through and the internal temperature reaches 180°F. Remove from the oven or air fryer and serve.

4. Store in an airtight container in the refrigerator for up to 3 days. To reheat, place in a preheated 400°F oven or air fryer for 5 minutes, or until warmed through.

Per Serving:

Calories: 637   Fat: 38 g   Protein: 68 g   Carbs: 1 g

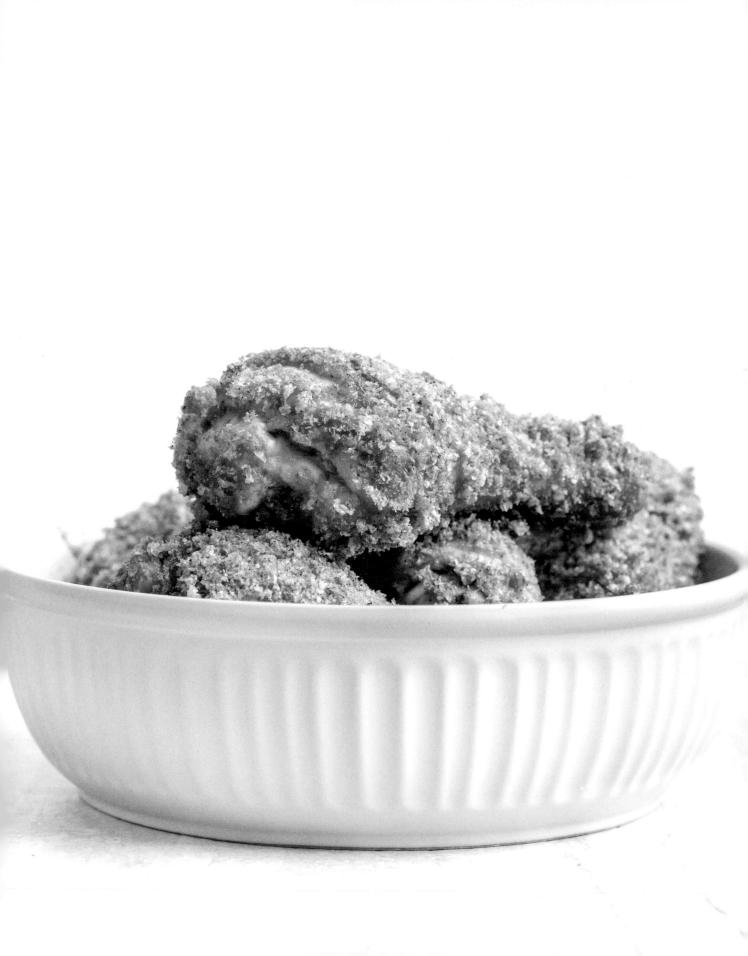

CHICKEN FINGERS

Yield: 4 servings
Prep Time: 8 minutes   **Cook Time:** 10 minutes

My boys love these chicken fingers, which have a delicious crispy coating. I like to make a double batch and store the extras in the fridge for easy lunches for them.

Duck fat or lard, for greasing the air fryer

2 large eggs, beaten

1 cup powdered Parmesan cheese or pork dust (for dairy-free)

1 pound boneless, skinless chicken breasts, cut into 3 by 1½-inch pieces

1. Preheat the oven or an air fryer to 400°F. If using the oven, line a rimmed baking sheet with parchment paper. If using an air fryer, grease the air fryer basket with duck fat.

2. Place the eggs in a medium bowl and lightly beat with a fork. Place the powdered Parmesan cheese in another medium bowl. Dip the chicken fingers into the eggs, then into the Parmesan. Use your hands to press the cheese onto the chicken to form a nice crust.

3. Place the chicken fingers on the lined baking sheet or in the greased air fryer basket. Cook for 10 minutes, flipping after 5 minutes. Remove from the oven or air fryer and serve.

4. Store in an airtight container in the refrigerator for up to 4 days. To reheat, place in preheated 400°F oven or air fryer for 3 minutes, or until heated through.

Per Serving:

Calories: 329   Fat: 16 g   Protein: 42 g   Carbs: 1 g

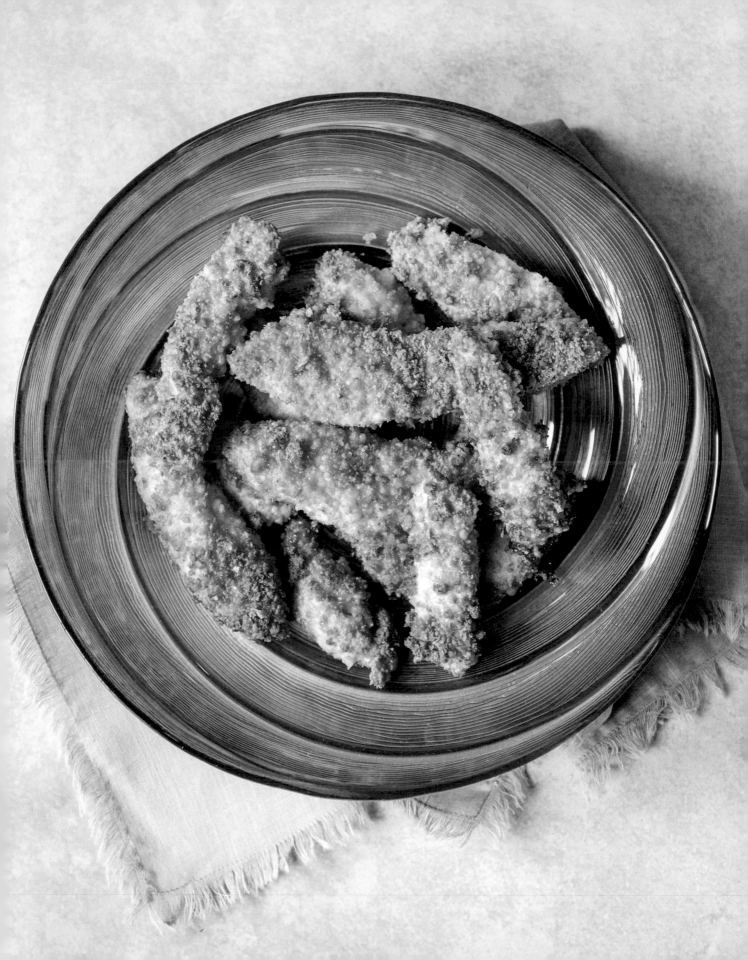

CHICKEN CORDON BLEU ROULADE

Yield: 4 servings
Prep Time: 10 minutes, plus 10 minutes to rest   **Cook Time:** 30 minutes

I ask my butcher to pound the chicken for me to make this roulade recipe very quick and easy to prepare.

4 small (4-ounce) boneless, skinless chicken breast halves, pounded to ¼-inch thickness

1½ teaspoons fine sea salt

4 thin slices deli ham

4 thin slices provolone cheese

1 tablespoon unsalted butter or ghee

1. Preheat the oven or an air fryer to 350°F. If using the oven, line a rimmed baking sheet with parchment paper.

2. Season the chicken on all sides with the salt. Lay a slice of ham and a slice of cheese on a chicken breast and roll up tightly. Secure with toothpicks and brush with melted butter. Repeat with the remaining chicken, ham, cheese, and butter.

3. Place the rolled chicken on the lined baking sheet or in the air fryer basket. Cook for 30 minutes, or until the internal temperature reaches 165°F. Remove the roulade from the oven or air fryer and allow to rest for 10 minutes before serving.

4. Store in an airtight container in the refrigerator for up to 4 days. To reheat, place in a preheated 350°F oven or air fryer for 5 minutes, or until warmed through.

Per Serving:

Calories: 318   Fat: 17 g   Protein: 38 g   Carbs: 1 g

1 2 3 CARNIVORE

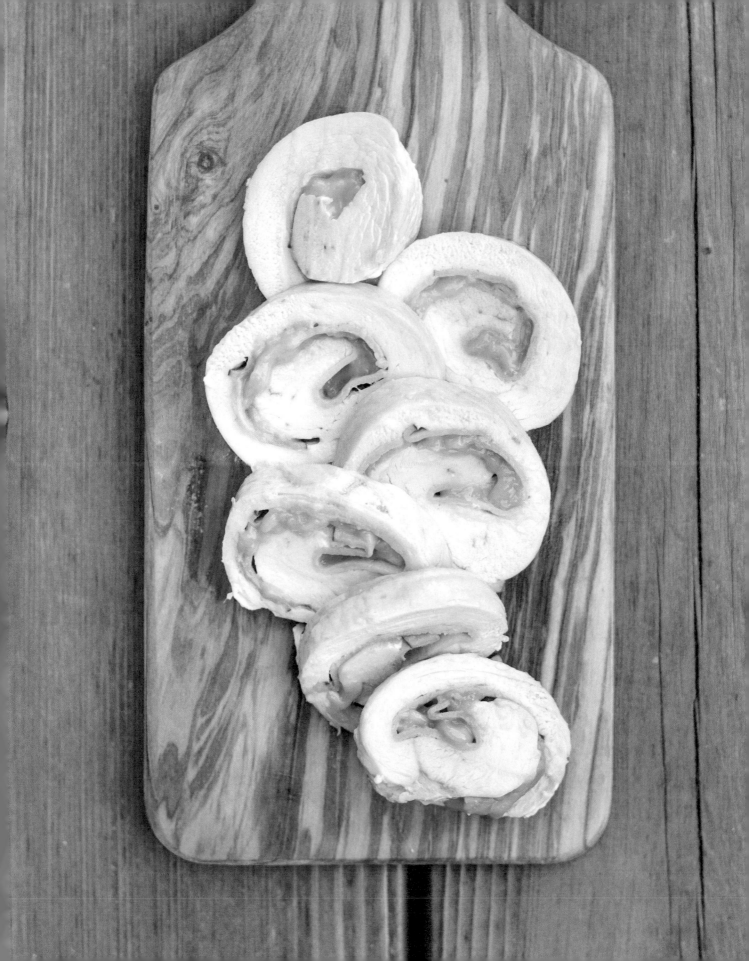

EASY BAKED CHICKEN LIVERS

OPTION

Yield: 4 servings
Prep Time: 5 minutes   **Cook Time:** 10 minutes

Chicken livers are readily available at most grocery stores. This baked version is delicious and very tender!

1 pound chicken livers

1 teaspoon fine sea salt

Bacon Mayonnaise (page 318), for serving (optional)

1. Preheat the oven or an air fryer to 400°F.

2. Rinse the chicken livers and pat dry with a paper towel. Season on all sides with the salt.

3. Place the livers on a rimmed baking sheet or in the air fryer basket and cook for 10 minutes, flipping after 5 minutes, or until cooked through. Properly cooked livers are pink in the center. Remove the livers from the oven or air fryer and serve with mayonnaise, if desired.

4. The livers are best served fresh; however, they can be stored in an airtight container in the refrigerator for up to 3 days. To reheat, place in a cast-iron skillet over medium-high heat for 3 minutes, or until warmed through.

Per Serving (without mayonnaise):

Calories: 154   Fat: 8 g   Protein: 19 g   Carbs: 0 g

CARNIVORE   WITH MAYO

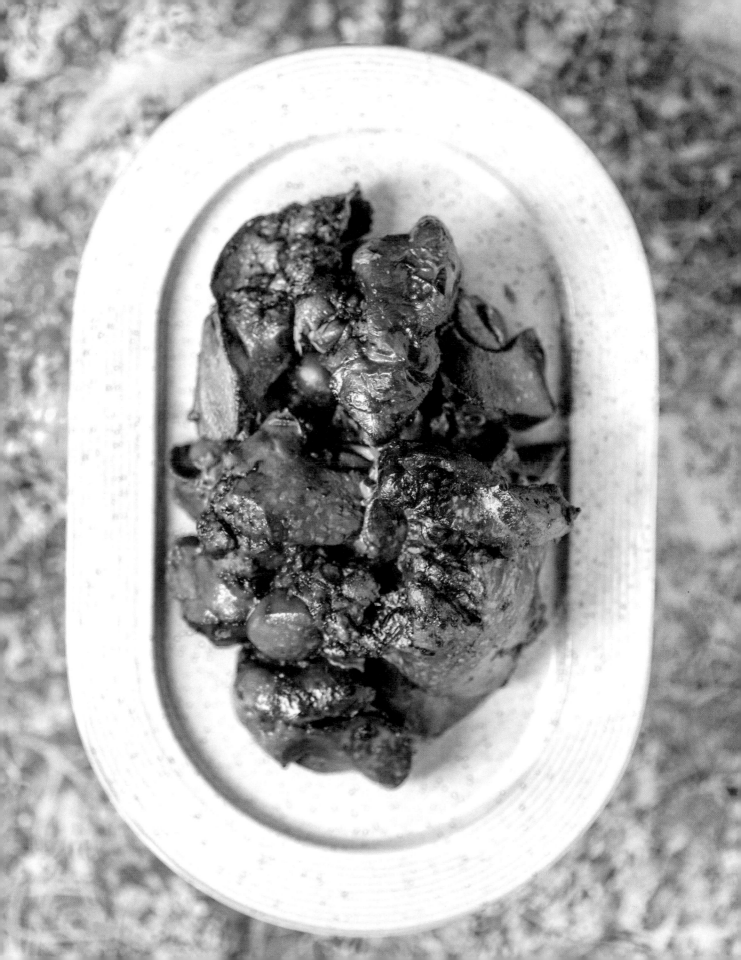

SLOW COOKER SHREDDED CHICKEN WITH CREAMY CHEDDAR AND BACON

Yield: 4 servings
Prep Time: 5 minutes   **Cook Time:** 4 to 8 hours

Often, after-school activities make it hard for everyone to sit down together for a family meal. I love using my slow cooker for easy dinners that my family can eat whenever they get hungry.

½ cup Carnivore Chicken Bone Broth (page 308)

½ cup heavy cream

2 ounces cheddar cheese, shredded (about ½ cup)

1 teaspoon fine sea salt

4 (6-ounce) boneless, skinless chicken breast halves, or 4 boneless, skinless chicken thighs

12 slices pork or beef bacon, diced

1. Place the broth, cream, cheese, and salt in a 4-quart or larger slow cooker. Stir well to combine. Add the chicken. Cover and cook on low for 6 to 8 hours or on high for 4 hours, until the chicken is fork-tender.

2. Meanwhile, cook the bacon: Heat a large cast-iron skillet over high heat. Place the diced bacon in the hot skillet and cook, stirring often with a wooden spoon, for 4 minutes, or until the bacon is crispy. Remove from the skillet, place on a paper towel–lined plate, and set aside.

3. Shred the chicken with two forks. Place the shredded chicken in serving bowls and top with the creamy cheddar sauce from the slow cooker. Garnish with the bacon crumbles.

4. Store in an airtight container in the refrigerator for 4 days. To reheat, place in a casserole dish in a 350°F oven for 7 minutes, or until heated through.

Per Serving:

Calories: 624   Fat: 45 g   Protein: 54 g   Carbs: 1 g

1 — 2 — 3 CARNIVORE

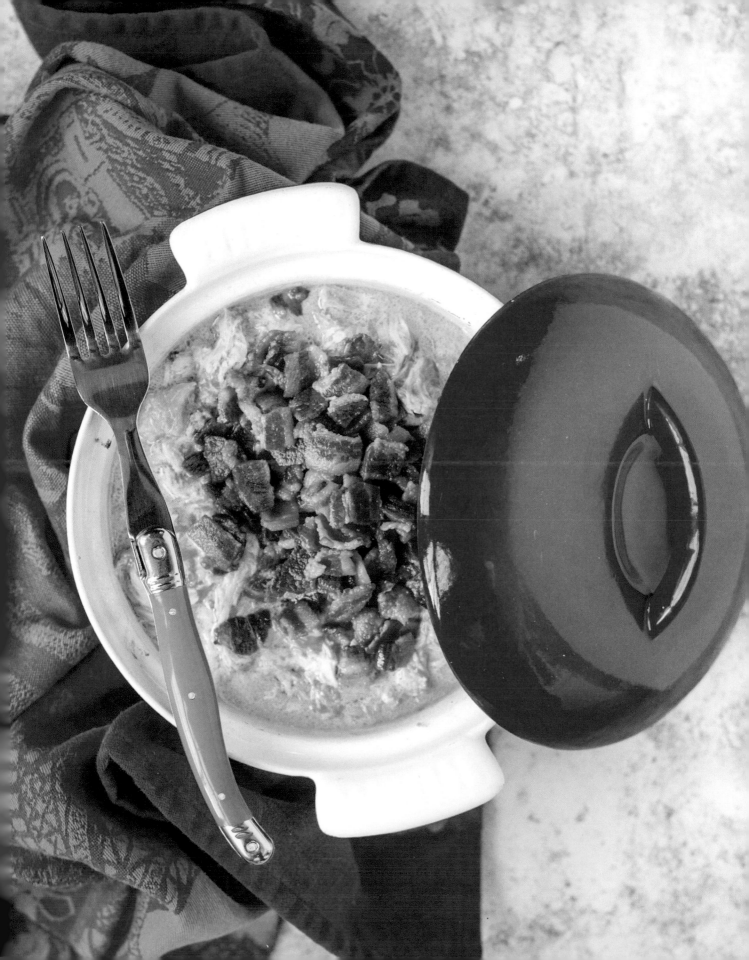

BRAISED RABBIT

Yield: 8 servings
Prep Time: 5 minutes   **Cook Time:** 55 minutes

Eating rabbit may be new to you. It reminds me of chicken—that's why I placed the recipe here in the poultry chapter. You can ask your butcher to cut the rabbit into portions for you, or it is quite simple to do at home. Start by removing the front legs. Next, place the rabbit belly side down and slice along one side of the spine and down the ribcage to cut each loin. Cut each loin in half and then cut the hind legs off so you have eight equal portions. If you don't want to try rabbit, you can prepare this recipe with a 2½-pound chicken instead.

¼ cup tallow (page 312) or bacon fat

1 (2½-pound) rabbit, cut into 8 equal portions

1 tablespoon fine sea salt

2 cups Carnivore Bone Broth (page 308), beef or chicken version

1. Heat the tallow in a large cast-iron skillet over medium-high heat. Season the rabbit pieces on all sides with the salt. Once the skillet is hot, add the meat and cook for 6 minutes, flipping after 3 minutes.

2. Pour in the broth and bring to a boil. Cover, reduce the heat to medium-low, and simmer for 35 to 40 minutes, until the rabbit is tender and the internal temperature reaches 160°F.

3. Remove the meat from the skillet and place on a serving platter to rest. Bring the pan juices to a boil over medium-high heat, whisking often. Reduce the heat to medium-low and simmer for 10 minutes, or until thickened. Spoon the sauce over the meat before serving.

4. Store in an airtight container in the refrigerator for 4 days. To reheat, place in a casserole dish with ½ cup of chicken broth in a preheated 350°F oven for 5 to 8 minutes, or until heated through.

Per Serving:

Calories: 360   Fat: 19 g   Protein: 44 g   Carbs: 0 g

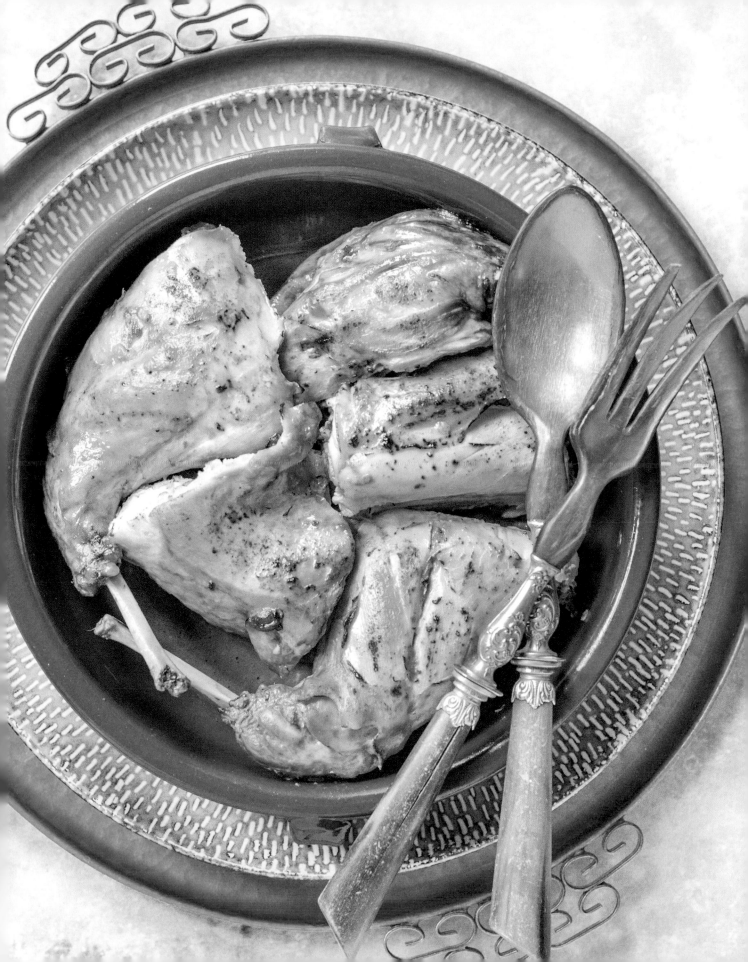

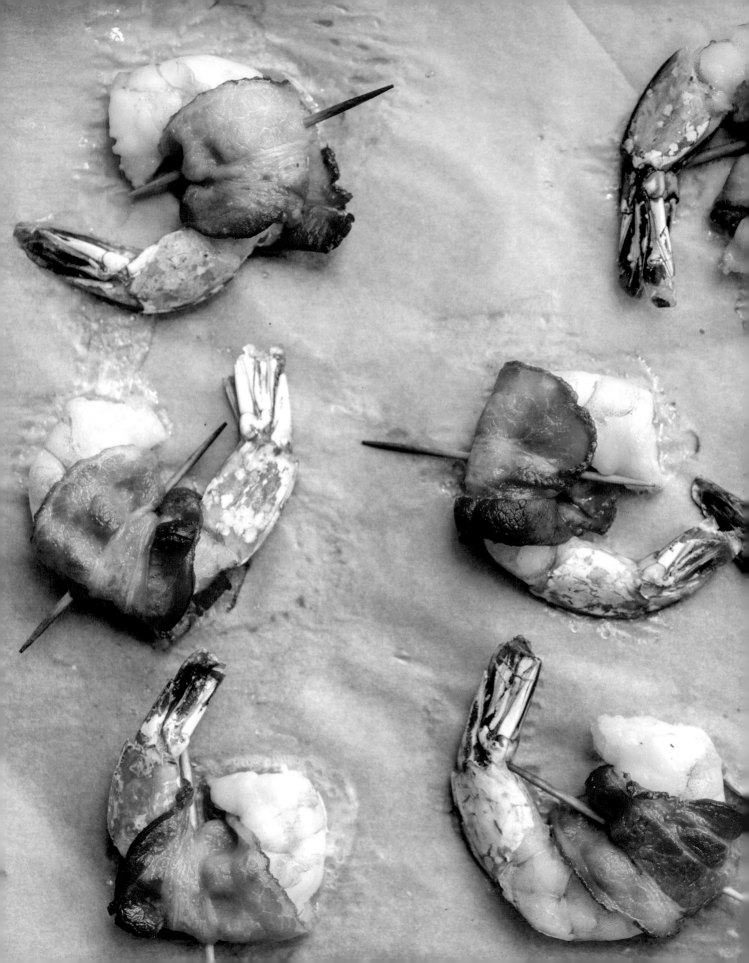

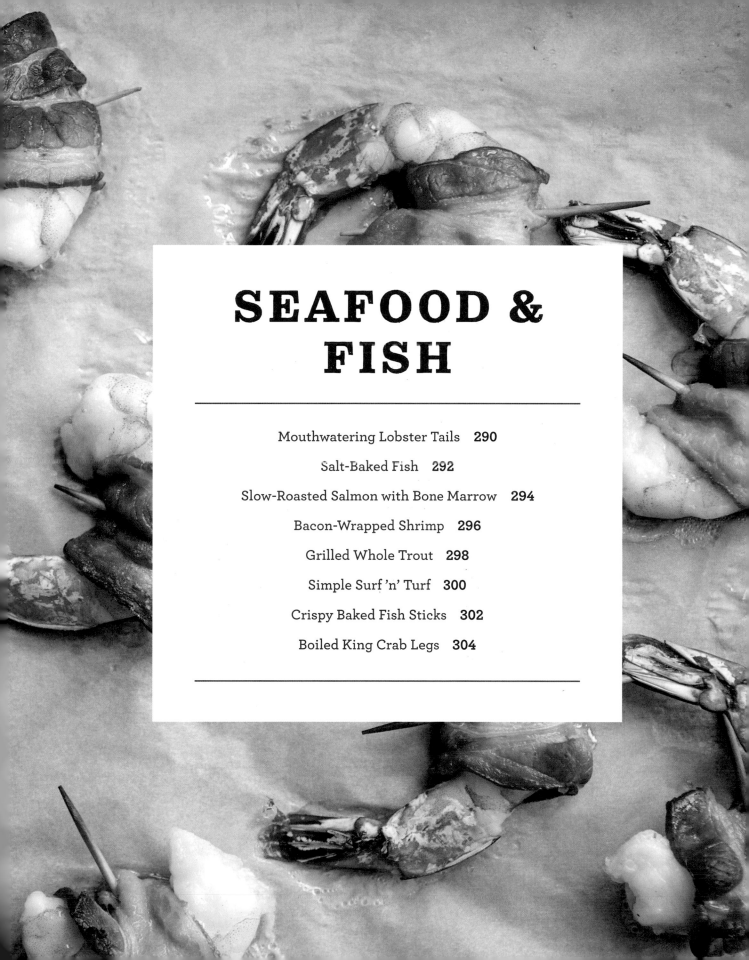

SEAFOOD & FISH

MOUTHWATERING LOBSTER TAILS

Yield: 2 servings
Prep Time: 5 minutes   **Cook Time:** 7 minutes

I get lobster in my monthly shipment from Sizzlefish. Lobster is very easy to cook, so this tasty dinner is fast from start to finish!

2 (2-pound) lobster tails

2 tablespoons melted lard or unsalted butter, plus more for serving

¾ teaspoon fine sea salt

1. Preheat the oven to broil.

2. Cut the shell of each lobster tail lengthwise with sharp kitchen scissors. Use your hands to pull the shells apart a little to expose the meat.

3. Place the lobster tails on a rimmed baking sheet. Drizzle with the lard and season with the salt.

4. Broil for 5 to 7 minutes, until the lobster meat is cooked through and no longer translucent. Serve with additional melted lard.

Per Serving:

Calories: 433   Fat: 18 g   Protein: 65 g   Carbs: 0 g

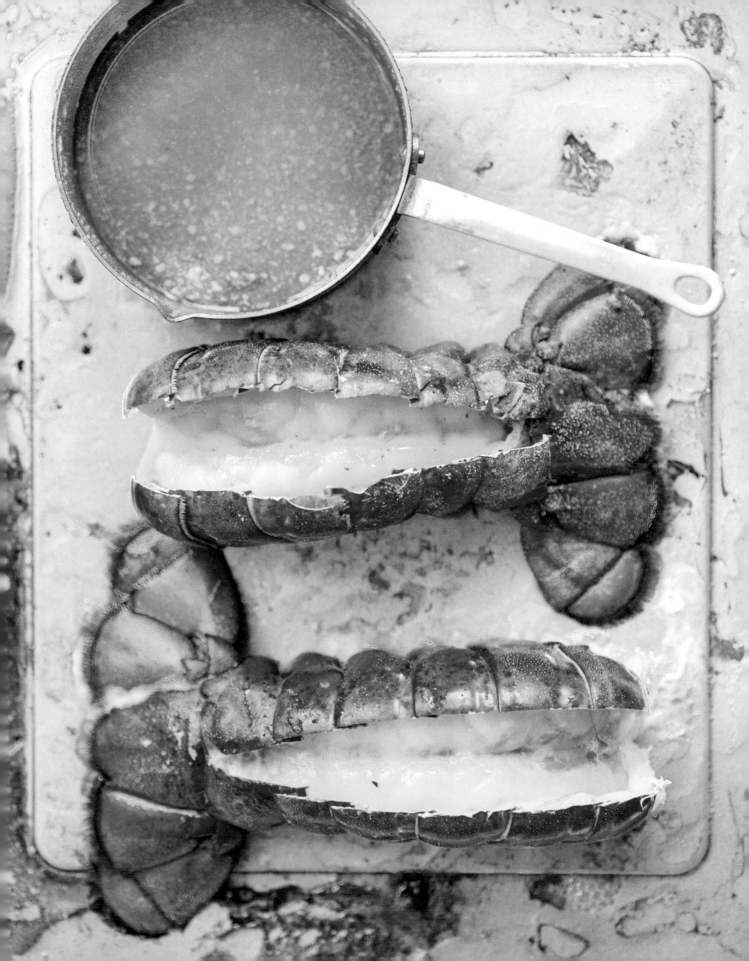

SALT-BAKED FISH

OPTION

Yield: 4 servings
Prep Time: 7 minutes, plus 10 minutes to rest   **Cook Time:** 25 minutes

If you really want to impress your family or dinner guests, you must try this recipe. You will look like a master chef, but in reality, this method of cooking fish is very simple, and it creates tasty, tender fish. To make this recipe even easier, I ask the fishmonger to remove the gills and fins from the fish for me.

4 large egg whites

2 cups coarse sea salt

1 whole (3-pound) sea bass or red snapper, gutted, gills and fins removed

Melted ghee or unsalted butter, for serving (optional)

1. Preheat the oven to 450°F.

2. Place the egg whites in a mixing bowl or the bowl of a stand mixer fitted with the whisk attachment. Whisk until soft peaks form. Gently fold the salt into the whites with a spatula.

3. Place about ¼ cup of the whipped egg whites on an ovenproof platter. Spread the whites into the size and shape of the sea bass. Place the fish on top of the whites, then top with the rest of the egg whites, covering the fish completely.

4. Set the platter on a rimmed baking sheet and bake for 25 minutes, or until the fish is no longer translucent and flakes easily with a fork.

5. Let the fish rest for 10 minutes before serving. For a dramatic presentation, move the platter to the dinner table and crack the salt crust open in front of your guests. Then place pieces of fish on serving plates. Serve with melted ghee, if desired.

6. Store in an airtight container in the refrigerator for up to 3 days. To reheat, place in a baking dish in a preheated 350°F oven for 5 minutes, or until warmed through.

Per Serving:

Calories: 568   Fat: 10 g   Protein: 112 g   Carbs: 0.2 g

2
1 3
CARNIVORE

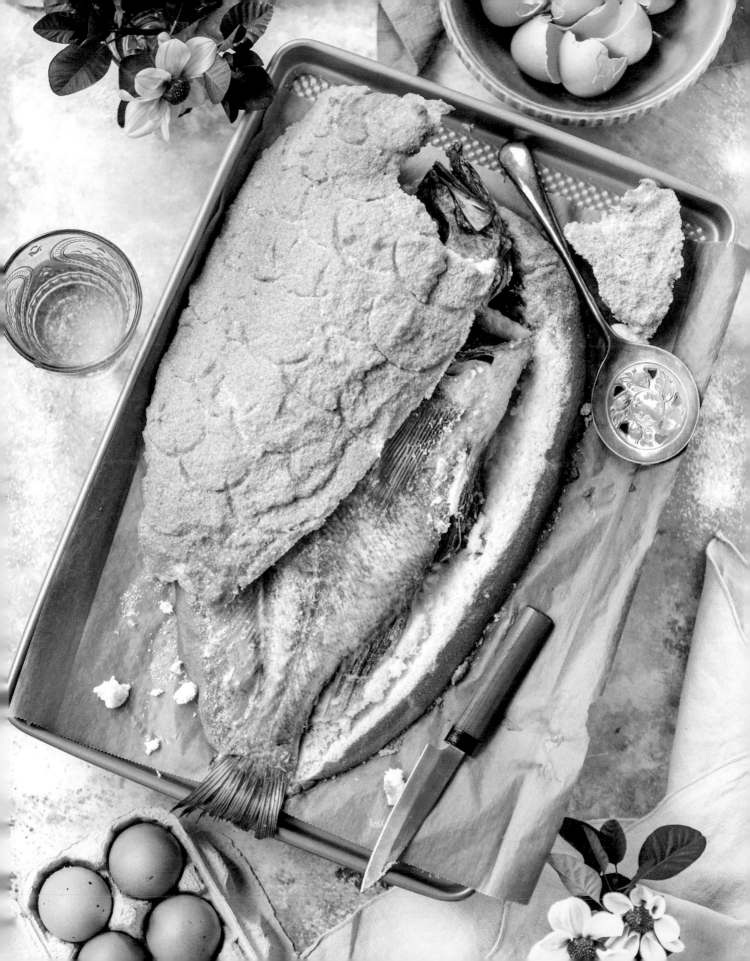

SLOW-ROASTED SALMON WITH BONE MARROW

Yield: 4 servings
Prep Time: 5 minutes **Cook Time:** 55 minutes

My son Micah's favorite meal is salmon, and bone marrow was one of the first foods I gave to my sons. It is basically a savory custard that is easy for babies to eat. I love to add bone marrow to foods for a creamy dairy-free addition.

4 large beef or veal marrow bones

3½ teaspoons fine sea salt, divided

1 (2-pound) skinless salmon fillet, preferably center-cut

¾ cup tallow (page 312) or ghee, melted

Flaked sea salt, for garnish

1. Preheat the oven to 450°F.

2. Rinse and drain the marrow bones and pat them dry with a paper towel, then season the bones with 1 teaspoon of the salt.

3. Place the bones in a roasting pan. If the bones are cut lengthwise, place them cut side up. If the bones are cut crosswise, place them standing up.

4. Roast for 15 to 25 minutes, until the marrow in the center has puffed slightly and is warm. (The exact timing will depend on the diameter of the bones; if they are 2 inches in diameter, it will take closer to 15 minutes.) To test for doneness, insert a metal skewer into the center of the bone. There should be no resistance when it is inserted, and some of the marrow will have started to leak from the bones. Remove from the oven and set aside.

5. Lower the oven temperature to 275°F. Season the salmon with the remaining 2½ teaspoons of salt and place in a casserole dish. Pour the melted tallow over the salmon. Bake for 30 minutes, or until the fish is cooked though and a tiny bit opaque in the middle for medium-rare doneness.

6. Remove from the oven and transfer the salmon to a serving platter. Use a spoon to scoop out the bone marrow and place it on top of the salmon. Garnish with flaked sea salt.

7. Store in an airtight container in the refrigerator for up to 4 days. To reheat, place on a rimmed baking sheet in a preheated 300°F oven for 5 minutes, or until the fish is heated through and the marrow is soft.

Per Serving:

Calories: 550   Fat: 39 g   Protein: 46 g   Carbs: 0 g

2
1 ⌄ 3   1 ⌄ 3
2
CARNIVORE   IF USING GHEE

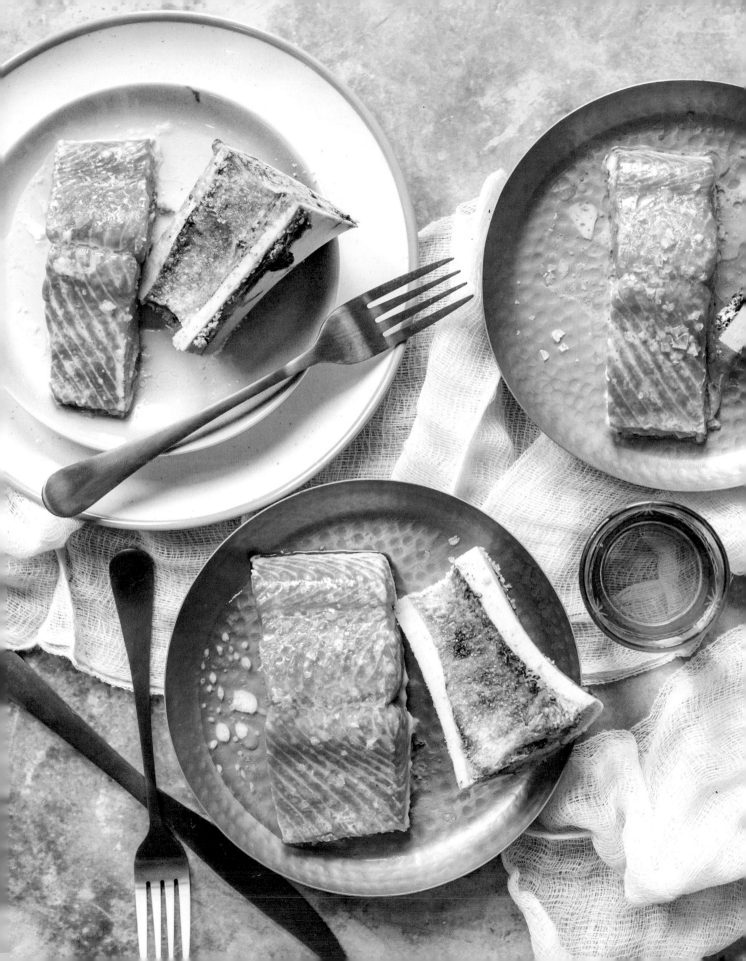

BACON-WRAPPED SHRIMP

Yield: 2 servings
Prep Time: 10 minutes   **Cook Time:** 8 minutes

I often make bacon-wrapped shrimp for family gatherings, and it is usually the first food to disappear! This dish can be a meal or an appetizer.

12 large raw shrimp, tails on, peeled and deveined

12 thin slices pork or beef bacon

1. Preheat the oven or an air fryer to 400°F.

2. Wrap each shrimp tightly in a slice of bacon and secure with a toothpick. Place the wrapped shrimp on a rimmed baking sheet or in the air fryer basket and cook for 8 minutes, flipping after 5 minutes, or until the shrimp are no longer translucent.

Per Serving:

Calories: 490   Fat: 36 g   Protein: 41 g   Carbs: 0 g

CARNIVORE

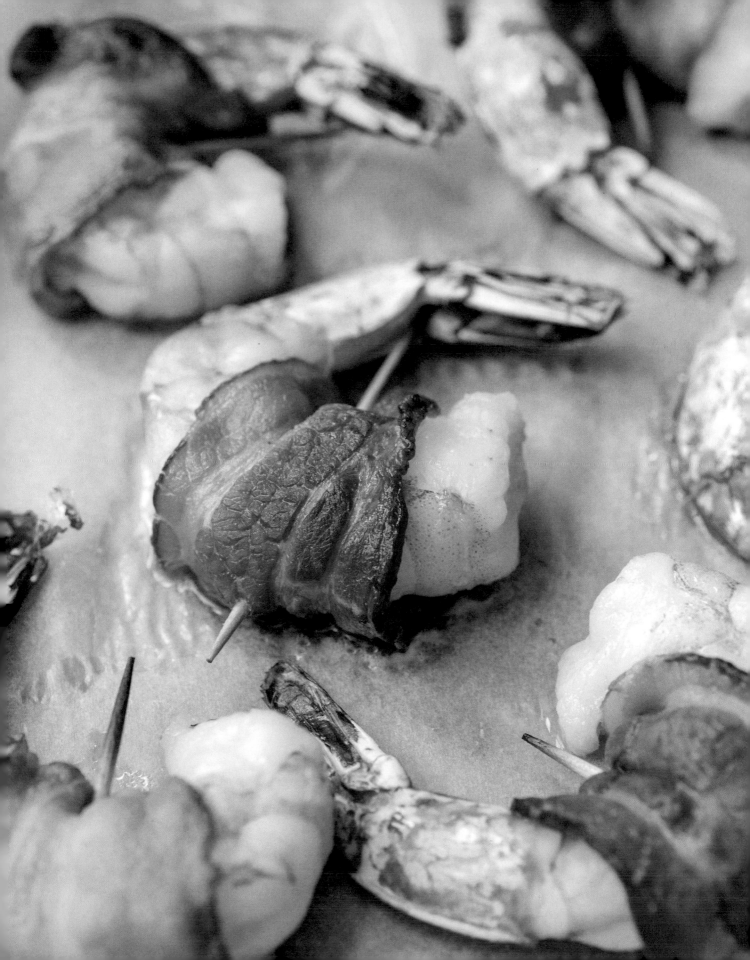

GRILLED WHOLE TROUT

Yield: 2 servings
Prep Time: 5 minutes **Cook Time:** 12 minutes

I spend summer evenings fly fishing on the river near our home. It is a class A trout stream. If you aren't able to catch your own trout, you can ask your fishmonger to order a whole trout for you. The fishmonger will often debone the fish for you, too.

1 (12-ounce) whole trout, gutted, gills and fins removed, or 12 ounces trout fillets

1 tablespoon lard or tallow (page 312), melted, plus more for greasing

1½ teaspoons fine sea salt

Melted salted butter, for serving (omit for dairy-free)

1. Preheat a grill to high heat. Lightly brush the grill grate with melted lard.

2. Brush the outside of the trout with the melted lard. Season the outside and the inside cavity of the fish with the salt.

3. Place the trout on the grill, away from the heat source, and cook for 6 minutes, then flip and cook for another 6 minutes, or until the fish is flaky and no longer translucent.

4. Remove the trout from the grill and serve with melted butter, if desired.

Per Serving:

Calories: 350   Fat: 22 g   Protein: 35 g   Carbs: 0 g

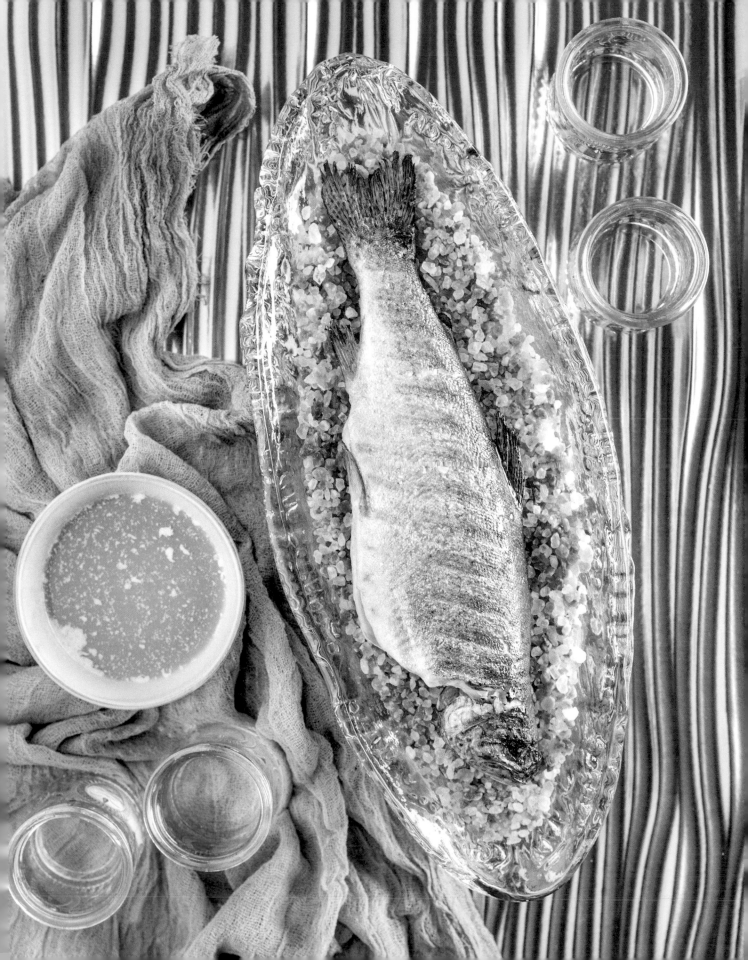

SIMPLE SURF 'N' TURF

Yield: 2 servings   **Prep Time:** 6 minutes, plus 25 minutes to rest
Cook Time: 16 minutes

I worked at a restaurant called High View when I was in high school. It was situated on a cute lake where I would often fish. One of our specialties was steak with jumbo shrimp. It was a big hit!

2 (5-ounce) rib-eye steaks, trimmed

1¾ teaspoons plus 1 pinch of fine sea salt, divided

2 raw jumbo prawns or jumbo shrimp, tails on, peeled and deveined

¼ cup tallow (page 312) or unsalted butter

1. Season the steaks well on both sides with 1 teaspoon of the salt. Let sit at room temperature for 15 minutes. Preheat the oven or an air fryer to 400°F.

2. Place the steaks on a rimmed baking sheet if using the oven, or in the air fryer basket, and cook for about 10 minutes for medium-rare steaks, or to your desired doneness (see the chart on page 180). Remove the steaks from the oven or air fryer and allow to rest for 10 minutes.

3. While the steaks are resting, cook the prawns: Season the prawns well with ¾ teaspoon of the salt. Place on a rimmed baking sheet if using the oven, or in the air fryer basket, and cook for about 6 minutes, flipping after 3 minutes, or until the prawns are cooked through and no longer translucent.

4. Meanwhile, season the tallow with a pinch of salt and melt in a small saucepan over low heat for 2 minutes.

5. Place each steak on a plate. Top with a prawn, pour the melted tallow over the steak and shrimp, and serve.

Per Serving:

Calories: 723   Fat: 62 g   Protein: 41 g   Carbs: 0 g

CARNIVORE   IF USING BUTTER

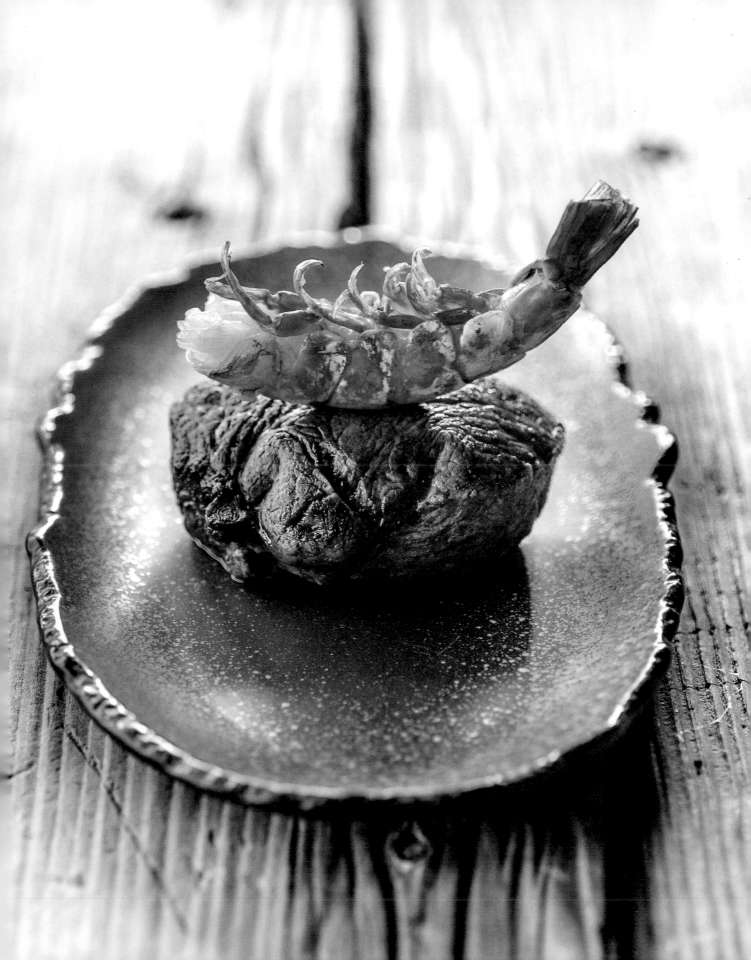

CRISPY BAKED FISH STICKS

Yield: 4 servings
Prep Time: 10 minutes   **Cook Time:** 8 minutes

OPTION

Melted lard or tallow (page 312), for greasing the air fryer

1 large egg

1 cup powdered Parmesan cheese or pork dust (for dairy-free)

1 pound cod fillets, cut into sticks about ½ inch wide by 2½ inches long

3 tablespoons unsalted butter or tallow, melted

Bacon Mayonnaise (page 318), for serving (optional)

1. Preheat the oven or an air fryer to 400°F. If using the oven, line a rimmed baking sheet with parchment paper. If using an air fryer, grease the air fryer basket with melted lard.

2. Crack the egg into a small shallow baking dish and beat lightly with a fork. Place the powdered Parmesan cheese in a separate medium-sized shallow baking dish.

3. Dip a piece of fish into the egg just enough to wet it, then dip it into the Parmesan cheese and coat the fish well. Use your hands to press the cheese around the piece of fish. Dip it in both dishes a second time for a thicker coating. Set the coated fish aside on a large plate. Repeat with the remaining pieces of fish, then brush the coated fish with the melted butter.

4. Place the coated fish in a single layer on the lined baking sheet or in the greased air fryer basket and cook for 8 minutes, flipping after 4 minutes, or until the fish is no longer translucent in the center. Work in batches if needed.

5. Transfer the fish sticks to a platter and serve with mayonnaise, if desired. Store in an airtight container in the refrigerator for up to 4 days. To reheat, place in a preheated 400° oven or air fryer for about 3 minutes, or until heated through.

Per Serving (without mayonnaise):

Calories: 194   Fat: 10 g   Protein: 22 g   Carbs: 0.1 g

1 2 3
CARNIVORE

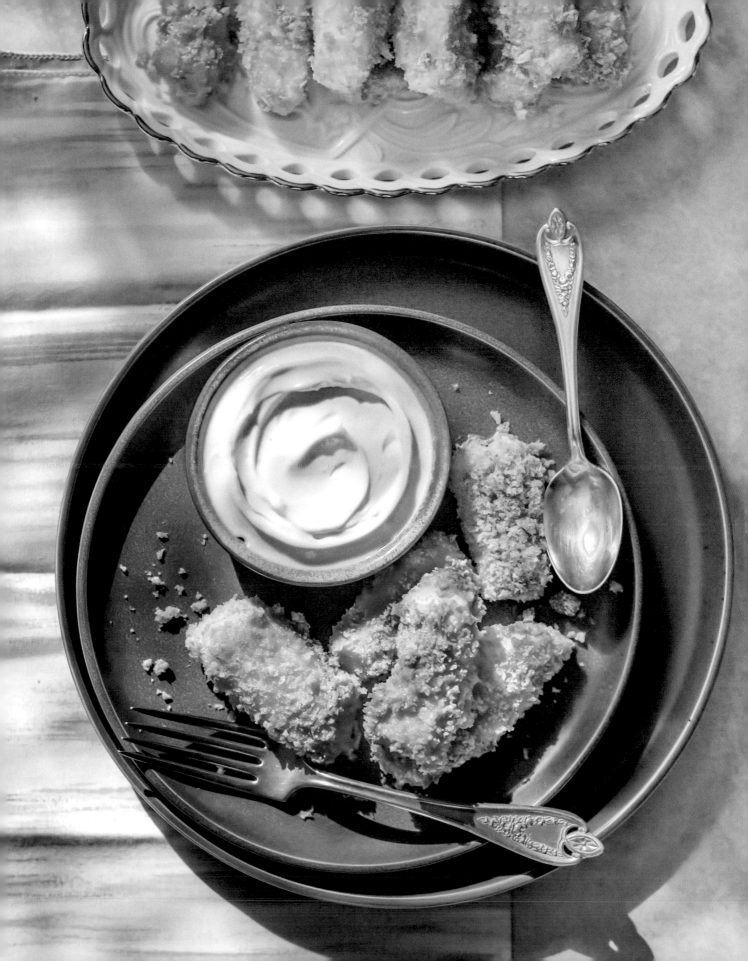

BOILED KING CRAB LEGS

Yield: 4 servings
Prep Time: 5 minutes   **Cook Time:** 3 minutes

I love crab legs—simple and delicious! I once ordered crab legs at a famous crab restaurant, and when my food arrived, I asked for plain butter. The server said all they had was a butter and vegetable oil mixture. There was no plain butter in the restaurant! Here, I give you the option of dipping your crab legs in melted duck fat instead of butter, which takes the recipe from Carnivore Level 3 to Level 2.

2 pounds king crab clusters, thawed if frozen

1 tablespoon fine sea salt

½ cup duck fat or unsalted butter, melted, for serving (optional)

1. Make a small cut lengthwise in the shell of each crab leg.

2. Fill a large pot with water. Add the salt and bring to a boil. Add the crab legs and reduce the temperature to a simmer for 3 minutes, or until the crab legs are heated through.

3. Transfer the crab legs to a serving platter and serve with the melted duck fat.

4. Store in an airtight container in the refrigerator for up to 2 days. To reheat, place in a pot of boiling water for 3 minutes, or until heated through.

Per Serving (with duck fat):

Calories: 497   Fat: 28 g   Protein: 53 g   Carbs: 0 g

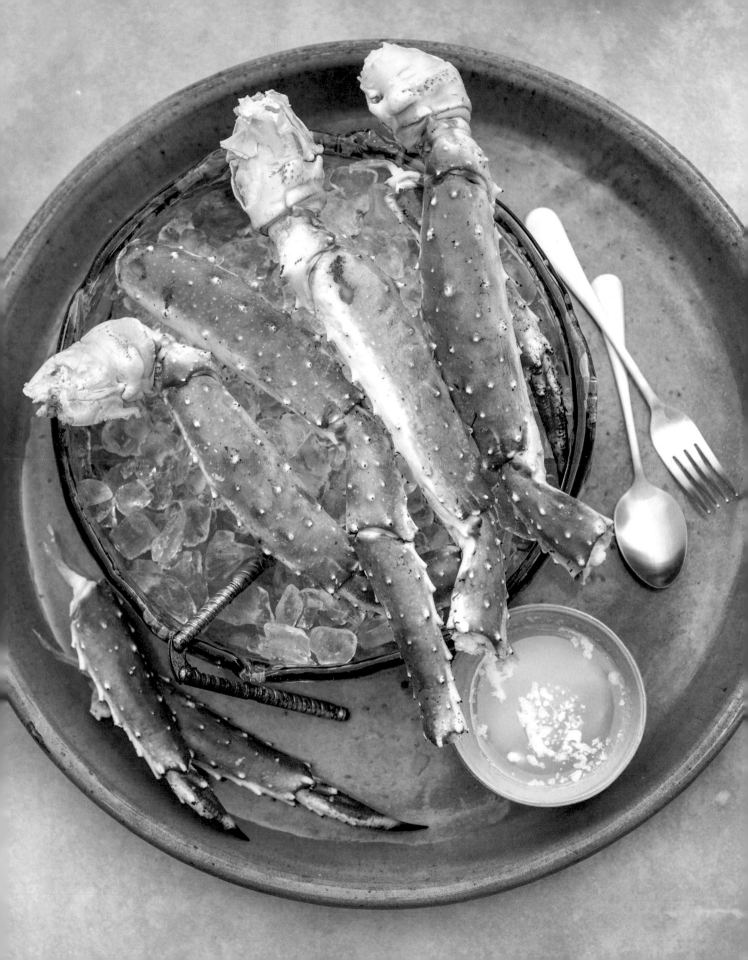

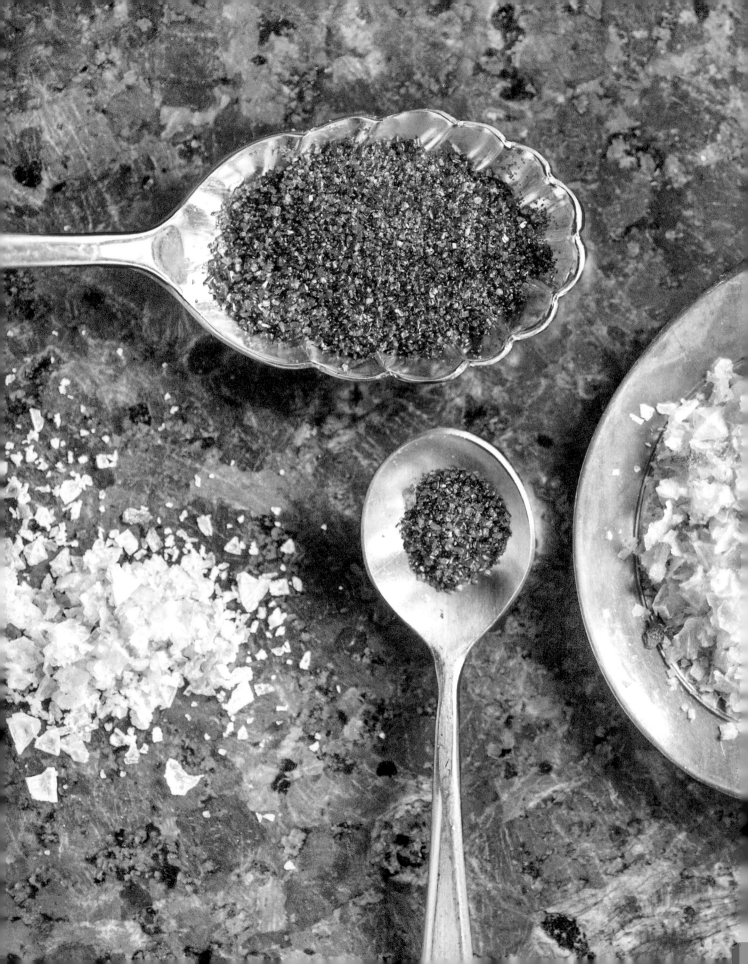

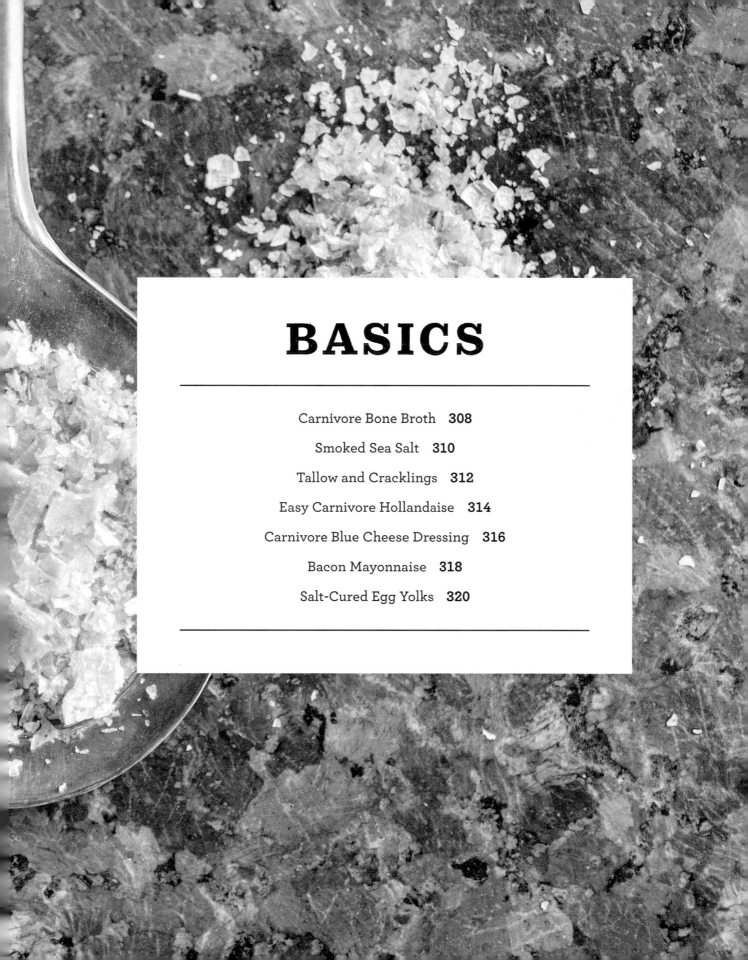

BASICS

CARNIVORE BONE BROTH

Yield: 4 quarts (1 cup per serving)
Prep Time: 10 minutes   **Cook Time:** 1 to 3 days

I add eggshells to my bone broth to provide additional calcium. If you use beef bones, the broth is Carnivore Level 1; using chicken or fish bones would make it Level 2.

4 quarts cold water (reverse osmosis water or filtered water is best)

4 large beef bones (about 4 pounds), or leftover bones and skin from 1 pastured chicken (ideally with the feet), or 4 pounds fish bones and heads

6 eggshells (optional)

2 teaspoons fine sea salt

1. Place all the ingredients in a 6-quart slow cooker. Cook on high for 1 hour, then turn the heat down to low and simmer for a minimum of 1 day or up to 3 days. The longer the broth cooks, the more nutrients and minerals will be extracted from the bones.

2. When the broth is done, pour it through a strainer and discard the bones. Store in an airtight container in the refrigerator for up to 5 days or in the freezer for up to several months.

Per Serving:

Calories: 50   Fat: 1 g   Protein: 10 g   Carbs: 0 g

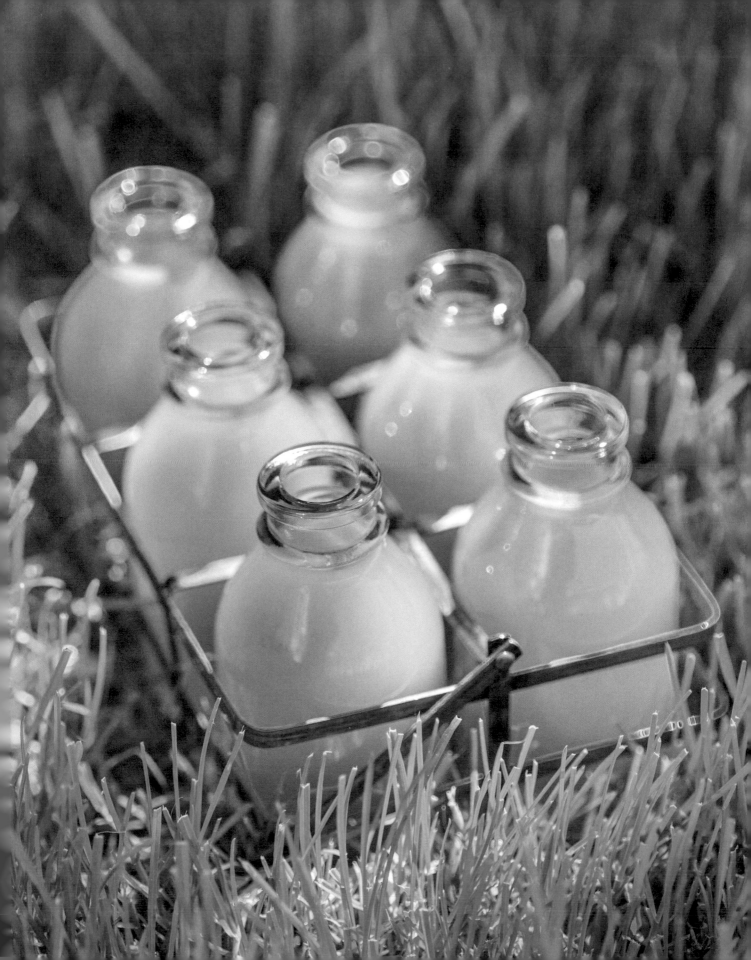

SMOKED SEA SALT

Yield: about 1½ cups   **Prep Time:** 5 minutes, plus 30 minutes to soak wood chips
(if using)   **Cook Time:** 8 to 12 hours

Smoked salt provides intense flavor, making it a real treat when eating carnivore. You can find smoked salt at most grocery stores, but smoking your own salt gives you the freedom to choose the type of smoke—hickory, applewood, or whichever wood you prefer—and how deep of a smoky flavor you want.

Be sure to read the manufacturer's directions for your smoker before you begin. There are wood, electric, propane, and charcoal smokers, and each type works differently. If you do not have a smoker, see page 79 for how to create a smoking technique using your oven or an outdoor grill.

1 pound fine sea salt

Special Equipment:
Spray bottle of water,
smoker, wood chips
(optional)

1. If using wood chips, cover them with water and allow to soak for 30 minutes.

2. Start the smoker, following the manufacturer's instructions. If the smoker came with a water bowl, add water to it.

3. Spread the salt on a rimmed baking sheet and spray it lightly with water. Place the baking sheet in the smoker and secure the lid so that it is airtight and no smoke can escape.

4. Smoke the salt for 8 to 12 hours; the longer you smoke it, the deeper the flavor becomes. Open the smoker and stir the salt every 2 hours to break up any clumps. Every so often, check the temperature and adjust the air vents to maintain a temperature of 225°F to 250°F. Add more fuel to the smoker if needed to maintain the temperature or more soaked wood chips if the smoke starts to dissipate.

5. Once finished, remove the salt from the smoker and allow to cool completely. Store in airtight containers in the pantry for up to a month.

Per Serving:

Calories: 0   Fat: 0 g   Protein: 0 g   Carbs: 0 g

1 2 3
CARNIVORE

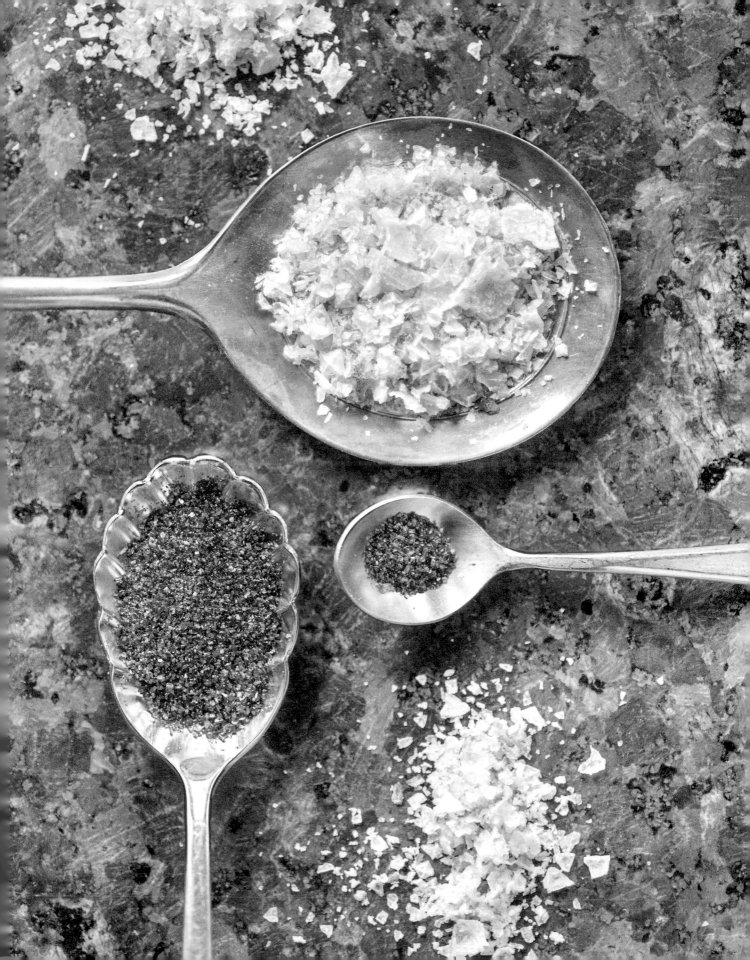

TALLOW AND CRACKLINGS

Yield: 16 servings
Prep Time: 5 minutes   **Cook Time:** 30 minutes

Making homemade tallow is wonderful because you also get delicious crispy cracklings for a snack! Tallow is the fat rendered from beef suet. Cracklings are the crispy bits of meat that are left behind. I get suet from a local farmer who raises grass-fed animals.

1 pound grass-fed beef suet

Fine sea salt

1. Chop the suet into 2-inch squares. Melt the suet in a large heavy stockpot over medium heat. Reduce the heat to low, cover the pot with the lid, and cook for 30 minutes, or until cracklings form.

2. Use a slotted spoon to remove the cracklings from the pot. Place on a paper towel–lined plate and sprinkle with salt. Set aside. Turn off the heat and allow the fat to cool a little.

3. Pour the tallow into mason jars and cover. Store the tallow in the refrigerator for up to 2 weeks or in the freezer for up to 3 months. Store the cracklings in an airtight container in the pantry for up to 3 weeks.

Per Serving (tallow):

Calories: 242   Fat: 27 g   Protein: 0.4 g   Carbs: 0 g

2
1 ◣ 3
CARNIVORE

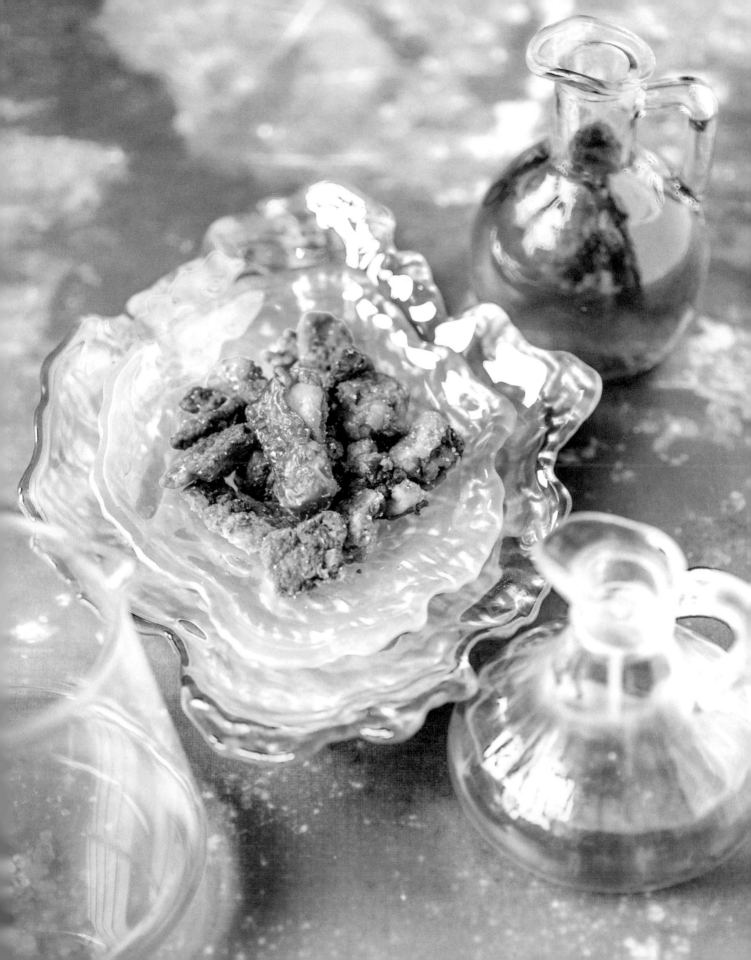

EASY CARNIVORE HOLLANDAISE

YIELD: 2 cups (about 2½ tablespoons per serving)
PREP TIME: 5 minutes   **COOK TIME:** 5 minutes

I love sauce, so when I went carnivore, I had to find a great sauce option for putting on a burger or steak. This hollandaise is a bit different from the traditional version since you don't want to use lemon juice or cayenne pepper when eating carnivore. You can use unsalted butter in place of the bacon fat if you don't need the hollandaise to be dairy-free.

½ cup bacon fat, lard, or duck fat

2 large egg yolks

2 teaspoons water or Carnivore Beef Bone Broth (page 308)

Up to ¼ teaspoon fine sea salt (optional)

Special Equipment:
Immersion blender

1. Heat the bacon fat in a small saucepan until very hot. Pour the hot fat into a measuring cup.

2. Place the egg yolks and water in a wide-mouth pint-sized jar. Place an immersion blender at the bottom of the jar and turn the blender on. Slowly add the hot fat and very slowly move the blender up to the top of the jar. Be patient! It should take you about a minute to reach the top. Moving the blender slowly is the key to getting the hollandaise to emulsify. Taste and add salt, if desired.

3. Use immediately or keep warm for up to 1 hour in a heat-safe bowl set over warm water.

4. Store in a covered jar in the refrigerator for up to 5 days. To reheat, place the sauce in a double boiler or a heat-safe bowl set over a pot of simmering water, whisking often, until the sauce is warm and thick.

Per Serving:

Calories: 86   Fat: 9 g   Protein: 0.5 g   Carbs: 0.1 g

1 — 2 — 3
CARNIVORE

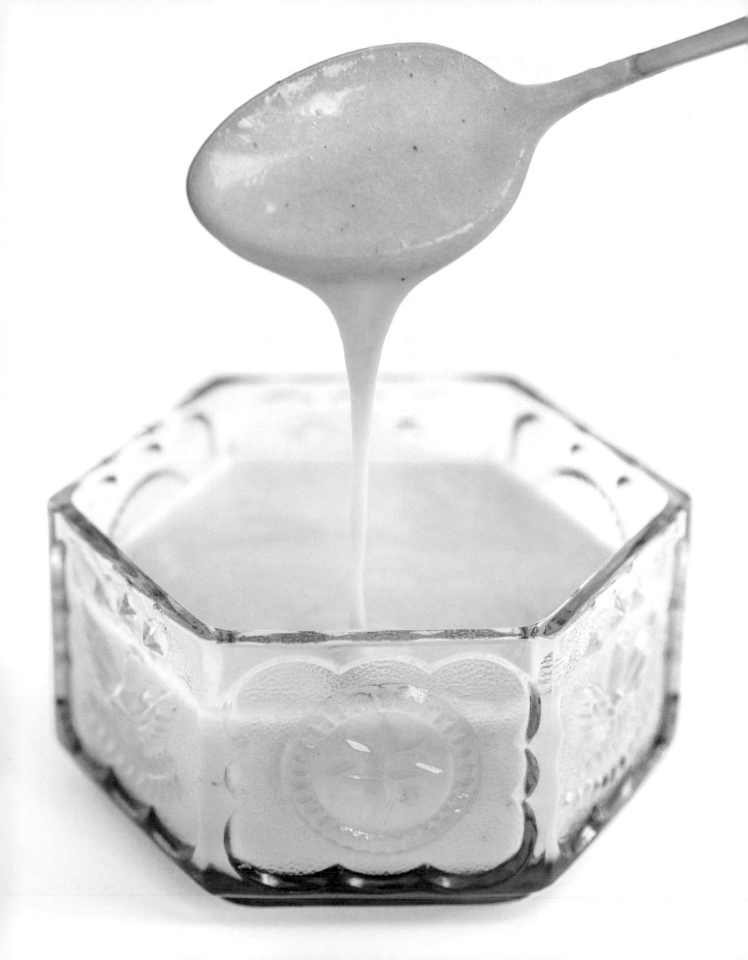

CARNIVORE
BLUE CHEESE DRESSING

Yield: 1½ cups (1½ tablespoons per serving)
Prep Time: 5 minutes   **Cook Time:** —

8 ounces blue cheese
crumbles, plus more if
desired for chunky texture

4 ounces cream cheese
(½ cup), softened

½ cup Carnivore Beef Bone
Broth (page 308), cold

Place all the ingredients in a food processor and process until smooth.
Pour into a mason jar. Stir in extra blue cheese, if desired. Store in a
mason jar in the refrigerator for up to 5 days.

Per Serving:

Calories: 78   Fat: 6 g   Protein: 4 g   Carbs: 0.2 g

1 — 2 — 3
CARNIVORE

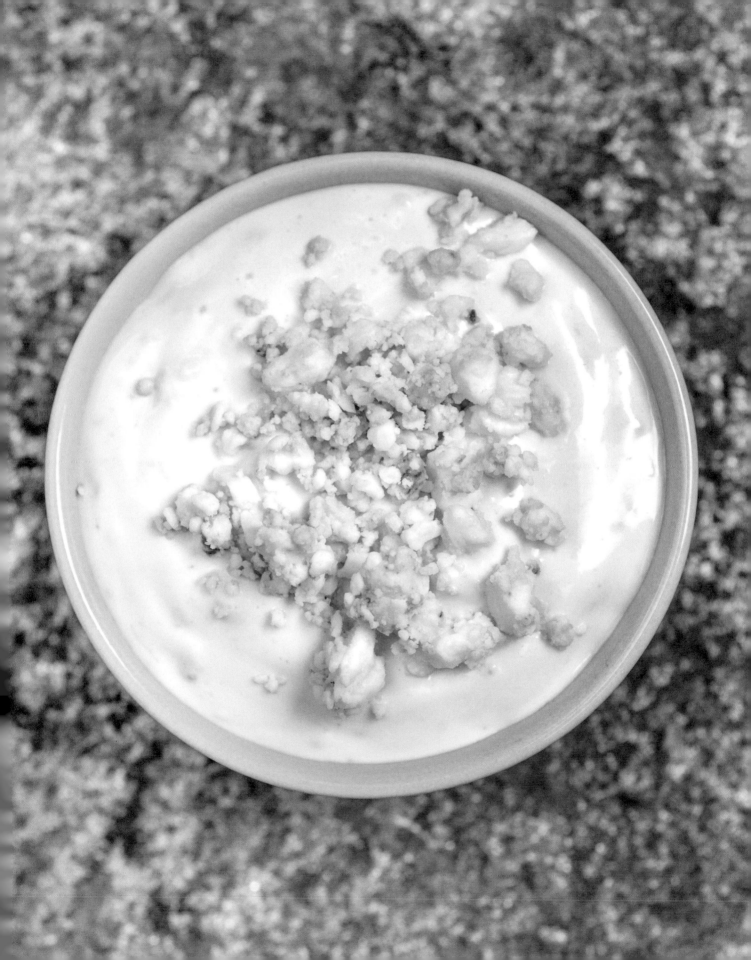

BACON MAYONNAISE

Yield: 1½ cups (about 1 tablespoon per serving)
Prep Time: 5 minutes **Cook Time:** —

2 large egg yolks

2 teaspoons water or Carnivore Beef Bone Broth (page 308)

1 cup melted bacon fat

½ teaspoon fine sea salt

Special Equipment:
Immersion blender

1. Put the ingredients in the order listed in a wide-mouth pint-sized jar. Place an immersion blender at the bottom of the jar. Turn the blender on and very slowly move it to the top of the jar. Be patient! It should take you about a minute to reach the top. Moving the blender slowly is the key to getting the mayonnaise to emulsify. Taste and add more salt, if desired.

2. Store in a covered jar in the refrigerator for up to 5 days.

Per Serving:

Calories: 82   Fat: 9 g   Protein: 0.2 g   Carbs: 0.1 g

1 — 2 — 3
CARNIVORE

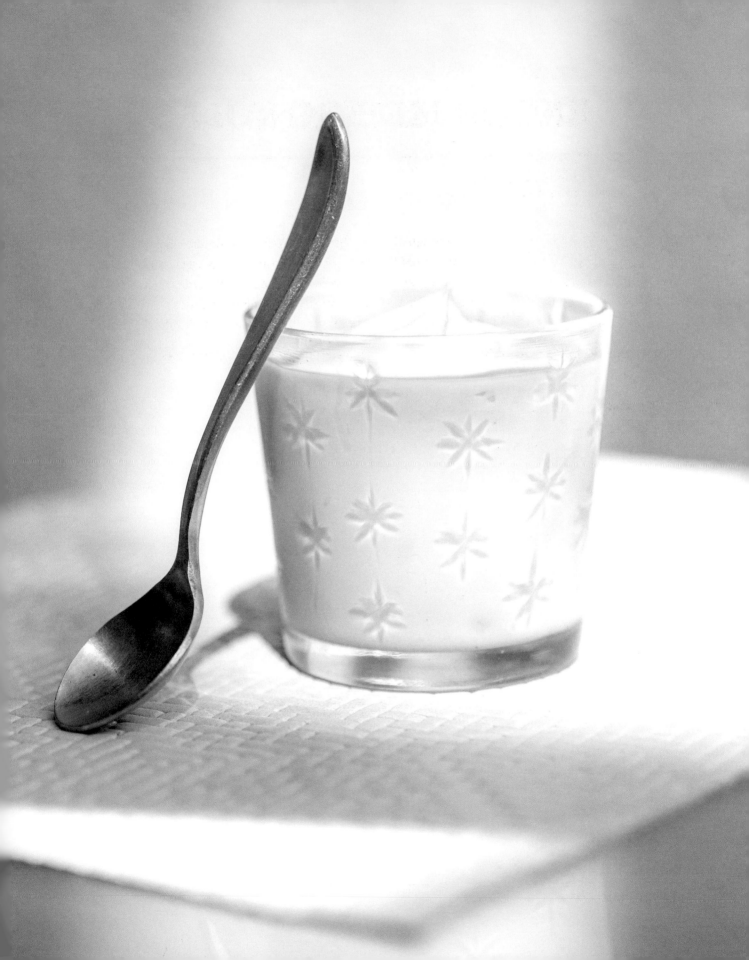

SALT-CURED EGG YOLKS

Yield: 6 servings
Prep Time: 10 minutes, plus 2 weeks to cure   **Cook Time:** —

Salt-cured egg yolks are a delicious way to add color, flavor, and texture to dishes. I love to grate them over a Butter Burger (page 218) or grilled steak or fish.

1 cup fine sea salt or smoked sea salt, store-bought or homemade (page 310)

6 large egg yolks

Special Equipment:
Cheesecloth

1. Place the salt in a small shallow casserole dish. The salt should be about ½ inch deep; add more if needed. Use a spoon to make a rounded indentation for each of the yolks. Gently place a yolk into each indentation, making sure not to break the yolks. Use your hands to gently cover all the yolks with the salt.

2. Place the dish in the refrigerator for 1 week. After a week, remove from the fridge and gently brush the salt off each yolk. Place the yolks in a piece of cheesecloth and hang the cloth in the fridge for another week, or until the yolks are dried. Store in the hanging cheesecloth in the fridge for up to a year.

Per Serving:

Calories: 55   Fat: 5 g   Protein: 3 g   Carbs: 1 g

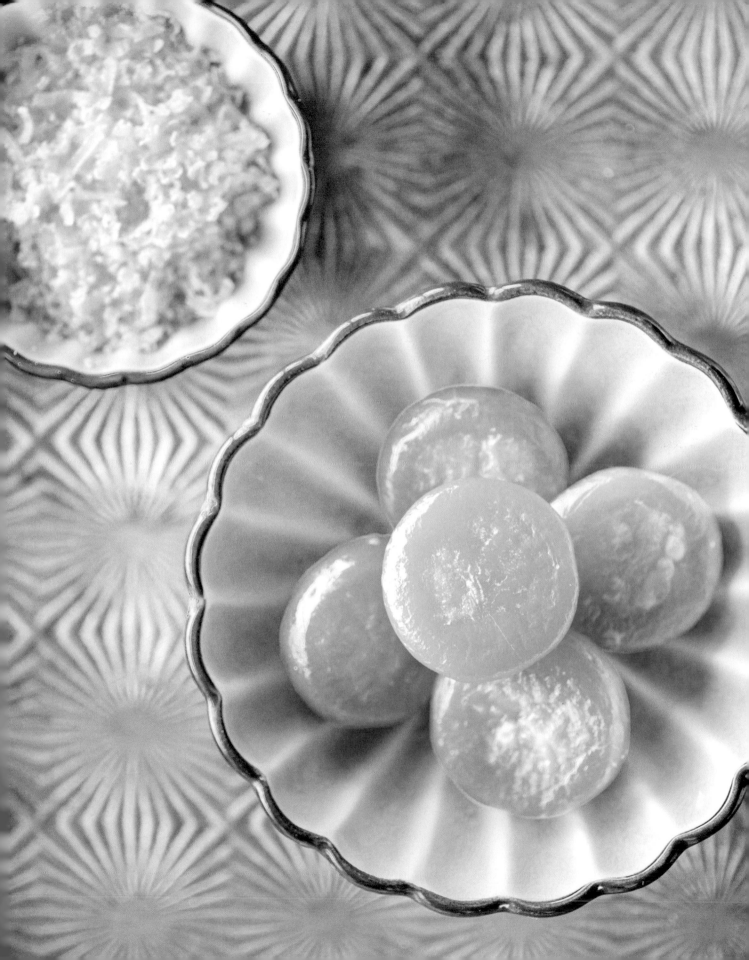

ADDITIONAL CARNIVORE REFERENCES

Carnivore Podcast: www.carnivorecast.com/podcast

Shawn Baker: www.shawn-baker.com/

Peter Ballerstedt: grassbasedhealth.blogspot.com/

Dr. Georgia Ede: www.diagnosisdiet.com/

Dave Feldman: cholesterolcode.com/

Sally Norton: sallyknorton.com/

Amber O'Hearn: www.empiri.ca/

Kevin Stock: www.kevinstock.io/

RECIPE INDEX

BREAKFAST

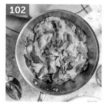

Salmon French Eggs

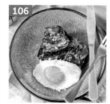

Bon Vie Scrambler

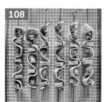

Ham Hocks and Fried Eggs

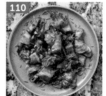

Breakfast Kabobs

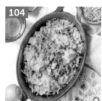

Bacon Knots

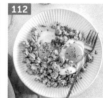

Pork Fried Eggs

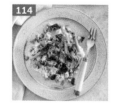

Bacon Cheeseburger Scrambled Eggs

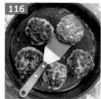

Breakfast Patties

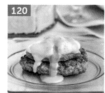

Breakfast Pie

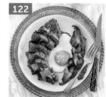

Carnivore Eggs Benedict

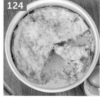

Steak and Eggs

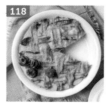

Ham 'n' Cheese Frittata

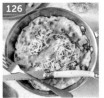 126 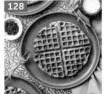 128 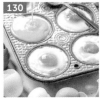 130 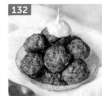 132 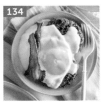 134

Carnivore Omelet Carnivore Waffle Carnivore Egg Cups Breakfast Meatballs Breakfast Burgers

APPETIZERS, SALADS & SIDES

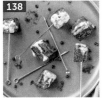 138 140 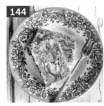 142 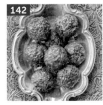 144 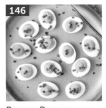 146 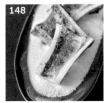 148

Meat Lollipops Braunschweiger Beef Pemmican Head Cheese Bacon Burger Lover's Deviled Eggs Bone Marrow

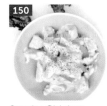 150 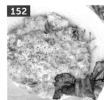 152 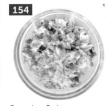 154 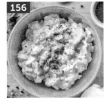 156 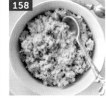 158 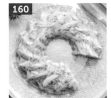 160

Smoky Chicken Salad Tuna Salad Smoky Salmon Salad Egg Salad Ham Salad Chicken in Aspic

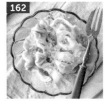 162 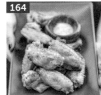 164 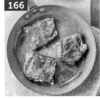 166 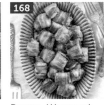 168 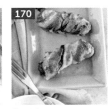 170 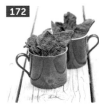 172

Chitterlings Chicken Wings Fried Goat Cheese Ravioli Bacon-Wrapped Chicken Nuggets Carnivore Mozzarella Sticks Venison or Beef Jerky

 174 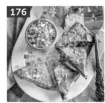 176 178

Carnivore Gummies Samosas Smoky Chicken Pâté

BEEF & LAMB

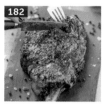
182
Reverse Sear
Long-Bone

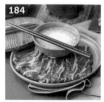
184
Carnivore
Shabu Shabu

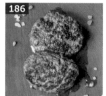
186
Salisbury Steak

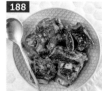
188
Slow Cooker
Short Ribs with
Brown Butter

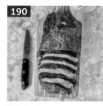
190
Brisket

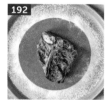
192
Grilled Lamb Chops

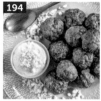
194
Meatballs

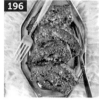
196
Smoked Meatloaf

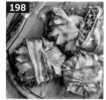
198
Bacon-Wrapped
Juicy Lucy

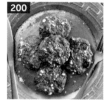
200
Baked Lamb and
Feta Patties

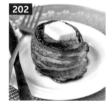
202
Bacon-Wrapped
Filet Mignons

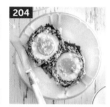
204
Egg-cellent
Meatloaf Cupcakes

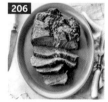
206
Roast Beef

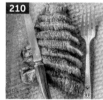
208
Bacon-Wrapped
Tenderloin

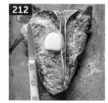
210
Basted Top Sirloin

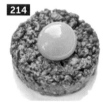
212
Air-Fried T-Bone
Steaks with
Smoked Butter

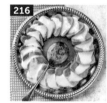
214
Smoky Beef Tartare

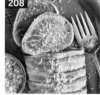
216
Beef Tongue

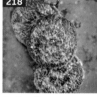
218
Butter Burgers

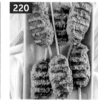
220
Grilled Lamb Kofta

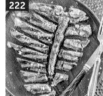
222
Grilled Porterhouse

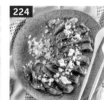
224
Black 'n' Blue Strip
Steak

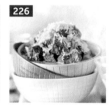
226
Creamy Parmesan
Beef Tips

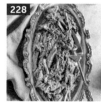
228
Shredded Beef with
Brown Butter Jus

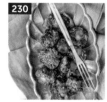
230
Oxtail

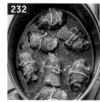
232
Rouladen

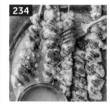
234
Grilled
Sweetbreads

236
Traditional Terrine

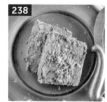
238
Short Rib Terrine

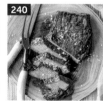
240
Smoked Beef Roast

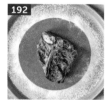

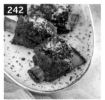
Smoked Short Ribs

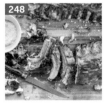
Beef Heart Steaks

PORK

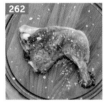
Smoked Baby Back Ribs

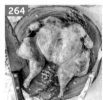
Homemade Brats

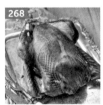
Scotch Eggs

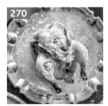
Bacon-Wrapped Pork Chops

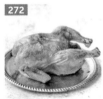
Riblets

Sous Vide Pork Chop

POULTRY

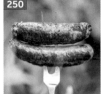
Chicken Confit

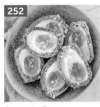
Brick Chicken

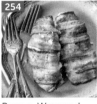
Braised Pheasant with Soft-Boiled Eggs

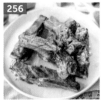
Smoked Turkey

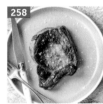
Cornish Game Hens

Roast Chicken

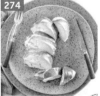
Prosciutto-Wrapped Stuffed Chicken

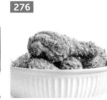
Crispy Chicken Legs

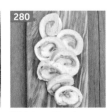
Chicken Fingers

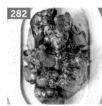
Chicken Cordon Bleu Roulade

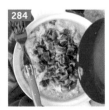
Easy Baked Chicken Livers

Slow Cooker Shredded Chicken with Creamy Cheddar and Bacon

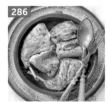
Braised Rabbit

SEAFOOD & FISH

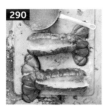
290
Mouthwatering Lobster Tails

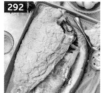
292
Salt-Baked Fish

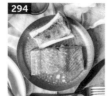
294
Slow-Roasted Salmon with Bone Marrow

296
Bacon-Wrapped Shrimp

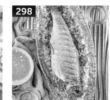
298
Grilled Whole Trout

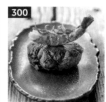
300
Simple Surf 'n' Turf

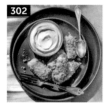
302
Crispy Baked Fish Sticks

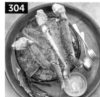
304
Boiled King Crab Legs

BASICS

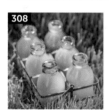
308
Carnivore Bone Broth

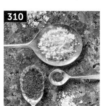
310
Smoked Sea Salt

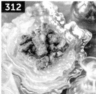
312
Tallow and Cracklings

314
Easy Carnivore Hollandaise

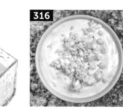
316
Carnivore Blue Cheese Dressing

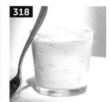
318
Bacon Mayonnaise

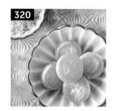
320
Salt-Cured Egg Yolks

ALLERGEN INDEX

Recipe	Page	🥛	🥚	1 – 2 – 3 CARNIVORE
Salmon French Eggs	102			3
Bon Vie Scrambler	104			3
Ham Hocks and Fried Eggs	106	✓		3
Breakfast Kabobs	108	✓	✓	2
Bacon Knots	110	✓	✓	1, 2
Pork Fried Eggs	112	✓		3
Bacon Cheeseburger Scrambled Eggs	114			3
Breakfast Patties	116	✓	✓	1, 2
Breakfast Pie	118			3
Carnivore Eggs Benedict	120	✓		3
Steak and Eggs	122	✓		3
Ham 'n' Cheese Frittata	124			3
Carnivore Omelet	126			3
Carnivore Waffle	128	✓		3
Carnivore Egg Cups	130	○		3
Breakfast Meatballs	132	✓	○	2, 3
Breakfast Burgers	134	✓		3
Meat Lollipops	138		✓	3
Braunschweiger	140	✓	✓	2
Beef Pemmican	142	✓	✓	1
Head Cheese	144	✓	✓	2
Bacon Burger Lover's Deviled Eggs	146	✓		3
Bone Marrow	148	✓	✓	1
Smoky Chicken Salad	150	○		3
Tuna Salad	152	✓		3
Smoky Salmon Salad	154	✓		3
Egg Salad	156	✓		3
Ham Salad	158	✓		3
Chicken in Aspic	160	✓	✓	2
Chitterlings	162	✓	✓	2
Chicken Wings	164	✓	✓	2
Fried Goat Cheese Ravioli	166		✓	3
Bacon-Wrapped Chicken Nuggets	168	✓	✓	2
Carnivore Mozzarella Sticks	170		✓	3
Venison or Beef Jerky	172	✓	✓	1, 2
Carnivore Gummies	174	✓	✓	1, 2
Samosas	176	✓	✓	2

Recipe	Page	🥛⃠	🥚⃠	1 2 3 CARNIVORE
Smoky Chicken Pâté	178	✓	✓	2
Reverse Sear Long-Bone	182	O	✓	2,3
Carnivore Shabu Shabu	184	O	✓	1, 3
Salisbury Steak	186	O	O	1, 3
Slow Cooker Short Ribs with Brown Butter	188		✓	1, 3
Brisket	190	✓	✓	1
Grilled Lamb Chops	192	✓	✓	2
Meatballs	194	✓		3
Smoked Meatloaf	196	✓		3
Bacon-Wrapped Juicy Lucy	198		✓	3
Baked Lamb and Feta Patties	200		✓	3
Bacon-Wrapped Filet Mignons	202	O	✓	2, 3
Egg-cellent Meatloaf Cupcakes	204	✓		3
Roast Beef	206	✓	✓	1
Bacon-Wrapped Tenderloin	208	✓	✓	1, 2
Basted Top Sirloin	210	O	✓	1, 3
Air-Fried T-Bone Steaks with Smoked Butter	212	O	✓	1, 3
Smoky Beef Tartare	214	✓		3
Beef Tongue	216	✓	O	1, 3
Butter Burgers	218		✓	3
Grilled Lamb Kofta	220	O	✓	2, 3
Grilled Porterhouse	222	✓	✓	1
Black 'n' Blue Strip Steak	224		✓	3
Creamy Parmesan Beef Tips	226		O	3
Shredded Beef with Brown Butter Jus	228		✓	1, 3
Oxtail	230	O	✓	1, 3
Rouladen	232	O	✓	2, 3
Grilled Sweetbreads	234	✓	✓	1, 3
Traditional Terrine	236	✓		3
Short Rib Terrine	238	✓	O	2, 3
Smoked Beef Roast	240	✓	✓	1
Smoked Short Ribs	242	✓	O	1, 3
Beef Heart Steaks	244	✓	✓	1, 3
Smoked Baby Back Ribs	248	✓	✓	2
Homemade Brats	250	✓	✓	2
Scotch Eggs	252	✓		3
Bacon-Wrapped Pork Chops	254	✓	✓	2
Riblets	256	✓	✓	2
Sous Vide Pork Chop	258	✓	✓	2
Chicken Confit	262	✓	✓	2

Recipe	Page	🚫🥛	🚫🥚	CARNIVORE
Brick Chicken	264	✓	✓	3
Braised Pheasant with Soft-Boiled Eggs	266	✓		3
Smoked Turkey	268	✓	✓	2
Cornish Game Hens	270	✓	✓	2
Roast Chicken	272	✓	✓	2
Prosciutto-Wrapped Stuffed Chicken	274		✓	3
Crispy Chicken Legs	276	O		2, 3
Chicken Fingers	278	O		2, 3
Chicken Cordon Bleu Roulade	280		✓	3
Easy Baked Chicken Livers	282	✓	O	2, 3
Slow Cooker Shredded Chicken with Creamy Cheddar and Bacon	284		✓	3
Braised Rabbit	286	✓	✓	2
Mouthwatering Lobster Tails	290	O	✓	2, 3
Salt-Baked Fish	292	O		3
Slow-Roasted Salmon with Bone Marrow	294	✓	✓	2, 3
Bacon-Wrapped Shrimp	296	✓	✓	2
Grilled Whole Trout	298	O	✓	2, 3
Simple Surf 'n' Turf	300	O	✓	2, 3
Crispy Baked Fish Sticks	302	O		3
Boiled King Crab Legs	304	O	✓	2, 3
Carnivore Bone Broth	308	✓	O	1
Smoked Sea Salt	310	✓	✓	1
Tallow and Cracklings	312	✓	✓	1
Easy Carnivore Hollandaise	314	✓		3
Carnivore Blue Cheese Dressing	316		✓	3
Bacon Mayonnaise	318	✓		3
Salt-Cured Egg Yolks	320	✓		3

GENERAL INDEX